"This volume highlights a transtheoretical approach to psychotherapy, most relevant to therapists of all orientations, and deals with the importance of needs in influencing how patients think, feel, and act. At the core of this approach is the role that the satisfaction of a person's interpersonal and intrapersonal needs plays in psychological well-being. The interventions described are not school-based in nature, and are richly illustrated with clinical material that brings to life key conceptual issues that speak to therapists of varying theoretical orientations."

**Marvin R. Goldfried** *is a distinguished professor of Psychology at Stony Brook University, Stony Brook, New York, USA*

"A truly integrative model of psychotherapy from conceptualization through treatment! With illustrative case studies, Dr. Meier and Ms. Boivin's developmental model of Self in Relationship Psychotherapy goes beyond symptom management, guiding therapists to a deeper understanding of their clients' presenting issues, enhancing their ability to help make meaningful lasting change. This book will be a frequent reference for our team!"

**Dr. Rebecca Moore** *is a clinical psychologist and director of the Kanata Psychology and Counselling Centre*

"This is a truly refreshing and remarkable piece of work. The Self-in-Relationship Psychotherapy approach identifies core unmet self, relational and physical intimacy needs as the root of psychological dysfunction. It is a developmental and relational approach to psychotherapy that integrates complex theories to promote an understanding of how early developmental relationships and experiences impact later adult functioning. The theory underlying the approach provides clinicians with an effective lens to conceptualize and treat the most difficult cases presented in therapy. Of the numerous approaches I have learned throughout my career, the Self-in-Relationship Psychotherapy approach has been game changing in my academic, supervision and clinical practice."

**Shelley Briscoe-Dimock** *is a clinical professor and supervisor based in Ottawa, Ontario, Canada*

"When I started graduate studies in psychotherapy, I was curious about understanding the client's struggles in-depth whilst having a structure in place that is rooted in theory and is easy to grasp. This book came at the right time, and I can confidently say that it has been extremely helpful in grounding me in addressing clients' core struggles with a special focus on clients' core needs. In this way, this book helped me look beyond behavioral challenges and aided me in addressing the heart of the matter in a timely manner. I highly recommend this book, as a must read, to clinicians and to graduate students in psychotherapy."

**Sogol Kafi** *is a Ph.D. candidate at Saint Paul University, Ottawa, Ontario, Canada*

# Self-in-Relationship Psychotherapy

In this innovative book, the authors set out their theory of Self-in-Relationship Psychotherapy (SIRP), advocating for the integration of relational, self, and physical intimacy needs in the conceptualization and treatment of psychological problems, placing human needs at the center of treatment.

This marks a shift in how psychological and relational problems are understood, currently being perceived in terms of affects, cognitive processes, and behaviors. Using numerous illustrations from their own clinical practice, Meier and Boivin contend that this understanding overlooks the pivotal role that needs play in all aspects of peoples' personal lives and relationships. Children, adolescents, and adults do not live primarily from feelings and thoughts, but from basic psychological and relational needs, such as wanting to be in a meaningful relationship, having the autonomy and freedom to make decisions about their lives, experiencing being competent, being regarded as a significant and important person and experiencing emotional, intimate and sensual and/or sexual contacts. By taking such an approach, this book stands out among other books on psychotherapy theories.

Authored by two seasoned psychologists, who have provided therapeutic services to children, adolescents, and adults for 40 years, this book comprises the foundational theory for practicing Self-in-Relationship Psychotherapy, making it of interest to graduate students, clinicians in training, and practicing psychologists, social workers, and psychotherapists alike.

**Augustine Meier** is a certified clinical psychologist, individual, couple, and family therapist, researcher, author, and Professor Emeritus at Saint Paul University, Ottawa, Ontario, Canada. He is the founder of the Institute for Self-in-Relationship Psychotherapy.

**Micheline Boivin** is a certified clinical psychologist, child, parent, and family psychotherapist, researcher, and author based in Ottawa, Ontario, Canada. She is a board member of the Institute for Self-in-Relationship Psychotherapy.

# Self-in-Relationship Psychotherapy

## A Complete Clinical Guide to Theory and Practice

Augustine Meier and
Micheline Boivin

Routledge
Taylor & Francis Group
LONDON AND NEW YORK

Cover image: Anna Efetova; gettyimages

First published 2022
by Routledge
4 Park Square, Milton Park, Abingdon, Oxon OX14 4RN

and by Routledge
605 Third Avenue, New York, NY 10158

*Routledge is an imprint of the Taylor & Francis Group, an informa business*



*British Library Cataloguing-in-Publication Data*
A catalogue record for this book is available from the British Library

*Library of Congress Cataloguing-in-Publication Data*
Names: Meier, Augustine, 1933- author. | Boivin, Micheline, 1950- author.
Title: Self-in-relationship psychotherapy: a complete clinical guide to theory and practice / Augustine Meier and Micheline Boivin.
Description: Milton Park, Abingdon, Oxon; New York, NY: Routledge, 2022. | Includes bibliographical references and index. |
Identifiers: LCCN 2022002478 (print) | LCCN 2022002479 (ebook) | ISBN 9781032224121 (hardback) | ISBN 9781032224152 (paperback) | ISBN 9781003272502 (ebook)
Subjects: LCSH: Self psychology. | Psychoanalysis.
Classification: LCC BF175.5.S44 M45 2022 (print) | LCC BF175.5.S44 (ebook) | DDC 150.19/5--dc23/eng/20220120
LC record available at https://lccn.loc.gov/2022002478
LC ebook record available at https://lccn.loc.gov/2022002479

ISBN: 978-1-032-22412-1 (hbk)
ISBN: 978-1-032-22415-2 (pbk)
ISBN: 978-1-003-27250-2 (ebk)

DOI: 10.4324/9781003272502

Typeset in Times New Roman
by MPS Limited, Dehradun

This book is Dedicated

To our Parents

Leopold Meier & Rosa Meier, née Bineider

Raymond Boivin & Rita Boivin, née Tremblay

# Contents

# Acknowledgments

It is impossible to acknowledge all of the people who have, in their own way, contributed to our thinking about and articulation of psychotherapy, which ultimately led to the development of Self-in-Relationship Psychotherapy. Nevertheless, we are heartily grateful to the many people who have supported our work and have contributed to it through their insightful questions and comments.

Appreciation is expressed to the graduate students who attended the training on Self-in-Relationship Psychotherapy and to the psychotherapists who invited us to supervise their clinical practice. Their questions and discussions were stimulating and help us more clearly define our therapeutic approach.

Appreciation is expressed to the children, adolescents, and adults and to the couples, parents, and families who sought our services to help them address their concerns. Our experience in providing these services challenged us to continually refine our theoretical constructs and techniques, and more clearly link theory, techniques, and research to their lived experiences.

The authors wish to express their appreciation to their professors, clinical supervisors, and dissertation directors at the University of Ottawa, Canada, who have been instrumental in the authors' theoretical research and professional development as clinical psychologists. Appreciation is also expressed to the senior administrators and to the director of the Research Department at Saint Paul University, Ottawa, Canada, for their support in our academic activities by funding our research projects and annual travels to international conferences to present our research results.

The authors want to express their appreciation to the members of the Society for Psychotherapy Research and to the members of the Society for the Exploration of Psychotherapy Integration. Attending the annual conferences of these societies and exchanging ideas with its members made us aware of the cutting edge in psychotherapy research and theory. These experiences inspired us to try and make a contribution to the advancement of psychotherapy theory, practice, and research.

We wish to express our appreciation to our families, particularly, our parents, who provided constant support to us and inspired us to be of service to others by setting an example in their own lives.

We express our deepest appreciation to our daughter, Molisa, for the warm and thoughtful relationship that we have developed over the years. Our relationship has brought to light the significant place that self- and relational needs have in an enduring open and healthy relationship. This awareness has supported our theorizing, professional work, research and writing. For all of these we are extremely grateful.

Lastly, we would like to acknowledge the support of the senior editor, Ms. Kate Hawes, at Routledge, England, for her keen interest in our book and for her help in making its publication possible. We wish to thank the assistant editor, Ms. Georgina Clutterbuck, at Routledge, England, whose expertise, guidance and dedication helped bring this project to fruition.

# Introduction

In 1980 the American Psychological Association (APA) held its annual convention in Montréal, Québec. At the convention, the APA Division 17, The Society of Counseling Psychology, held a meeting to discuss the future of research. For the meeting there were formal presentations and position papers. The participants were also invited to submit written comments to the organizers of the meeting. The formal presentations and the participants' comments were published in *The Coming Decade in Counseling Psychology* by Whitley, Kagan, Marmon, Fretz, and Tanney (1984). In our comments, which comprised one-half page, we wrote that "papers which attempt to propose a new orientation should be encouraged … we are ready for some synthesis in theories concerning counselling." To this we added "that we once again rediscover the client and his inner world of experiences" which is constituted by "feelings, thoughts, needs" (p. 194). At the time that we offered these comments we recently graduated from the university and were beginning our careers. These thoughts, however, were the beginning of our formulation of an integrated model of therapy which led to the development of Self-in-Relationship Psychotherapy.

Self-in-Relationship Psychotherapy is an innovative, integrative and insight-action oriented approach that integrates explanatory constructs from psychoanalysis, ego psychology, object relations theory, relational psychology, self-psychology and developmental psychology, and interventions from action-oriented therapies such as Gestalt therapy, experiential therapy, behavior therapy, and cognitive-behavioral therapy. A core theme of Self-in-Relationship Psychotherapy is that the paradigm of affects, cognitive processes, and behaviors that informs current psychotherapy approaches needs to be expanded to include core relational, self, and physical intimacy needs.

The authors arrived at the significance of human needs from their research and from their 40 years of clinical work with children, adolescents, and adults in the context of individual, couple, family, and child-parent therapy. For example, they observed that children crave the love and affection of their parents and want to be included by their peers. They noticed that teenagers want to have a voice in matters that relate to their lives and the freedom and autonomy to choose and make decisions. They observed in adults, particularly in couples, how one partner wants to spend more time with their partner while their partner wants more time for himself.

Based on these observations, the authors formed a taxonomy of core needs that include relational, self, and physical intimacy needs. Core relational needs include the need for emotional bonding and autonomy; core self needs include the need for competency and significance; and core physical intimacy needs include the need for sensual contact and sexual intimacy.

When a person's needs go unmet for an extended period, the authors observed that it affects all aspects of a person's psychological functioning and relational patterns and leads to emotional and psychological problems. When needs are not met in the appropriate relationships, including in infancy, childhood, and adolescence, the person seeks to have her needs met in compensatory behaviors that provide the nurturance and validation not provided for by the significant persons in her life. These observations led to the formulation of a Self-in-Relationship Psychotherapy that gives priority to human needs.

The goal of therapy is for individuals to recognize, accept, and to appropriately assert their core needs in significant relationships. It is equally important for individuals to learn how to be in an intimate relationship and at the same time maintain their sense of self and autonomy. Self-in-Relationship Psychotherapy focuses both on the relationship and on the self, that is, it helps individuals to be intimately bonded in a relationship and at the same time to maintain their sense of selfhood and autonomy.

Self-in-Relationship Psychotherapy pays equal attention to an individual's subjective experiences which include thoughts/beliefs, affects, and motives and to an individual's external behaviors such as relational patterns, communication style, and defensive strategies. It is assumed that a client's subjective experiences significantly affect both functional and dysfunctional behaviors, relational patterns, and communication style. More precisely, Self-in-Relationship Psychotherapy assumes that unmet core needs underlie psychological and relational problems.

Self-in-Relationship Psychotherapy stands alone among psychotherapy approaches, be they for individual, couple, child, or family therapy. It differs from these approaches as it alone focuses on the role that core human needs – relational, self, and physical intimacy needs – play in the etiology of emotional problems and in the recovery from them. The present approaches to therapy focus either on unexpressed emotions and their release, on correcting cognitive processes and irrational beliefs that one might have, or changing behaviors. Self-in-Relationship Psychotherapy incorporates these aspects but goes further and makes core relational, self, and physical intimacy needs the center piece of its approach. This is the distinguishing characteristic of Self-in-Relationship Psychotherapy.

This book is divided in three parts. The first part presents the seven theorists whose principal constructs have been incorporated in Self-in-Relationship Psychotherapy. It provides as well a thorough review of the literature on human needs and the importance to include them in a theory of psychotherapy. This is followed by a presentation of the major constructs of Self-in-Relationship Psychotherapy. The second part addresses the procedure to formulate a conceptualization using Self-in-Relationship Psychotherapy constructs, presents an assessment form to code the Self-in-Relationship Psychotherapy constructs, and illustrates the use of the form with an actual case. The third part addresses the topic of psychotherapy, which includes the Self-in-Relationship Psychotherapy approach, working with needs and the relational and self issues that present themselves. It concludes with the application of Self-in-Relationship Psychotherapy in the assessment, conceptualization and treatment of a clinical case.

To make the text of this book more reader friendly, the male form of third person noun and pronoun are used in the odd numbered chapters and the female form of third person noun and pronoun are used in the even numbered chapters.

# Part I

# Theoretical Aspects

Chapter 1

# Theoretical Foundations

In the development of Self-in-Relationship Psychotherapy the authors were influenced by the written works of many theoreticians and psychotherapists. This chapter limits itself to the theoretical contributions of seven major authors, namely, Sigmund Freud, Melanie Klein, William R. D. Fairbairn, Donald W. Winnicott, Margaret Mahler, Heinz Kohut, and Edith Jacobson. The contributions from other writers representing different orientations such as experiential, Gestalt and cognitive behavioral are presented in the chapters that follow and particularly in Chapter 7. The purpose of this chapter is to present the major theoretical concepts and processes that have become part of the SIRP approach. Freud's theory is presented in greater detail since it provides the foundation for the elaborations of the theoretical and practical contributions of those who expanded Freudian theory.

## SIGMUND FREUD (1856–1939)

Sigmund Freud was born on May 6, 1856, in Frieberg, Moravia. When Sigmund was three years of age, his family moved back to Vienna where he remained until 1938 when he fled Austria to England because of the persecution of the Jews. He died in London England at the age of 83 on September 23, 1939 (Fancher, 1973).

Freud was initially interested in the humanities, but after listening to an essay on nature written by Goethe, he decided for a career in natural sciences. At the age of 17, he entered medical school at the University of Vienna and in his third year he entered the Physiological Institute and became a distinguished neurologist. Realizing that there was no future in research, he began his medical training with accomplished physicians (Fancher, 1973).

Freud's interest in neurology led him to work with patients struggling with hysteria. As a method of treatment, he replaced hypnosis with free association, which led to the development of psychoanalysis that he continued to elaborate and revise over a 50-year period.

DOI: 10.4324/9781003272502-2

Freud's ideas about emotional problems came from two sources. The first source came from neurology, the discipline in which he was trained, that tended to picture the psyche as a mechanism and a homeostatic organism. The second source came from the new psychodynamic science which he was developing that tended toward a personal psychology of the influence that people have on each other's lives, especially parents on children (Guntrip, 1973, p. 30).

## Freud's Psychoanalytic Theory

Freud laid out a plan for a comprehensive study of personality in terms of the conscious and unconscious continuum, motivating factors, psychic organization, personality development, psychopathology, and treatment of emotional disorders. He addressed these topics from a person's biological (genetic) inheritance and his social/cultural heritage.

### *Conscious and Unconscious Continuum*

In his work with patients diagnosed with hysteria, Freud (1900) observed the power of the unconscious in the formation of symptoms. Through his explorations of these symptoms, Freud discovered and formulated the conscious system which comprised the conscious, preconscious, and unconscious that he presented in *The Interpretation of Dreams*. This system has come to be called the *Topographical Model* or the *Instinctual Model* (Bellak et al., 1973, pp. 7–8).

Freud's main discoveries were about the unconscious, which embraced all that which is inherited and that which has been repressed because it was not acceptable. The repressed feelings and memories strive constantly to become conscious; however, the person spends much energy to keep them repressed. The repressed material leaks out and expresses itself in slips of the tongue, nightmares, and dreams. The unconscious system is a dynamic system. The task of the therapist is to link the current symptoms and behaviors to the unacceptable thoughts and/or impulses (Freud, 1923).

### *Motives – Instincts*

The unconscious embraces all of that which is inherited which Freud (1923) described in terms of instincts. The instincts act as innate motives and impulses and impart direction to human actions, thoughts, and feelings and to the development of personality and emotional disturbances. Freud used the word instinct to refer to animal behavior and the word drives/impulses (i.e., *Trieb*) to refer to human behavior. Instincts are "inborn, unconscious, and basically unalterable" whereas a drive/impulse is "an impelling force; a sudden inclination to act, without conscious thought; a motive or tendency coming from within" (Bettleheim, 1984, pp. 105–106).

Freud (1923) recognized two groups of instincts, the *life instincts* collectively referred to as *libidinal instincts* and the *death instincts* referred to as *non-libidinal instincts*. Among the libidinal instincts, the sexual instinct (*Eros*) held primary importance and among the non-libidinal instincts, the death instinct (*Thanatos*) held primary importance. In his reformulation of the instincts, Freud (1938) perceived the aim of Eros is "to establish ever greater unities and to preserve them" and the aim of Thanatos "is to undo connections" (p. 148). The concept to undo connections includes the thrust toward psychological separation and to being assertive and not complying with the needs of others (Blanck & Blanck, 1979).

Libidinal drives can be turned inward and invested in oneself, referred as *ego-libido*, or can be turned outward and be invested in others, referred to as *object-libido* (Freud, 1914, p. 77). The primary investment of energy in oneself and in one's interests is referred to as *primary narcissism*. When there is a withdrawal of a massive amount of object-libido which propels the person back to self-absorption, this is referred to as *secondary narcissism* (p. 75). In normal development, the move is from the investment of energy in oneself to the investment of energy to that which is outside of self (e.g., parents, toys). Freud (1912) believed that psychoanalysis was not an effective treatment for persons struggling with secondary narcissism because they were not able to develop transference (p. 108).

### Psychic Organization

An infant/child organizes its experiences and perceptions of the significant other, the self, and the real world to form structures of the mind. These have come to be named the *id*, *ego*, and *superego* (Freud, 1923). Freud did not use the terms mind, id, ego, and superego but in place of them he used the common words of *seele* (soul), *das es*, (the thing), *das ich* (I), and *über-ich* (the one above me), respectively (Bettleheim, 1984, p. 76).

#### The id

The id is believed to contain "everything that is inherited," is "present at birth" and "laid down in the constitution" (Freud, 1938, p. 145). It is the inaccessible part of the personality (Freud, 1933). The instincts are the chief components of the id and the main source of energy (Freud, 1915a). They impart direction to psychological processes and play a role in adaptation. The id also comprises mental material that has been repressed because it was unacceptable. The id's main function is to satisfy the individual's innate needs (Freud, 1938).

### *The ego*

Freud (1923) described the ego as a "coherent organization of mental processes" (p. 17). It is innate, present at birth, and distinguished by innate characteristics such as the capacity for perception, memory, and motility (Freud, 1937). The ego has come to signify a cluster of perceptual and cognitive processes and functions, and defense mechanisms. In terms of perceptual and cognitive processes (e.g., perception, memory), the ego "seeks to present the influence of external world to bear upon the id and its tendencies" (Freud, 1923, p. 17). As for defense mechanisms, the ego serves to mediate between the instinctual demands of the id, the internalized parental inhibitions and prohibitions of the superego and the demands of reality.

The ego also possesses capacities to adapt to the environment. The adaptive capacities which are present before the experience of conflict are referred to as "primary autonomous ego functions" (e.g., motility, perception, intelligence) and the defensive functions which emerge to deal with frustrations and conflicts are referred to as "secondary autonomous ego functions" (Hartmann 1939, p. 101).

The ego evolves across space and time. The factors that contribute to its evolution include the maturation of the primary autonomous ego apparatuses, the catalytic influence of the maternal object, and the psychic mechanism of internalization that include introjection and identification. Through introjection, the ego identifies with a lost object (e.g., mother) and retains it as part of the internal structure of the psyche. Through identification, the ego modifies the subject's self or behavior to more closely resemble an object taken as a model (Freud, 1923).

The superego represents the morals and standards of the society that have been internalized and become part of an individual's internal world (Freud, 1938). It represents a regulatory agent for the ego similar to that of the parents and thus has available similar means to punish or reward the person. The punishing or inhibiting functions include prohibition, self-judgment, and sense of guilt, disapproval of actions and wishes, and demand for reparation for wrong doing. The rewarding functions include self-love, self-praise, and self-esteem as a reward for desirable thoughts and actions (Freud, 1923).

The superego is considered as having two major branches, namely, the *ego-ideal* and the *conscience*. The ego-ideal corresponds to the child's conceptions of what his parents consider to be morally good and admirable and represent the positive aspects of striving toward ideals. The conscience corresponds to the child's conceptions of what his parents feel is morally bad and represents the negative aspects characterized by prohibitions (Freud, 1933).

The superego is formed with the resolution of the Oedipus complex through the mechanisms of sublimation and repression of the instinctual needs (sexual) and through the mechanism of identification, especially with the father, who is seen as the preferred parent (Freud, 1923).

When the id, ego, and superego are compared as to how they are governed, the id is governed by the pleasure principle, the ego by the reality principle, and the superego by the ideal principle. In terms of their mode functioning, the id functions in terms of the primary process and the ego in terms of the secondary process (Freud, 1900, p. 604). The id, ego, and superego are perceived to interact, consciously or unconsciously, in all human thoughts, feelings, motives, and behaviors.

### Personality Development and Its Dynamics and Stages

Freud presented the development of personality in terms of its dynamics and stages. Personality dynamics comprise psychic energy, conflict and anxiety, defense mechanisms, changing objects, and identifications and internalizations. Freud presented the psychosexual stages in biological and psychological terms.

#### *Personality dynamics*

*Psychic energy:* The development of personality involves two sources of psychic energy that are derived from the id, namely, *Eros* and *Thanatos*. Eros is sexual and love energy and leads to bonding and emotional connection. Thanatos is aggressive energy that leads to self-protection, assertive behavior, and attacking behavior (Freud, 1938). The energy is cathected (invested), decathected (withdrawn), and transformed or displaced for the purpose of connecting and bonding with others or for the purpose of self-protection and assertive behavior. In addition to the id-energy, there is also ego-energy derived from the ego and used for adaptation (e.g., thinking, planning, and action) and for creative activities such as the literary, arts, and music (Hartman, 1939, p. 51).

*Conflict and anxiety:* The internal conflicts between the quest for the immediate satisfaction of instinctual demands of the individual and his environment are another source of personality dynamic. The intensity of the conflict depends on the extent to which the environment exercises censorial controlling functions that impede the immediate expression of the child's impulses (Freud, 1933).

Freud distinguished between neurotic anxiety and moral anxiety. Neurotic anxiety arises when a person fears that his instincts will get out of control and cause him to do things for which he will be punished. Moral anxiety occurs when the person feels guilty about unacceptable things that he feels that he has done (Freud, 1923). In his revised (affect) model, anxiety represented the anticipation of danger whether from an inner structure (e.g., superego) or from an external source (Freud, 1926).

*Defense mechanisms:* The development of one's personality is also influenced by the mode of coping with problems encountered at each stage of psychosexual development. When realistic methods of handling anxiety and conflict are ineffective, the person may develop elaborate defenses to avoid anxieties and come to terms with instinctual impulses seeking release. The defenses serve to protect the person from psychological harm. The manner in which a person protects himself is reflected in the nature of character formation, symptoms, and defense mechanisms. Defense mechanisms can be grouped according to whether they are more primitive and biological in nature and operate by blocking off some idea, emotion, or memory (e.g., repression, dissociation) or more cognitive in nature (e.g., rationalization, displacement, sublimation).

*Changing objects:* Personality development is also reflected in terms of the changing objects which satisfy the instinctual needs (Freud, 1909). In the course of development, the libido becomes manifest in increasingly more organized ways; there is a movement from a general pleasure orientation to a specific sexual and genital orientation and there is a progression from an autoerotic infantile sexuality to more object-directed relationship where sexual feelings are focused in a sexual person rather than in oneself. As the personality grows, there is also a change in the nature and quality of objects that the ego chooses. The early choices are that of self (e.g., sucking of thumb) whereas the later mature choices are others as love objects (e.g., a boy/girlfriend) (Freud, 1909).

*Identifications and internalizations:* Identification refers to a person modifying his subjective self or behavior, or both, in order to increase his resemblance to an object taken as a model (Schafer, 1968). The mechanism of identification plays a key role in both the development of the ego and ego-ideal and in the resolution of the Oedipus complex (Freud, 1923). Identifications help the ego to expand and to broaden; they aid in the integration of personality, serve as incentives for continuous learning, and help in the determination of sex-roles in the child. When compared to an introject, which operates as a function of instinctual forces, identification functions relatively autonomously from drive derivatives (Freud, 1916).

### Freud's Theories of Affect

During his career, Freud offered three distinct theories of affect. In his first theory, Freud equated affect with the energetic forces (i.e., libido, aggression) which became dammed up in neurotic disorders and were discharged (Freud, 1894). With the introduction of his topographical model and the theory of instinctual drive, Freud (1915a, 1915b) defined affect as a "subjective, conscious experience" but not "as identical with drive" (Jacobson, 1953, p. 39).

> Affect is a consciously perceived expression of the underlying instinctual process; it is the non-ideational part of the drive representation that must be distinguished from the ideational part of the drive representation (Jacobson, 1971, p. 4).

In his third theory of affect, with the introduction of the structural model, Freud (1926) held that all affects with the exception of anxiety originate within the system conscious, that is, in the ego. It is only the ego that can feel affective states, the id cannot have anxiety. However, processes can begin or take place in the id which causes the ego to produce anxiety (p. 140). The ego uses anxiety as a signal in situations of danger triggered by external events. Freud considered that all affects are "inherited, once purposeful, and adaptive reactions to traumata imposed by reality" (p. 9).

### *Psychosexual Stages of Personality, Fixations, and Regressions*

Freud (1909) viewed the developmental process in term of psychosexual stages. The stages were regarded as successive phases in the maturation of the sexual instinct: oral, anal, phallic (or preadolescent genital), and genital. Libido was the basic sexual energy and each of the organic zones was regarded as possessing its own inherent libidinal drive for the pleasure of detensioning (Guntrip, 1973, p. 60).

The defining characteristics of each stage are the ways in which the libido manifests itself and the different quality of relationship with objects. The infant/child proceeds through the developmental stages beginning with that which it can incorporate through its mouth and arriving at a final stage where he relates to loved-person in a mature way. As the person moves along the developmental path, he detaches libido from one object and one mode of gratification and attaches the libido to a new object and to a new way of gratification. Infantile sexuality is oral, anal, or phallic; genital libido is mature sexuality and represents the ability to relate to a whole person (Guntrip, 1973, p. 60).

In the course of personality development, the person might experience fixations and regressions. Fixation refers to an arrest in sexual impulses at an early stage of psychosexual development. Regression refers to reversion to behaviors characteristic of an earlier age of development and the return of the libido to its former halting place in development. This may occur when the demands placed on a child are greater than its resources to respond to them (Freud, 1909, p. 48). The person's experience at each psychosexual stage leaves a characteristic imprint that influences his future development.

### *Psychopathology*

Freud viewed all of psychopathology in terms of conflicts within the psychic organization. The etiology of psychopathologies reflects a failure in the functioning of the ego to reconcile the various demands made on it by its agencies and by reality (Freud, 1938, p. 172). Freud believed that neuroses and psychoses share in common a frustration which is a consequence of the non-fulfillment of a childhood wish. The frustration proceeds from the superego which has taken over representation of the demands of reality.

In the case of neurosis, the ego remains true to its dependence on reality and refuses to accept the powerful impulses in the id, and tries to find an acceptable motor outlet for them, or it forbids the impulse the sought-after object (Freud, 1924a). Consequently, the ego defends itself against the impulse by repressing it. The repressed material struggles against the repression and creates for itself a substitutive representation, a symptom, over which the ego has no power and therefore is forced to compromise.

Regarding psychoses, the ego lets itself be overcome by the id and therefore is torn away from reality. Either the ego does not perceive the external world or the perception of it has no effect on it. New perceptions are refused and the internal world loses its significance. The ego creates, autocratically, a new external and internal world constructed in accordance with the id's wishful impulses which results in a disconnect from reality (Freud, 1924a).

As for narcissism, it entails directing libidinal energy toward the subject's own ego (Freud, 1924b). This energy was referred to as "narcissistic" or "ego-libido." This differs from transference neuroses where the energy is directed outward to a person or a thing (pp. 203–204). Regarding melancholia, Freud (1921) understood it as representing anger turned inward due to the loss of a loved one. The person identifies with the lost object and sets it up within his ego. The grieving person than treats the ego as if it were abandoned or lost and will inflict upon himself the disappointments and anger that he feels because of the loved one's leaving.

### *Treatment*

Freud provided a broad outline of the essential components of effective treatment. These components have become the foundation for the extensions of psychoanalysis such as ego psychology, object relations therapy, and self-psychology.

The goal of treatment was to strengthen the ego by advancing the client's insight into his problem through critical examination of the underlying causes of the symptom. Therapy was to continue as long as new unconscious material relevant to the symptoms continued to come to light, regardless of whether or not the symptoms themselves were constantly present. Treatment was not complete by the mere removal of symptoms (Freud, 1910, p. 144).

The therapeutic relationship included a contract called the "formation of a pact" (Freud, 1938, pp. 173–174). As part of the pact the client was asked to be candid and report everything that came to his mind without censoring it whether it was agreeable or disagreeable. On his part, the psychoanalyst exercised the strictest discretion and to put at the client's service his experience in interpreting material influenced by the unconscious so as to provide the ego with more mastery over his own mental life.

Freud indicates five fundamental therapist qualities that affect the outcome of treatment. These qualities are that the therapist: (a) not mold the client into an image of himself (Freud, 1938); (b) exercise empathy which is a form of "emotional knowing" (Freud, 1913, p. 320); (c) refrain from actively intervening in a patient's life by giving advice or imposing his values (Blanck & Blanck, 1979); (d) be able to manage countertransference (Freud, 1920); and (e) exercise good judgment and timing by providing interventions at appropriate moments (Freud, 1938).

Freud (1938) utilized two therapeutic techniques, namely, free association and interpretation. Free association was used to elicit unconscious material. Interpretation was used to help the client intellectualize and replace superego functions with ego functions with the therapist playing the role of the alter-ego.

The content for analysis comprised the client's transference, resistance and dreams and parapraxis and slips of the tongue (Freud, 1901, 1938). Dreams were considered to be the "most favourable object of study" and the royal vehicle to the unconscious (Freud, 1938, p. 167). Freud did not interpret dreams but elucidated the meaning behind them (Bettleheim, 1984). Freud (1938) differentiated the "manifest dream material" (i.e., dream remembered) from the "latent dream thoughts" (symbolic meaning); he viewed dreams to be governed by the laws of condensation and displacement (p. 165).

In summary, Freud "opened the door" for a comprehensive study of personality and for understanding and treatment of emotional problems. Guntrip (1973) stated that Freud's greatness was that he could not let his emotional intuition and his intellectual urge for exploration be bound by his professional scientific education and that he had the courage to change his theories as he gathered new experiences and experimented with new hypotheses (p. 33). According to Guntrip, the question to ask about Freud is not so much "What did Freud say?" but "What has Freud's work led on to?" (p. 5).

## MELANIE KLEIN (1882–1960)

Melanie Klein was born in 1882 in Vienna. Her desire was to study medicine but her engagement at 17 and marriage at 21 closed the door to this dream. Early in her marriage she struggled with depression during which time she happened to read Freud's *Interpretation of Dreams* which motivated her to go into psychoanalysis with Sandor Ferenczi in Budapest to where the family moved. Observing her talent in handling disturbed children, he encouraged her to work in the field of child psychoanalysis. She began to formulate her approach to child psychoanalysis in Budapest, developed it further at the Berlin Psychoanalytic Institute and consolidated it in England where she trained others to work with children (Grosskurth, 1986; Lindon, 1972; Segal, 2004).

In her work with children, Klein (1952a) observed that children devoted more energy to constructing their interpersonal worlds than to controlling libidinal impulses. She investigated how infants/children form relationships, internalize them to develop an inner world populated by relationships, and how these relationships unfolded across time to become more mature relationships. The importance of relationships became the center piece around which she constructed her theory.

## Theoretical Constructs

To investigate relationships, Klein adopted Freud's concept of the life and death instincts and the mechanisms of introjection and projection. She modified his concept of phantasy and added the defense of splitting. As for treatment, she developed the play technique and interpreted the child's fantasies in the same manner that Freud interpreted adult verbalizations from free associations.

### *Instincts and Human Motive*

In her study of infants/children, Klein (1946, 1948) began with the Freud (1923) assumption that they are born with two innate forces, namely, the life force (i.e., *Eros*) represented by the sexual instinct, and the death force (i.e., *Thanatos*) represented by the aggressive instinct. The two instincts do not emerge from an infant's interaction with real objects, rather they are part of his constitution with which he is born; they are at war with each other. The infant/child lives in terror that the death instinct will destroy him and to protect himself from annihilation he projects the aggressive instinct onto the outer world (e.g., bad mother). At the same time, he also projects the life instinct outward (e.g., good mother) as he needs the object to protect him.

Klein differed from Freud in terms of human motives. Freud (1920) held that the fundamental motive in life was pleasure and that others were important to an individual only through their function to satisfy the infant's needs and to reduce tension. Drives were not keyed to any specific object and whatever appeared to satisfy their need became its object. Klein's (1952a) findings led her to contend that children were less driven by a compulsive need to control erotic impulses than by a need to control feelings directed at significant figures in their lives. She altered Freud's definition of drive which was objectless to saying that drives are inherently directed toward objects; that is "libido is object seeking" (Cashdan, 1988, pp. 4–5).

### *Inner World of Phantasy*

Through his contact with the real world (e.g., mother) on to which he projects both the death instincts and life instincts, he forms perceptions of his world. His perception of the real world, however, is modified by his feelings (e.g., feeling of persecution) and beliefs and knowledge (Klein, 1937, p. 308). His perceptions are an amalgam of reality and projected feelings. Such perceptions are referred to as phantasies. Klein defines a phantasy as a "mental corollary, the psychic representation of an instinct" and the "mental expression of the activity of both the life and death instincts" (Klein, 1952b, p. 58). Phantasies are perceptions that have been modified by the infant/child's feelings and instincts. Phantasies are distorted perceptions of people who are seen through the infant/child's emotional state (Segal, 2004).

In this internal world of phantasy and feeling, life is viewed as a matter of ego-object relationships. These ego-object relationships are formed from the infant/child's perception of reality, which is distorted by his projected instincts. The infant cannot experience the outer world; it knows the outer world through its projection of the innate death instinct and its struggle against it. The internal bad objects first come into being as an introjection of the infant's projected version of his own innate badness and destructiveness (Guntrip, 1973).

In this internal world, the child lives fantasied and highly emotion-laden relationships with a great variety of good and bad objects which are mental images of aspects or parts of persons. At the primitive level, they are part-objects (e.g., breast images) and later they develop into whole-objects that are good or bad in the infant's experience.

### *Good Mother and Bad Mother and Splitting*

The infant/child first works out the two instincts in its encounter with the mother who is perceived to be "good" or "bad" depending on whether or not she was able to respond to its needs and relieve the child of its distress and frustrations. When she gives the child pleasure, the mother is considered to be a good mother and when she is the source of displeasure, the mother is a bad mother. To describe these two experiences Klein referred to them as the "good breast" and the "bad breast." The child, however, saw the two mothers (breasts) as being different persons. It accomplished this through the defense of splitting which means to separate the good from the bad experiences of the mother. This was needed for survival as the child could not think of mother as being bad as he relied on her. Within the first year of life, the child begins to see the mother as the one and same person who can be "good and bad" rather than "good or bad" (Klein, 1945, p. 377).

### Division of World into Benevolent and Malevolent Objects

The infant/child, because of the two instincts, is predisposed to react to others from the position of aggression and/or love. It projects its aggression outward to create bad objects (people) and it projects its love outward to create good objects (people). The child then internalizes the bad and good people to create good and bad internal objects (internal representations). The child also develops good and bad representations of itself; it is good when mother is pleased and bad when mother is not pleased. The infant, thereby, creates an external world that is divided into good and bad people and an inner world that is divided into good and bad objects (representations of others) and of good and bad selves. The dynamic interplay of the good and bad objects makes up the infant's psyche (Klein, 1940).

### Projective Identification

This involves a phantasy in which some unbearable and undesirable aspect of self is expelled by projecting it into someone else (Klein, 1952a). The infant/child no longer feels that the unbearable and undesirable qualities of himself and the feelings associated to them belongs to him. The relationship with others is deeply colored by the investment of the part of self in the other person. For example, powerful feelings of jealousy may be quite intolerable but relatively easy to attribute to someone else: "s/he is jealous, not me!" (Segal, 2004, p. 37). A consequence of a projective identification is that a person tries to draw the other into his way of relating. Thus, if the person has learned to depend on others, he will try to draw the other into caretaking behaviors (Cashdan, 1988).

### Developmental Positions

As the infant/child works out his love and hate relationships with the object world, Klein (1952a, 1959) perceives him to move between two major problem positions which she named the *paranoid-schizoid position* and the *depressive position*. The infant/child does not pass through and grow out of one position to leave it behind, rather, he continues to move between the two positions for most of his life.

The infant/child begins in the paranoid-schizoid position wherein he feels that the world is hostile toward him. He projects the death instincts and life instincts on to the outer world and divides the world into malevolent and benevolent people; he sees persons in terms of being either all good (i.e., idealization) or all bad (i.e., devaluation) or in being bad at one time and good at another time; his greatest fear is to be annihilated from which fear he protects himself.

The infant progresses to the depressive position where he begins to view the person that he thought to be good or bad as being the same person, he fears losing the love object, becomes empathic toward the person that he might have hurt, and desires reparation for the damage done. Klein (1952a) observed that highly troubled and aggressive children moved between the paranoid-schizoid position and the depressive position with the latter being a higher level of development.

### *Greed, Envy, and Gratitude*

The infant/child can emerge from the early relationships with significant others being greedy/envious or grateful or a combination of both. In his relationship with the first object, the mother's breast, the greedy/envious child can respond to it in one of two ways (Klein, 1957, 1959). First, the greedy child might enjoy what he receives at the moment but soon becomes dissatisfied and desires to appropriate the breast for its own needs; to possess and control it. He is driven to exploit initially the mother and later anyone who can give him attention. Second, the envious child does not wish to gain access to the breast and to possess it, but to spoil it. The child cannot tolerate the very existence of something that is so powerful and important and outside of his control. He would rather destroy the good rather than remain helplessly dependent on it. Envy and greed are characteristics of the paranoid-schizoid position.

A second way that a child can emerge from the relationship with significant others is to feel joy for what he has received and to experience gratitude toward the person who gives it (Klein, 1959). The infant/child's gratitude and devotion, first of all toward his mother, develops into devotion to various causes that are felt to be good and valuable. Gratitude, a component of love, mitigates hateful feelings and the child experiences both the real external world and his psychic inner world as friendlier environments. An infant/child with a strong capacity for love and gratitude, having a deep-rooted relationship with a good object, can withstand temporary states of envy and hatred without being fundamentally damaged (Klein, 1957).

### *Play Therapy and the Goal of Therapy*

In her work with children, Klein (1927) introduced play therapy, a form of a projective, which encouraged the externalization and displacement of the child's inner world and inner conflicts and phantasies on the outer world, particularly through the transferences. She interpreted the expressions and phantasies observed in play in the same way that Freud interpreted the verbalizations of adults. She also observed that children were more concerned about their relationships with peers than with regulating their sexual impulses and drives.

The goal of therapy is to elicit and work through transference. The transference embodies the child's phantasies, fears, and feelings experienced in previous relationships. The transferences are explored, analyzed, and interpreted for their instinctual basis. In the child's transferences, the therapist can represent many different figures from his early life. According to Klein, healing takes place within the context of relationships, that is, the client-therapist relationship.

In summary, Klein was the first to apply psychoanalysis to working with children. She discovered that the pursuit of relationships is a fundamental human motive, she presented a clearer view of the inner world that is populated by ego-objects, she underlined the importance of the prototypical nature of the infant-mother relationship, and she emphasized how greed, envy, and gratitude can act as predispositions toward the relationships that one chooses. Lastly, she introduced the play technique and modified the concepts of transference and countertransference.

## WILLIAM R. D. FAIRBAIRN (1889–1964)

Fairbairn was born on August 11, 1889, in Edinburgh, Scotland, where he spent his entire professional career as a physician and psychoanalyst. In his studies, he was influenced by Aristotelian philosophy that viewed human nature as integral and participatory striving for integration and reciprocity between subject and object. The idea that the subject and the object are participants led him to become absorbed with the individual's subjective experience and with the process whereby individuals differentiate from the environment (Scharff & Fairbairn Birtles, 1994). Following his military service during the First World War, he studied medicine and obtained his MD in 1927. Without formal training he began to practice psychoanalysis in 1925 with patients who were diagnosed with schizoid and hysterical conditions.

### Theoretical Concepts

Fairbairn's major work focused on how the infant/child's experience of his mother was internalized to form the psychic organization (i.e., endopsychic situation) that is constituted by the relationship of split-off subsidiary ego states to the characteristic of the internalized split object. This position led to the formulation of supporting constructs including that the libido is object seeking, energy and structure are inseparable, the splitting of the object and the ego, and the endopsychic situation. He proposed that developmental stages are about working through dependency and that therapy comprises the releasing of the bad object.

### The Object-Seeking Libido, Energy, and Structure

Borrowing from Klein (1952a), Fairbairn (1951) postulated that "libido is essentially object-seeking" (p. 162) and that "the ultimate goal of libido is the object" (1941, p. 31). Libido is seen as being directional and relational with the object always being a person (Mitchell & Black, 1995).

Unlike Freud who stated that the energy is derived from both the id and ego, Fairbairn (1944) located the libido solely in the ego. By locating the energy in the ego and viewing it as a drive toward relationships, Fairbairn eliminated the id, modified the superego, and changed the ego which for him became a dynamic structure (p. 88).

Fairbairn (1954) viewed instinct as a "characteristic dynamic pattern of behavior" (p. 218). Instincts were not "forces invading the ego from outside itself ... but dynamic reactions of 'person-ego,' sexually or aggressively, and to an object-relational situation" (Guntrip, 1973, p. 34). Fairbairn also gave up the use of the term libido and always spoke of the libidinal ego.

### The Splitting of the Object and Establishing a World of Internal Object Relations

Fairbairn (1941) viewed the mother to be the first and primary object sought by the infant and stated that the mother-child relationship was the most significant relationship. The child experiences the mother predominantly as good. She fulfills his needs and gratifies his wishes. When the mother ignores the child, rejects his advances, and frustrates his desires, the mother is seen as bad (Fairbairn, 1944). To deal with an inconsistent and ungratifying mother and to change it and improve it, the child, through the mechanism of splitting, constructs an inner world inhabited by different aspects of the mother. The mother is divided into good and bad components which are psychically split off one from the other. The result is the creation of an inner world that is split into good and bad internal objects with each corresponding to the gratifying and ungratifying aspects of the real mother (Fairbairn, 1946).

Fairbairn (1944) refers to the good internal object as the "*ideal object*" that embodies the rewarding and comforting aspects of the mother (pp. 110–111). According to Fairbairn (1949), the bad object has two characteristics, namely, an exciting aspect and a rejecting aspect (p. 159). The bad internal object, consequently, is split into the "*exciting object*" and the "*rejecting object*" (Fairbairn, 1944, p. 104). Guntrip (1969) suggested a third object to this split in the bad object, namely, an "*impingement object*" which Fairbairn accepted (p. 67).

The *exciting object* refers to the alluring, tantalizing, and promising features of the mother but who does not bring closure to these actions.

The infant/child is left feeling frustrated and empty. The *rejecting object* refers to the frustrating and disappointing features of the mother who is hostile and withdrawing. The infant/child is left feeling unloved and unwanted and chronically angry (Fairbairn, 1944). The *impingement object* is formed by the mother forcing herself on the child in ways that he does not want. The child feels pressured and exploited in the interests of the mother.

By mentally splitting the object into good and bad aspects, the infant/child internalizes its bad aspects. The result is that the environment is made to be good and the child is made to be bad. The child can now deal with the outer world as it has been made good.

### *The Splitting of the Ego*

Each of the four internal objects (ideal, exciting, rejecting, and impinging) gives rise to idiosyncratic ego states through a process of parallel ego splitting (Fairbairn, 1944). Part of the central ego becomes attached to the bad object through the process of identification and therefore takes on the same qualities as the bad object and becomes like the bad object. The consequence is that the person has internalized the same pattern of relating that he experienced with the external object.

Fairbairn (1944) postulates three ego states, namely, *infantile libidinal ego state* (ILES), *antilibidinal libidinal ego state* (ALES), and *central ego state* (CES) (pp. 101–105). To these was added a fourth ego state, namely, a *regressive libidinal ego state* (RLES) (Guntrip, 1969, p. 77).

The ILES is described as the oral needy libidinal ego. The child feels perpetually frustrated and deprived and thirsts for more but is never satisfied (Fairbairn, 1944). This ego state corresponds to the exciting object.

The ALES is the attacking ego; it is aggressive especially toward the needy part of the self. It is hateful and vengeful and rails against the denial it has experienced. It desperately yearns for acceptance and connectedness that it feels it deserves. It is controlled by the fear that it is unwanted and unlovable. The ALES arises from the rejecting object and functions in a way similar to the superego (Fairbairn, 1944). The ALES is characterized by an undeveloped childish conscience and by self-persecuting behaviors (Guntrip, 1973). The ALES is not identical to the superego, a term that Fairbairn (1949) retains, to "describe an internal object which is cathected and accepted as 'good' by the central ego, and which appears to function as an ego-ideal … and provides the basis for the establishment of moral values in the inner world" (pp. 159–160).

The RLES is that part of the self that fears the overpowering outer world and evokes withdrawal as a flight into the inner world. The child feels overwhelmed by fear and is in a state of exhaustion. It feels that it will be fit to live only if it "can escape into a mental convalescence where it can lie quiet, protected and be given a chance to recuperate" (Guntrip, 1969, p. 76).

This ego state arises due to the hostile and aggressive object or situation and corresponds to the impingement object.

The CES derives from the good object and the ideal ego. This part of the ego is still connected to those parts of the mother that were gratifying (Fairbairn, 1944). The CES, or the "I," comprises conscious and unconscious elements and relates to the environment. It aggressively severs subsidiary egos from itself and represses them. When the disturbing parts of the other ego states have been split off and repressed, the CES engages in conforming behavior with the idealized parents. The splitting off of these parts leaves the inner world fragmented and forms the basis for the development of psychopathology. The compromised CES is a depleted ego (Guntrip, 1973).

### *Endopsychic Situation*

In place of Freud's (1923) concept of psychic structure which comprised the id, ego, and superego, Fairbairn (1944) used the term *endopsychic situation* which refers to the multiple substructures of the ego in relation to the internalized objects that have become structures (pp. 109, 112). The endopsychic situation includes the internal bad objects and the parts of the ego associated with them but it does not include the CES and the good object. The child internalized bad objects partly with a view to controlling them (an aggressive motive) and because he experienced a libidinal need of them (Fairbairn, 1949).

Fairbairn considers the internal objects to be structures that are dynamic and capable of acting as independent agencies within the mind. Thus, the internal objects are not merely mental representations, but they are agencies capable of psychological activity (Fairbairn, 1944).

### *Developmental Process and Its Stages*

Unlike Klein who viewed the development of the child-mother relationship as working out a love and hate relationship, Fairbairn believes that the task for the infant is to resolve its dependency needs and to move from dependency to independency. According to Fairbairn (1941) every child progresses through three broad stages of development, namely, *infantile dependence stage*, *the transition stage*, and *mature dependence stage* (p. 39).

The *infantile dependence stage* is characterized predominantly by an attitude of taking and incorporating. This comprises two sub-stages, namely, a pre-ambivalent (i.e., sucking or rejecting) and an ambivalent (i.e., sucking or biting) stage. In this stage, the child is psychologically merged with the primary caregiver and there is very little differentiation and a poorly developed sense of self. The child is bound to the mother in a very primitive way which Fairbairn (1946) refers to as "primary identification" (p. 145).

The *transition stage* is characterized by a lifelong process of breaking away from the child's dependency of early relationships and a move toward interdependence. The conflict of this stage is "between a progressive urge to surrender the infantile attitude of identification with the object and a regressive urge to maintain that attitude" (Fairbairn, 1946, p. 145).

The *mature dependence stage* is marked by mutuality and exchange. The participants are able to acknowledge each other's differences and are aware of the healthy dependence that underlies their interaction. This stage is characterized by a "capacity on part of the differentiated individual for co-operative relationships with differentiated objects" (Fairbairn, 1946, p. 145).

### The Analytic Situation

According to Fairbairn, treatment entails the development of the capacity to relate and to the release of bad objects. This is to be achieved with the psychoanalyst becoming a good object (Fairbairn, 1944). Analytic change was not located "in the dawning of insight, but in a changed capacity for relatedness, an ability to connect with the analyst in new ways" (Mitchell & Black, 1995). The goal is to restore the capacity to make direct and full contact with others. A second goal of analysis is the release of bad objects from the unconscious and following that to rediscover what remains of the "original pristine unitary ego" (Eagle, 1984, pp. 82–83). The bad objects were internalized because they once seemed indispensable and were repressed because they were not tolerable (Fairbairn, 1943).

To help the analysand release the bad objects, the psychoanalyst must provide a secure environment since the analysand is predisposed to view him as an old and bad object. Within the secure environment, the analysand renounces "old, transferential forms of connection to the analysand … [and begins] … to believe in new, less constrained patterns of relatedness" (Mitchell & Black, 1995, p. 122). In this manner, the transference relationships are worked through until they give way to good realistic relationships between therapist and client.

In brief, Fairbairn's contribution consists in his clear articulation of the relationship between the various experiences of the mother and how these experiences contribute to the formation of the ego states that act like dynamic structures that influence how he relates to self and to others. The other contributions comprise his view of the developmental process in terms of a movement away from dependency toward interdependency and his understanding that the goal of psychotherapy is to develop the capacity to relate and to release of the bad object.

## DONALD W. WINNICOTT (1896–1971)

Winnicott was born on April 7, 1896, in Devon, England. He studied medicine at Cambridge and completed his medical degree in 1920 and began to work as a pediatrician in 1923. In the same year, he entered psychoanalysis which he completed in 1933 and immediately began to practice as a child psychoanalyst. Intellectually and professionally, he was influenced by classical psychoanalysis, ego psychology, and Kleinian theory (Rodman, 2003).

### Theoretical Constructs

In his work as a child psychoanalyst, Winnicott observed how the infant develops and grows within the context of "good enough" mother-child relationship. From these observations he formulated his ideas about the sort of mother and child relationship that facilitates healthy development. Winnicott described the essentials of the mother-child relationship and the process of child development using constructs that include maturational process, parental care, transitional objects, true and false self, and the origin and treatment of emotional and mental disturbances.

#### *Maturational Process*

The infant is endowed with innate (maturational) tendencies to move forward and with capacities to become a "whole person" and to relate to self and to the world in a real way (Winnicott, 1963a, pp. 180–181). Conceptually, maturational processes refer to "the evolution of the ego and of the self, and includes the whole story of the id, of instincts and their vicissitudes, and of the defenses in the ego relative to instinct" (Winnicott, 1963b). Four of the maturational processes include integration, personification, personal reality, and object relating.

Integration refers to the increased organization of the individual into a unit. An infant, at birth is made up of a number of motility phases and sensory perceptions. Integration develops gradually out of the state of disintegration. Under favorable environmental conditions, the infant grows into a completed whole (Winnicott, 1965).

Personification entails the process whereby the psyche (i.e., ego) and the soma, with its various id drives and satisfactions, become intimately related to each other (Winnicott, 1963c). Parental care fosters a firm union of the baby's ego and body by providing a reasonable degree of adaptation to the needs of the child. When there is a failure of adaptation, there is a tendency for the psyche to develop an existence that is only loosely related to bodily experience (Winnicott, 1965).

Personal reality connotes the existence of an inner world composed of images, feelings, thoughts, and so on. Positive elements of the inner world are derived from the pattern of personal experience interpreted in a personal way and ultimately based on the infant's inborn inherited characteristics. By the end of the first year, the infant's inner world is organized according to complex mechanisms which have as their purpose

> the preservation of what is felt to be "good" (i.e., ego), the isolation of what is felt to be "bad" (i.e., trauma), and the preservation of an area in the personal psychic reality in which objects have living interrelationships, exciting, and even aggressive, as well as affectionate. (Winnicott, 1965, pp. 8–9)

Object relating refers to the infant being capable to "relate to an object and join up the idea of the object with a perception of the whole person" (Winnicott, 1963c, p. 224). It comprises feeling real and relating to real people and to real objects in the environment. In the early state, the relationships "are of the nature of a union of part with part" (Winnicott, 1965, p. 11), that is, to part objects. The capacity to relate to an object develops as a result of a good enough adaptation of the mother which lasts over a long period of time.

### Parental Care

The environment, in the form of parental care, interacts with the maturational processes of the child. Winnicott coined the term, *good-enough mother*, to describe the parental function of providing sufficiently for the child to get a good start in life (Winnicott, 1962, p. 57). The good enough mother repeatedly meets the "omnipotence of the infant and to some extent makes sense of it" (Winnicott, 1960b, p. 145). Other functions of parental care include holding, handling, and object presenting.

Holding denotes both the actual physical holding of the infant and also the total environmental provision prior to the concept [and stage] of living with (Winnicott, 1960a). The holding period sees the infant merged with the mother and not yet capable of perceiving objects as external to the self. The infant becomes a person in his own right with an inside and an outside, "a me" and a "not-me" (p. 45). The infant's capacity for object relationships changes from a relationship with a subjectively conceived object to a relationship with an objectively conceived object. This is closely linked to the infant's change from being merged with his mother to be being separate from and relating to her as separate and not-me.

Handling refers to the manner in which the parent handles (e.g., touches) the baby's body. It describes "the environmental provision that corresponds loosely with the establishment of psycho-somatic partnerships" (Winnicott, 1962, p. 62). Handling facilitates the formation of psychosomatic partnership in the infant. It contributes to the sense of being "real" as opposed to a sense of being "unreal" (Winnicott 1965, p. 19).

Object presenting refers to that form of parental care which characterizes how objects (e.g., breast, bottle) are presented to the child and it shapes how the child will relate to external reality and external objects. Object presenting initiates the infant's capacity to relate to external objects. Faulty object presenting blocks the way for the infant to develop the capacity to feel real in relating to the actual world of objects (Winnicott, 1962, p. 59).

### *Transitional Phenomena and Objects*

As the infant/child develops and matures within the facilitating environment, he dwells in two realms of experience, the one psychical, subjective, and located inside of self and the other objective and environmental located outside of oneself. Between these two realms of experience, there is an intermediate area of experience to which both the infant's inner reality and external contribute (Winnicott, 1951). In this realm, the subjective and objective are fused. To designate this intermediary experience, Winnicott (1971) used the terms "transitional phenomena" and "transitional objects" (pp. 2–3). It is in this intermediary area that the infant/child learns to renounce the tendency to hallucinatory wish-fulfillment in favor of adaptation to the environment and passes from omnipotent control to control by physical manipulation (i.e., reality testing).

Transitional phenomena include an infant's babbling or some part of the child's own body (e.g., thumb) that is not yet recognized as belonging to external reality. A transitional object is the first "not-me" possession. It is something inanimate but valued (e.g., soft blanket) which the child uses in the course of separation from the other and often uses it in times of distress and in going to sleep. The transitional object, symbolically, stands for the breast or the object of the first relationship (Winnicott, 1951).

### *True Self and False Self*

In the course of his interaction with his environment and its adaptation to his needs, the infant may develop either a true self or a false self (Winnicott, 1960b). The true self, or the central self, is the "inherited potential" that constitutes the "kernel" of the child which is experiencing "a continuity of being, and acquiring in his own way and in his own speed a personal psychic reality and a personal body-scheme" (Winnicott, 1960b, p. 46). The true self is brought in by the mother responding to the infant's omnipotence and in providing a healthy environment and a meaningful responsiveness to the young infant's sensorimotor and postural self. The infant's task in developing a true self is the letting go of omnipotence and illusion (Winnicott, 1960b).

The false self is built up by an infant's compliance to the wishes of a mother who is not able to attune herself to the infant's needs and to implement his omnipotence (Winnicott, 1960b). The false self is "an aspect of the true self; it hides and protects it" by complying with environmental demands (Winnicott 1955–1956, p. 296). The organized false self is characterized by rigid defenses, which prevent growth and development (Winnicott, 1960b). A false self builds up a false set of relationships, feels unreal, and is unable to act spontaneously and be genuine in relationships. A false self is an existence that is only loosely related to bodily experience (Winnicott, 1965).

### Mental and Emotional Disturbances

Winnicott (1963c) viewed mental and emotional disorders in terms of environmental deficits which prevent the development and growth of the maturational processes. The environmental deficits interfere with the normal growth processes that normally lead to the establishment of an integrated self, the embodiment of the psyche, and the capacity to relate as a real person to real objects. These disorders are perceived as being compromises between the individual's immaturity and the actual social reactions, not as diseases.

Winnicott (1959–1964) classified mental and emotional disorders and their origin according to the degree and quality of environmental deficiency or distortion. However, he cautioned the use of this method of classification since there is a great overlap among the disorders (Winnicott, 1963c). One of the disorders that was of interest to Winnicott was the false self disorder, which connotes an individual who feels "unreal or futile in spite of apparent success of the defence" (Winnicott, 1959–1964, p. 134). False self disorders originate at the later infancy phase and prior to the Oedipal phase.

### Treatment and Controlled Regression

The primary goal of therapy is for the client to develop a genuine and healthy true self. This is accomplished by reproducing in therapy the early mothering process which provides the client with those provisions necessary for maturation. An added goal is to unfreeze an early environmental failure situation by providing a successful experience of omnipotence (Winnicott, 1954).

For Winnicott (1955–1956), therapy is a process of controlled regression to early dependence and to the stage of early environmental failure. The purpose of regression is for the client to revisit and relive earlier infantile experiences, which provides him with the opportunity for the correction of earlier developmental deficits (Winnicott, 1954). In regression, the client gives up the false self and the true self emerges. The client is perceived to bring about his own psychological healing which may occur within the context of controlled regression toward dependency and to a dependent relationship (Winnicott, 1959–1964).

Winnicott (1963c) believes that it is important for the therapist to enter into the subjective experience of the client and know how it feels to be his client. As well, it is important for the therapist to be the object of the client's transference of feelings and to meet them with strength rather than with revenge. A profound insight on part of Winnicott was the connection that he drew between false self disorders in adult patients and the subtle variations he observed in the mother and infant interactions from the beginning of the infant's life (Mitchell & Black, 1995).

In summary, Winnicott's significant contribution is his study of the interaction of maturational processes and of parental care in child development. In his study, Winnicott identified the innate potentials with which an infant begins life and how the infant depends on good enough parental care to bring the potentials to full realization. Lastly, his therapeutic approach that consists of the therapist entering into the subjective experience of the client and the technique of controlled regression is helpful in working with clients who present with problems that can be traced back to childhood disturbances.

## MARGARET MAHLER (1897–1985)

Margaret Schonberger Mahler was born on May 10, 1897, in a small western Hungarian town of Sopron close to Vienna. She completed a degree in medicine with specialization in pediatrics but began immediately to transition to psychiatry and to train as a psychoanalyst and upon its completion she started her career as a child psychoanalyst.

Before the beginning of World War II, Mahler and her husband moved to New York City where she established a therapeutic nursery at the Masters Children Center in New York. She and her associates used the nursery to study the development of normal and psychotic children and traced their development from birth to three to four years of age. They were interested to understand how a child that is emotionally connected with its mother moves out of the emotional bond, toward psychological separation and individuation. Mahler and associates studied emotional bonding and the separation and individuation process along the lines of information processing systems (e.g., coenesthetic, sensory, perceptual systems), motor development, language development, and the characteristics of the mother-child relationship (Mahler et al., 1975; Stepansky, 1988).

### Phases of the Developmental Process

By their careful observation of the interaction between mother and child in the first months of life, Mahler and associates were able to layout the nature of early bonding. This bonding, together with the child's early efforts to establish a separate identity, was seen as the beginning of a lifelong process called separation-individuation. It is within the separation-individuation phase that "life's major conflict – the longing for autonomy versus the urge to stay fused with the mother – is played out most intensely" (Cashdan, 1988, p. 13). The separation-individuation process is characterized by three major developmental phases, namely, autistic phase, symbiotic phase, and the separation-individuation phase with the latter comprising a series of subphases. Mahler and associates did not study the normal autism phase but accepted the thoughts about this phase as described by previous psychoanalysts.

### Phase of Normal Autism

In normal autism, which extends from birth to the second month, the infant is in a state of non-differentiation between self and other and not able to differentiate his mother's ministrations in reducing tension from his own efforts (Mahler et al., 1975). The infant's task is to "achieve physiological homeostasis" which he accomplishes by the use of mechanisms that are predominantly somatopsychic and physiological in nature (Bergman & Ellman, 1985, p. 240). As well, the infant is equipped to perform tasks, such as seeking out the breast for sustenance, by his innate reflex capacities as sucking, rooting, grasping, and clinging. These early inner body experiences contribute, ultimately, to the development of the body-ego and the body-self, forming the very core of the self (Mahler & Furer, 1968).

In personal communication with Stern, Mahler mentioned that the phase of autism might have been called "awakening" which is close to Stern's (1985) concept of "emergence" (p. 235). The concepts of "awakening" and "emergent relatedness" assume that the infant from the moment of birth is deeply social and is being designed to engage in interactions with other humans.

### Phase of Normal Symbiosis

In the phase of normal symbiosis, which extends from the second to the fourth month, the infant has an awareness of the need-satisfying object and perceives the small part of reality represented by the mother's breast, face, and hands. With the dim awareness of an external object, the infant's coenesthetic system shifts to a sensorioperceptive system. As well, there is a shift of libidinal energy from him to a need-gratifying object and symbiotic object.

At the beginning of the normal symbiosis phase, the infant "behaves and functions as though he and his mother were an omnipotent system, a dual unity, within one common boundary" (Mahler et al., 1975, p. 44).

This phase represents a state of fusion with the other, a state of undifferentiation in which the "I" is not yet differentiated from the "Not-I," and in which the inside and the outside are only gradually coming to be sensed as different" (p. 45). At the same time, the mother promotes a physiological and sociobiological dependency of the child on her. It is within the matrix of this dependency that differentiation between id and ego functions and between the drives takes place. As well, the infant acquires object-representation and self-representation, the first being a body-ego and a body-image. All of this leads to the functioning of the ego and to the individual's organization for adaptation. During this phase it is essential that the mother attune herself to the needs of the child through empathy and adaptive regression of the ego (Mahler & Furer, 1968).

### *Phase of Separation-Individuation*

The separation and individuation phase comprises four subphases, namely, Differentiation and Body Image, Practicing, Rapprochement, and Consolidation/Object Constancy.

#### *Differentiation and Body Image Subphase*

This subphase extends from the fourth or fifth month to the eight month and is signaled by the "smiling response." In this subphase there is a maturation of the "sensorium – the perceptual-conscious system – which enables the infant to have a more permanently alert sensorium whenever he is awake" (Mahler et al., 1975, p. 53) and there is a development in motor skills. There is a shift from inward-directed attention to outward-directed attention and alertness and the infant's behavior becomes more outward and goal directed.

Around the seventh month, the infant takes its first tentative steps in breaking away from the passive lap-babyhood of the symbiotic phase. This is observed in the infant's tactile and visual exploration of his mother's face and the clad and unclad parts of her body, pulling away behavior while on her lap to observe her more carefully, sliding off the mother's lap only to immediately return or remain there and to play close to her feet, and "checking back to mother" and the experience of "stranger anxiety" (Mahler et al., 1975, pp. 52–60).

#### *Practicing Subphase*

The practicing subphase is divided into early practicing period (from eighth to tenth month) and practicing period proper (from 10th to 18th month). The early practicing period is characterized by quadrupedal locomotion, such as crawling. There is a shift in libidinal investment from mother and self to include objects of the external world, his body, and his own autonomous functions. However, the mother always remains the child's important object. The child takes a more active role in determining closeness and distance from the mother.

The practicing phase proper is characterized by free upright (i.e., bipedal) locomotion. With a spurt in autonomous function in cognition and locomotion, the child begins a "love affair with the world" (Mahler et al., 1975, pp. 70–71). This leads to great strides in human individuation and identity formation. The elation that the child experiences are related to both the exercise of his ego apparatuses and to his escape from the fusion with and engulfment by the mother. Even though the child might show disinterest in the mother, he needs her emotional support. It is important for the mother to provide a "secure base" to which the child can return for "emotional refueling" (p. 69).

It is important for the mother to support the child in his endeavors to pursue the pleasure of separateness and autonomy. Disturbances can occur if the child is pushed to grow up too quickly and the child, in response, might find it hard to grow apart and actively demand closeness with his mother, or when the mother finds it hard to give up her symbiotic holds on their child, and so on (Mahler et al., 1975).

### *Rapprochement Subphase*

The rapprochement subphase extends from the 18th to about the 36th month and is divided into three parts, namely, beginning rapprochement, rapprochement crisis, and individual patterning of rapprochement. During this subphase, there is a marked growth in his cognitive faculties and use of language, increased differentiation of his emotional life and greater abilities to physically separate, and a heightened awareness of his growing separation from his mother and the fear of losing her. The main characteristic of this subphase is the child's need for the mother to share with him every new acquisition of skill and experience. This is brought about by the child's decline in his sense of omnipotence and by the increased sense of identity.

During the early stages of rapprochement, the child wishes to be reunited with the mother and yet fears being re-engulfed by her. This is indicated by "shadowing" and in "darting-away" behaviors (Mahler et al., 1975, pp. 76–77). The failure to enlist the mother into all of his activities, leads to the rapprochement crisis which refers to the conflicts in which the child works out his increased need for the mother while at the same time protecting his own autonomy. The struggle for the child is between his own separateness, grandiosity, and autonomy and his wish for mother to magically fulfill his desires without acknowledging the need for help. In place of the rapprochement struggle, the child eventually finds an optimal distance at which he can function the best.

During this subphase, a period of great vulnerability, it is essential for the mother to be present emotionally to accept his ambivalence and at the same time to encourage normal individuation by letting him go and when appropriate, to nudge him. When a child is preoccupied with mother's emotional availability, he is unable to invest energy in the development of important skills and may revert to earlier splitting mechanisms; serious developmental arrest can result in pathological narcissism and borderline phenomena (Mahler et al., 1975).

### *Consolidation/Object Constancy Subphase*

The last phase, which begins in the third year of life, is referred to as the "Consolidation of Individuality and the Beginnings of Emotional Object Constancy" (Mahler et al., 1975, p. 109). "Object constancy" refers to maintaining the representation of the absent love object in which the "good" and "bad" object have been integrated into one whole representation (p. 110). It refers to the internalization of the mother's functions in dealing with the frustrations. The internalized functions become his internal capacities used to deal with separation and anxiety and to self-soothe and self-comfort.

The attainment of affective object constancy permits the child to substitute for the mother, during her physical absence, a reliable internal image that remains constant irrespective of inner discomfort. This allows the child to function separately despite moderate degrees of tension.

The establishment of affective object constancy depends upon the gradual internalization of a constant and positively cathected symbolic inner representation of the mother as well as maturation and tolerance of frustration and anxiety. Object constancy is built on the establishment of trust and confidence through the regularly occurring relief of needs which is referred to as "confident expectation" (Mahler & Furer, 1968, pp. 8–9).

In addition to developing object constancy, the child also develops "self constancy" which is described as a stable individuality that comprises an awareness of being separate and of individual identity and an awareness of gender identity (Mahler et al., 1975, pp. 110, 224). The achievement of individuality is facilitated by the establishment of a mental representation of self as distinctly separate from representation of others. During this subphase, there is an unfolding of complex cognitive functions and capacity for verbal communication that replace other forms of communication. As well, superego precursors begin and there is a considerable development of ego functions such as reality testing.

In brief, the separation-individuation process entails two complementary but distinct processes. Separation is the process by which the infant emerges from the symbiotic fusion with the mother and individuation marks the achievement of autonomous functions such as locomotion and language and the development of a stable experience of self. Mahler's contribution consists in her ability to document these abilities and demonstrate how they are rooted in the child's early object relations (Cashdan, 1988). Difficulties in the process of psychological separation and individuation have been applied by Kernberg (1975), Masterson (1976, 1980), Masterson and Klein (1995), and Cashdan (1988) to the etiology and the treatment of borderline personality disorders, self-disorders, and serious relational problems.

## HEINZ KOHUT (1913–1981)

Kohut was born in Vienna on May 3, 1913. He was introduced, by his elementary school tutor, to the writings of Plato and Kant. Kohut was deeply impressed with Kant's concept of the transcendental self which influenced his future thinking and writing about the self. Kohut obtained a medical degree in neurology in 1938 from the University of Vienna. In 1939, Kohut left for England and then for the University of Chicago. Kohut completed his training in psychoanalysis in 1949 and then joined the Chicago Institute of Psychoanalysis (Cocks, 1994; Kligerman, 1985; Simpson, 2001).

### Theoretical Aspects

In his clinical practice, Kohut observed that some patients presented with defective self-organizations that manifested emptiness, depression, self-esteem, and a craving for validation for being competent and lovable. Using "empathic immersion" and "vicarious introspection" (Kohut & Wolfe, 1982), Kohut investigated the self in terms of its development, constituents, disorders, and treatment. Constructs that form Kohut's theory of self include basic human striving and narcissism, selfobjects and their functions, the bipolar nuclear self, disorders of the self, and treatment of self disorders.

#### *Basic Human Striving and Narcissism*

Kohut (1977) considered the fundamental human striving to be the push toward "self-realization" and "self-expression" (p. 40). This entailed the experience of being well-put together, holding sameness over time, and containing and balancing the varied emotional states. Kohut emphasized "the capacity to feel one's life experience as energized, creative, and personally meaningful" (Mitchell & Black, 1995, p. 164).

Kohut (1971) considered the child to be basically narcissistic in nature because it was naturally concerned with developing a positive and rewarding self-structure. The child turns its energy inward toward itself. The child, through its early primary relationships, seeks to satisfy two basic narcissistic needs. One is to exhibit the developing capabilities and be admired for them (i.e., *nuclear ambitions*). The other is to form an idealized image of one of its parents so as to experience a sense of merger (i.e., *nuclear ideals*). Both needs are considered to be normal (p. 27). The first constitutes a healthy need for omnipotence and the second a healthy desire for connectedness (Cashdan, 1988, p. 21).

### *Selfobjects and Their Functions*

The two basic narcissistic needs achieve full expression, in healthy infant development, within the context of the primary relationships which are referred to as selfobjects since the infant/child invests them with narcissistic libido (Kohut, 1971). Selfobjects are persons who are undifferentiated from the infant. The child's primitive self merges with the selfobject's mature psychic organization, participates in its organized experience, and has its needs satisfied by the actions of the selfobject (Kohut, 1977).

The selfobject's primary role and purpose is to serve the needs of the infant's nascent self (Kohut, 1971) which evolves within the developmental milieu of three specific kinds of selfobject experiences: (a) selfobjects "who respond to and confirm the child's innate sense of vigor, greatness and perfection," (b) the child's involvement with powerful others "to whom the child can look up and with whom he can merge as an image of calmness, infallibility, and omnipotence," and (c) selfobjects who evoke a sense of essential likeness between them and the child (Kohut & Wolfe, 1978, p. 414).

The selfobjects foster the development of the (nuclear) self through empathic attunement to the feelings and needs of the infant/child. Kohut (1973) defines empathy as "the recognition of the self in the other … [as] … the expansion of the self to include the other … [as] … the accepting, confirming, and understanding human echo by the self …" (p. 705). In brief, empathy means trying to understand the infant/child's experience by placing oneself in the shoes of the patient (Kohut, 1981).

### *The Bipolar Nuclear Self*

In his analysis of the self, Kohut (1971) observed that a firm self comprises three major constituents referred to as poles of the self. Kohut (1984) named these three poles "nuclear ambitions," "nuclear ideals," and "nuclear talents."

The nuclear ambitions comprise grandiose and exhibitionistic self-images, which are formed through the mother mirroring the infant/child's early grandiosity and omnipotence. From these interchanges, the child begins to form desires, ambitions, and potentialities. This pole, formed around the second or third year of life (Kohut, 1977), represents the part of self from which emanate the basic strivings for power and success. The infant/child's self-image is made up of messages that take the form: "I am perfect" (Kohut, 1971, p. 27) and you must admire me (Cashdan, 1988).

The nuclear ideals are made up of idealized images of the world and of the self. The nuclear ideals, which are incorporated between the ages of four and six, comprise self-images involving fusion that evolve from interchanges with "idealized selfobjects." This consists of messages that approximate: "You are perfect and I am a part of you" (Kohut, 1971, p. 27). The ideals begin to be formed when the child has awareness that the external object, the mother, provides the desired satisfactions. Through the mechanism of splitting, all of selfobject's good properties are incorporated into the self and all of its nonsatisfying bad properties are excluded as "not self." The child makes the incorporated characteristics a genuine part of self-image and enduring life aspirations (Monte & Sollod, 2003).

The nuclear talents and skills are activated by the tension between the ambitions and ideals (Kohut & Wolfe, 1982, p. 45). This pole connects the nuclear ambitions and the nuclear ideals and enables the ambitions to turn into achieved goals. Kohut (1984) considered the third pole to be more or less equal with ambitions and goals, consequently, he began to think of a "tripolar self." The third pole develops from the twinship/alter ego selfobject relationship (Baker & Baker, 1987, p. 5).

Kohut (1971) viewed the concept of the self as a "content of the mental apparatus," analogous to a representation of an object, but not as a constituent or an agent of the mind such as the id, ego and superego (p. xv). However, the self is considered to be a structure in the mind since it is cathected with libidinal energy and it has continuity in time and is enduring (p. xv).

### *Disorders of the Self*

Kohut (1971) viewed all of psychopathology in terms of a disintegration of a grandiose self and idealized parent imago and in terms of a regression to an archaic (i.e., lacking structure) self and an archaic idealized parent imago (selfobject). This disintegration is thought to be due to thc repeated empathic failures on part of the mirroring and idealized selfobjects to respond to the child's "grandiose and exhibitionistic" and "idealized parent imago" needs (pp. 9–11). The woundedness to the self can occur at the level of feeling inadequate and incompetent (i.e., nuclear ambitions) and at the level of feeling unlovable and insignificant (i.e., nuclear ideals) or on the level of both (pp. 11, 171).

Kohut's main interest was the narcissistic personality disorder which he differentiated from the narcissistic behavior disorder. Narcissistic behavior disorders are characterized by a temporary breakup, enfeeblement and serious distortion of the self and are manifested in the form of words (alloplastic symptoms) and behaviors such as perversion, delinquency, or addiction (Kohut & Wolfe, 1982). In narcissistic personality disorders, the breakup, enfeeblement and serious distortion of the self is temporary and the symptoms primarily concern the person's psychological state (e.g., sexual fantasies) rather than his actions and interactions (e.g., sexual behaviors) (p. 48).

The nuclear psychopathology of the narcissistic personality disorder consists of defects in the pathological structure of the self and in the secondary-formations, acquired in childhood, which are related to the primary defect in one of two crucially different ways. These secondary-formations are referred to as "defensive and compensatory structures." A structure is referred to be defensive when its predominant function is to cover over the primary defect of the self. A structure is said to be compensatory when it compensates or makes up for the defect of the self. It accomplishes this by "making up for the weakness in one pole (i.e., nuclear ambition) through the strengthening of the other pole (i.e., nuclear ideal)" (Kohut, 1977, pp. 3–4).

The narcissistic personality disorder person relates to archaic selfobjects cathected with narcissistic libido which are still in intimate connection with the archaic self. Because of the connection of the defective self to the archaic objects, the individual remains fixated on archaic grandiose self configurations and/or on archaic, overestimated, narcissistically cathected objects (Kohut, 1971).

### *Treatment of Disorders of the Self*

Treatment consists in the acquisition of new structures in the self (Kohut & Wolfe, 1982). This is brought about by the creation of a "new kind of experience for the patient within the transference relationship" (Cooper, 1983, p. 5). The vehicle of change is the establishment and resolution of selfobject transference in therapy through which the client reworks the injuries to his sense of grandiosity and exhibitionism and to the idealized parental imago. Three types of transferences may occur in therapy, namely, idealizing, mirroring, and alterego/twinship transferences (Kohut, 1971, p. 114).

Idealizing transference develops when "the patient regards the analyst as being perfect and wonderful and feels himself to be increasingly strong and important" by virtue of his connection to the powerful and strong analyst (Mitchell & Black, 1995, p. 161). In the mirroring transference the "grandiose self is therapeutically reactivated in the transference like condition" (Kohut, 1971, p. 106) and the patient regresses to an early stage of development during which absolute narcissism prevails. In twinship transference, the "narcissistically cathected object is experienced as being like the grandiose self or as being very similar to it" (p. 115). The patient "yearns to feel an essential likeness with the analyst" in terms of "significance or function" (Mitchell & Black, 1995, p. 161).

The essential therapeutic interventions in helping a client to acquire new structures within the self are interpretation and empathy. Through these interventions, the therapist provides the missing selfobject functions which the client internalizes that allow him to overcome his trauma, grow, and assume his functions. The patient requires the self-functions of the therapist in order to internalize them and to self-activate (Masterson, 1991).

## EDITH JACOBSON (1897–1978)

### Introduction

Edith Jacobson was born in Haynau, a small town in the German province of Upper Silesia on September 10, 1897, and died on December 8, 1978, in Rochester, New York. She received her medical degree from Munich in 1922, began her training in psychoanalysis at the Berlin Psychoanalytic Institute and in 1930 became a member of the Berlin Psychoanalytic Society. She emigrated to the United States in 1941 where, as a member of the New York Psychoanalytic Society and Institute, she was a distinguished training analyst, trainer, and prolific writer (Tuttman, 1985).

### Theoretical Constructs

Jacobson's contribution is her reworking Freud's drive theory and integrating it with a relational approach. This was motivated mostly by her work with depressed patients. This section begins with a presentation of the undifferentiated representations. This is followed by presentations of the instinctual theory, the formation of identity and the superego.

#### *The Undifferentiated Representations*

Jacobson began reworking Freud's (1923) instinctual theory by building on Hartman's (1939) proposition that both the id and ego emerge from an undifferentiated psychophysical matrix with each having innate roots of its own. Jacobson proposed that not only the id and the ego were undifferentiated at birth, but that the two drives and self-representations and object representations were undifferentiated as well. Jacobson (1964) defined self-representations as "unconscious, preconscious, and conscious endopsychic representation of the bodily and mental self in the system ego" (p. 19) and object representations as an image of a person or of part of a person (p. 20). The concepts of self and other representations are at the core of Jacobson's theory as she proposes that it is these representations that are cathected with libido and aggressive energies and not the ego.

### *Instinctual Theory, Narcissism, and Masochism*

Jacobson revised, in relational terms, Freud's instinctual theory regarding the origin of the instincts and their investment. She proposed that "instinctual drives are not innate 'givens,' but rather are 'biological predisposed, innate potentials'" (Mitchell & Black, 1995, p. 50). They are contained and undifferentiated within a "psychosomatic matrix" which Jacobson (1964) calls the "primal psychophysiological self" (p. 6). Jacobson maintains that from the beginning of birth and under the influence of intrinsic and external stimulation, the undifferentiated energies "begin to develop into the libidinal and aggressive psychic drives" (p. 14). These potentials (i.e., drives) acquire their distinctive features in the context of the child's early libidinal stimulating and depriving experiences.

Jacobson (1964) revised Freud's concepts of primary and secondary narcissism and masochism by clarifying the distinctions among *ego*, which is a "structural mental system," *self*, which refers to "the whole person of an individual, including his body and body parts, as well as his psychic organization and its parts" (p. 6) and *self-representations*, which are "the unconscious, preconscious and conscious endopsychic representations of the bodily and mental self in the system ego" (p. 19). It is assumed that self-representations, particularly those that emerge from coenesthetic experiences, exist prior to the formation of the ego and therefore libidinal and aggressive energies are discharged toward the inside and invested in self-representations. These discharges are construed as primary narcissism and primary masochism.

With regards to secondary narcissism and masochism, Jacobson (1964) states that it is not the ego but the mental representation of the self, constituted in the course of ego formation, that becomes cathected with libido and aggression (p. 19). Assuming that the libidinal and aggressive energies are invested in the self-representation and not in the ego, Jacobson argued for the disposal of the "concept of primary narcissism" and for the disposal of the "concept of primary masochism" and for the disposal of the concepts of "secondary narcissism" and "secondary masochism" (p. 15). However, Jacobson retained the term primary narcissism for "the earliest infantile period, preceding the development of self and object images" (p. 15).

### *Identity, Identifications, and Sense of Identity*

Using Lichtenstein's (1961) definitions, Jacobson defines identity as "the capacity to remain the same in the midst of change" and the sense of identity as the "consciousness of such continuity of sameness" (p. 193). Identification refers to the process of internalizing the behaviors and admired traits of loved persons.

According to Jacobson (1964), the identification process begins with the infant's experiences during the primitive oral stage which include the feeding situation and also the gratifying and frustrating situations. The infant at this age is capable of retaining memory traces of pleasurable and unpleasurable experiences and to lay down engrams of these experiences. Lichtenstein (1961) refers to these engrams as an "identity theme" (p. 208).

Jacobson (1964) refers to the child's first identification as "primitive affective identification" which she links to a child's pleasurable experiences with its mother (p. 42). The infant's longing for food and physical merging with the mother is the origin of the first primitive identification. At about three months, the infant is able to perceive the mother as different from himself and because of maturing motor apparatus, he is able to begin imitative movements to maintain symbiotic merger. The identifications, however, are magical and found on the primitive mechanisms of introjection or projection which disregard for the realistic differences between the self and the object.

Emerging from the earlier primitive affective identification is a more active type of primitive identification where the child makes increasing efforts to imitate the love object. The child very early begins "to perceive, to respond to, and to imitate the gestures, the inflections of the voice and other visible and audible affective manifestations of the mother" (Jacobson, 1964, p. 42).

The primitive affective identifications are followed by selective identifications which are based on the internalization of the admired traits of objects into his wishful self-images (Jacobson, 1964, p. 50). This form of identification begins in the second year of life which is marked by changes that indicate a "gradual transition from early infantile symbiotic phase to the stage of individuation and of beginning secondary ego autonomy" (p. 49). The child's developing narcissistic strivings change from wishes to magically controlling the love object to the child making efforts for realistic achievements.

At the age of two and half years the child makes the "startling discovery of his own identity, the experience of 'I am I'" (Jacobson, 1964, p. 59). The sense of identity emerges from both the loving and frustrating experiences with the mother. By the end of the first year, the child begins to show feelings of envy and rivalry toward his father and others. In his relationship with rivals, the child experiences differences and similarities between himself and others (p. 26). The child's strivings and experiences of differences and similarities furnish the fuel that enables the child to develop his feeling of identity.

### *The Formation of the Superego*

Jacobson (1964) agreed with Freud (1938) that the superego is established as a "definite functional unit" with the resolution of the oedipal conflict but she believed that the superego begins to be formed much earlier within the pre-oedipal phase of development. (p. 123). In her exploration of the superego, Jacobson (1964) traced its formation in terms of stages which differed from each other based on the developmental stage of object relations within which they emerge. These stages have also been given the labels of a "three-tiered system" by Greenberg and Mitchell (1983, p. 316) and as "three broad layers" by Kernberg (1984).

The first stage begins at the end of the first year and at the beginning of the second year. This stage reflects the internalization of sadistically, prohibitive and punitive bad fused self and object representations that the infant projects onto the frustrating mother (Kernberg, 1984). It begins with the bowel training stage where the child learns the dos and don'ts and what is to be valued. There is a noticeable change in the infant's attitude which can show itself in three different ways: feces are dirty and belong in the toilet and children who soil, are bad; the feelings of disgust at the bowels, shame in loss of bowel control, and pride in achieving cleanliness; and active effort to punctually move the bowels on the toilet and to keep clean; the latter is the first value that the child learns (Jacobson, 1964).

The second stage extends from the second to the fifth year. It is characterized by the development of identifications that internalize the parental demands and prohibitions and the approvals and disapprovals (Kernberg, 1984). The object relations become more mature, realistic and affectionate and less archaic (i.e., lacking structure) and the child increasingly sees the parents as human, that is, as whole-objects that are less magical (Jacobson, 1964). A significant characteristic of this stage is the development of ego ideal which forms and shapes the enforcing qualities of the moral demands of the superego and the child's self-critical functions.

The third stage extends from the fifth to the seventh year. During this stage, self and object representations become more realistic and the child has internalized moral and behavioral codes and ideals, values and standards for self-criticism. Infantile demands lessen as drives become increasingly neutralized (Jacobson, 1954). A significant factor in the formation of the superego as a consolidated system is the development of the ego ideal which is largely formed following the establishment of a stable identity (Jacobson, 1964). All of these processes come together and produce the superego at the end of the oedipal period. With the resolution of the Oedipus complex, the superego is experienced as a "distinctly separate institution" (p. 123). Its main tools consist of the feelings of guilt and shame which help the individual to live in accordance to the mores of the society and his own urges and desires.

## Summary

This chapter presented the seven theorists whose constructs influenced the development of Self-in-Relationship Psychotherapy. The constructs have a unique meaning within the context of the theory as a whole rather than as separate from the theory and presented in abstract language. SIRP's goal is to adhere to the original meaning of the constructs that it incorporated. The following chapter provides a detailed review of the literature on psychological and social needs and the role that these needs play in human development and in healthy living.

## References

Baker, H. W., & Baker, M. N. (1987). Heinz Kohut's self psychology: An overview. *The American Journal of Psychiatry, 144*(1), 1–9.

Bellak, L., Hurvich, M., & Gediman, H. K. (1973). *Ego functions in schizophrenics, neurotics and normal: A systematic study of conceptual, diagnostic, and therapeutic aspects.* New York: John Wiley & Sons.

Bergman, A., & Ellman, S. (1985). Margaret Mahler: Symbiosis and separation-individuation. In J. Reppen (Ed.), *Beyond Freud: A study of modern psychoanalytic theorists* (pp. 231–256). London, UK: Lawrence Erlbaum Associates.

Bettleheim, B. (1984). *Freud and man's soul.* New York: Vintage Books.

Blanck, G., & Blanck, R. (1979). *Ego psychology II: Psychoanalytic developmental psychology.* New York: Columbia University Press.

Brenner, C. (1955). *An elementary textbook of psychoanalysis.* New York: International Universities.

Cashdan, S. (1988). *Object relations therapy: Using the relationship.* New York: W. W. Norton.

Cocks, G. (Ed.) (1994). *The curve of life: The correspondence of Heinz Kohut,* 1923–1981. Chicago, IL: University of Chicago Press.

Cooper, A. (1983). The place of self psychology in the history of depth psychology. In A. Goldberg (Ed.), *The future of psychoanalysis.* New York: International Universities Press.

Eagle, M. (1984). *Recent developments in psychoanalysis: A critical examination.* New York: McGraw-Hill.

Fairbairn, W. R. D. (1941). A revised psychopathology of the psychoses and psychoneuroses. In W.R.D. Fairbairn (Ed.), *Psychoanalytic studies of personality* (pp. 28–58). New York: Basic Books.

Fairbairn, W. R. D. (1943). The repression and the return of bad objects (with special reference to the "war neuroses"). In W. R. D. Fairbairn (Ed.), *Psychoanalytic studies of personality* (pp. 59–81). New York: Routledge.

Fairbairn, W. R. D. (1944). Endopsychic structure considered in terms of object relationships. In W. R. D. Fairbairn (Ed.), *Psychoanalytic studies of personality* (pp. 82–136). New York: Routledge.

Fairbairn, W. R. D. (1946). Object-relationships and dynamic structure. In W. R. D. Fairbairn (Ed.), *Psychoanalytic studies of personality* (pp. 137–161). New York: Basic Books.

Fairbairn, W. W. D. (1949). Steps in the development of an object-relations theory of personality. In W. R. D. Fairbairn (Ed.), *Psychoanalytic studies of personality* (pp. 152–161). London, UK: Routledge.

Fairbairn, W. R. D. (1951). A synopsis of the development of the author's views regarding the structure of personality. In W. R. D. Fairbairn (Ed.), *Psychoanalytic studies of personality* (pp. 162–179). London, UK: Routledge.
Fairbairn, W.R.D. (1954). *An object relations theory of personality*. New York: Basic books.
Fancher, R. E. (1973). *Psychoanalytic psychology: The development of Freud's thought*. New York: W. W. Norton & Company.
Freud, S. (1894). The neuro-psychoses of defense. *Standard Edition, 3*, 43–61.
Freud, S. (1900). Interpretation of dreams. *Standard Edition, 4*, xxiii–751.
Freud, S. (1901). The psychopathology of everyday life. *Standard Edition, 6*, vii–279.
Freud, S. (1909). *Five lectures on psycho-analysis. Sigmund Freud, two short accounts of psych-analysis*. Great Britain: Penguin Books.
Freud, S. (1910). The future prospect of psychoanalytic therapy. *Standard Edition, 11*, 141–151.
Freud, S. (1912). The dynamics of transference. *Standard Edition, 12*, 99–108.
Freud, S. (1913). The disposition to obsessional neurosis: A contribution to the problem of choice of neurosis. *Standard Edition, 12*, 317–326.
Freud, S. (1914). On narcissism: An introduction. *Standard Edition, 14*, 67–102.
Freud, S. (1915a). Instincts and their vicissitudes. *Standard Edition, 14*, 117–140.
Freud, S. (1915b). Repression. *Standard Edition, 14*, 141–158.
Freud, S. (1916). Some character types met with in psychoanalytic work. *Standard Edition, 14*, 311–333.
Freud, S. (1920). Beyond the pleasure principle. *Standard Edition, 18*, 3–64.
Freud, S. (1921). Group psychology and the analysis of the ego. *Standard Edition, 17*, 69–143.
Freud, S. (1923). The ego and the id. *Standard Edition, 19*, 12–63.
Freud, S. (1924a). Neurosis and psychosis. *Standard Edition, 19*, 147–153.
Freud, S. (1924b). A short account of psycho-analysis. *Standard Edition, 19*, 191–209.
Freud, S. (1926). Inhibitions, symptoms and anxiety. *Standard Edition, 20*, 87–174.
Freud, S. (1933). New introductory lectures on psycho-analysis. *Standard Edition, 22*, 1953, 7–182.
Freud, S. (1937). Analysis terminable and interminable. *Standard Edition, 23*, 216–253.
Freud, S. (1938). An outline of psychoanalysis. *Standard Edition, 23*, 144–207.
Greenberg, J. R., & Mitchell, S. A. (1983). *Object relations in psychoanalytic theory*. Cambridge, MA: Harvard University Press.
Grosskurth, P. (1986). *Melanie Klein: Her world and her work*. New York: Knopf.
Guntrip, H. (1969). *Schizoid phenomena, object-relations, and the self*. New York: Universities Press.
Guntrip, H. (1973). *Psychoanalytic theory, therapy and the self*. New York: Basic Books.
Hartmann, H. (1939). *Ego psychology and the problem of adaptation*. New York: International Universities Press.
Hartmann, H. (1950). Comments on the psychoanalytic theory of the ego. *The Psychoanalytic Study of the Child, 5*, 74–96.

Jacobson, E. (1953). The affects and their pleasure-unpleasure qualities in relation to the psychic discharge process. In R. M. Loewenstein (Ed.), *Drives, affects, behaviors.* New York: International Universities Press.

Jacobson, E. (1954). The self and the object world: Vicissitudes of their infantile cathexes and their influence on ideational and affective development. *Psychoanalytic Study of the Child, 9*, 75–127.

Jacobson, E. (1964). *The self and the object world.* New York: International Universities Press.

Jacobson, E. (1971). *Depression: Comparative studies of normal, neurotic, and psychotic conditions.* New York: International Universities Press.

Kernberg, O. F. (1975). *Borderline conditions and pathological narcissism.* New York: Jason Aronson.

Kernberg, O. (1984). *Severe personality disorders: Psychotherapeutic strategies.* New Have, NJ: Yale University Press.

Klein, M. (1927). Symposium on child-analysis. In M. Klein (Ed.), *Love, guilt and reparation and other works, 1921–1945* (pp. 139–169). New York: Delacorte Press/Seymour Lawrence.

Klein, M. (1937). Love, guilt and reparation. In M. Klein (Ed.), *Love, guilt and reparation and other works, 1921–1945* (pp. 306–343). New York: Delacorte Press/Seymour Lawrence.

Klein, M. (1940). Mourning and its relations to manic-depressive states. In M. Klein (Ed.), *Love, guilt and reparation and other works, 1921–1945* (pp. 344–369). New York: Delacorte Press/Seymour Lawrence.

Klein, M. (1945). The Oedipus complex in light of early anxieties. In M. Klein (Ed.), *Love, guilt and reparation and other works, 1921–1945* (pp. 370–419). New York: Delacorte Press/Seymour Lawrence.

Klein, M. (1946). Notes on some schizoid mechanisms. In M. Klein (Ed.), *Envy and gratitude and other works 1946–1963* (pp. 1–24). London, UK: Hogarth Press.

Klein, M. (1948). On the theory of anxiety and guilt. In M. Klein (Ed.), *Envy and gratitude and other works 1946–1963* (pp. 25–42). London, UK: Hogarth Press.

Klein, M. (1952a). Some theoretical conclusions regarding the emotional life of the infant. In M. Klein (Ed.), *Envy and gratitude and other works 1946–1963* (pp. 61–94). London, UK: Hogarth Press.

Klein, M. (1952b). The mutual influences in the development of the ego and id. In M. Klein (Ed.), *Envy and gratitude and other works 1946–1963* (pp. 57–60). London, UK: Hogarth Press.

Klein, M. (1957). Envy and gratitude. In M. Klein (Ed.), *Envy and gratitude and other works 1946–1963* (pp. 176–235). London, UK: Hogarth Press.

Klein, M. (1959). Our adult world and its roots in infancy. In M. Klein (Ed.), *Envy and gratitude and other works 1946–1963* (pp. 247–263). London, UK: Hogarth Press.

Kligerman, C. (1985). The memorials of Heinz Kohut, M.D., October 31, 1981. *The annual of psychoanalysis* (pp. 9–15). New York: International Universities Press.

Kohut, H. (1971). *The analysis of self.* New York: International Universities Press.

Kohut, H. (1973). The psychoanalyst in the community of scholars. In P. H. Ornstein (Ed.), *The search for the self: Selected writings of Heinz Kohut: 1950–1978* (Vol. 2, pp. 685–724). New York: International Universities Press.

Kohut, H. (1977). *The restoration of the self.* New York: International Universities Press.

Kohut, H. (1981). On empathy. In P. H. Ornstein (Ed.), *The search for the self: Selected writings of Heinz Kohut: 1978–1981* (Vol. 4, pp. 525–535). New York: International Universities Press.

Kohut, H. (1984). *How does analysis cure?* Chicago, IL: University of Chicago Press.

Kohut, H., & Wolfe, E. S. (1978). The disorders of the self and their treatment: An outline. *International Journal of Psycho-Analysis, 59*, 413–425.

Kohut, H., & Wolfe, E. S. (1982). The disorders of the self and their treatment. In S. Slipp (Ed.), *Curative factors in dynamic psychotherapy* (pp. 44–59). Toronto: McGraw-Hill.

Lichtenstein, H. (1961). Identity and sexuality: A study of their interrelationships in man. *Journal of American Psychoanalytic Association, 9*, 179–260.

Lindon, J. A. (1972). Melanie Klein's theory and technique: Her life and work. In P. L. Giovacchini (Ed.), *Tactics and techniques in psychoanalytical therapy* (pp. 33–61). U.S.A.: Science House Incorporated.

Mahler, M. S., & Furer, M. (1968). *On human symbiosis and the vicissitudes of individuation, Vol. 1, Infantile psychoses.* New York: International Universities Press.

Mahler, M. S., Pine, F., & Bergman, A. (1975). *The psychological birth of the human infant* (pp. xii–308). New York: Basic Books.

Masterson, J. F. (1976). *Psychotherapy of the borderline adult: A developmental approach.* New York: Brunner/Mazel.

Masterson, J. F. (1980). *From borderline adolescent to functioning adult: The test of time.* New York: Brunner/Maze.

Masterson, J. F. (1991). Comparing psychoanalytic psychotherapies. In J. F. Masterson, M. Tolpin, & P. E. Sifneos (Eds.), *Comparing psychoanalytic psychotherapies* (pp. 285–294). New York: Brunner/Mazel.

Masterson, J. F., & Klein, R. (Eds.) (1995). *Disorders of the self: New therapeutic horizons, the Masterson approach.* New York: Brunner/Mazel.

Mitchell, S. A., & Black, M. J. (1995). *Freud and beyond: A history of modern psychoanalytic thought.* New York: Basic Books.

Monte, C. F., & Sollod, R. N. (2003). *Beneath the mask: An introduction to theories of personality* (7th ed.). Toronto, Ontario: John Wiley & Sons.

Rodman, F. R. (2003). *Winnicott: A portrait of the man and his contributions.* Cambridge, MA: Perseus.

Schafer, R. (1968). *Aspects of internalization.* New York: International Universities Press.

Segal, J. (2004). *Melanie Klein.* London, UK: SAGE.

Scharff, D. E., & Fairbairn Birtles, E. F. (1994). Introduction. In W. R. D. Fairbairn (Ed.), *Psychoanalytic studies of the personality* (pp. ix–xxi). London, UK: Routledge.

Simpson, P. (2001). *Heinz Kohut: His enduring influence today.* Retrieved from http Influence: www.sfu.ca/~psimpson

Stepansky, P. E. (Compiler & Editor) (1988). *The memoires of Margaret Mahler.* New York: The Analytic Press.

Stern, D. N. (1985). *The interpersonal world of the infant.* New York: Basic Books.

Tuttman, S. (1985). Edith Jacobson's major contributions to psychoanalytic theory of development. *American Journal of Psychoanalysis, 45*, 135–147.

Winnicott, D. (1951). Transitional objects and transitional phenomena. In D. Winnicott (Ed.), *Through paediatrics to psychoanalysis* (pp. 229–242). New York: Basic Books.

Winnicott, D. (1954). Metapsychological and clinical aspects of regression within the psychoanalytical setup. In D. Winnicott (Ed.), *Through paediatrics to psychoanalysis* (pp. 278–294). New York: Basic Books.

Winnicott, D. (1955–1956). Clinical varieties of transference. In D. Winnicott (Ed.), *Through paediatrics to psychoanalysis* (pp. 295–299). New York: Basic Books.

Winnicott, D. (1959–1964). Classification: Is there a psycho-analytic contribution to psychiatric classification. In D. Winnicott (Ed.), *The maturational processes and the facilitating environment* (pp. 124–139). New York: International Universities Press.

Winnicott, D. (1960a). The theory of the parent-infant relationship. In D. Winnicott (Ed.), *The maturational processes and the facilitating environment* (pp. 37–55). New York: International Universities Press.

Winnicott, D. (1960b). Ego distortion in terms of true and false self. In D. Winnicott (Ed.), *The maturational processes and the facilitating environment* (pp. 140–152). New York: International Universities Press.

Winnicott, D. (1962). Ego integration in child development. In D. Winnicott (Ed.), *The maturational processes and the facilitating environment* (pp. 56–63). New York: International Universities Press.

Winnicott, D. (1963a). Psychiatric disorders in terms of infantile maturational processes. In D. Winnicott (Ed.), *The maturational processes and the facilitating environment* (pp. 230–241). New York: International Universities Press.

Winnicott, D. (1963b). From dependence towards indepedence in the development of the individual. In D. Winnicott (Ed.), *The maturational processes and the facilitating environment* (pp. 83–92). New York: International Universities Press.

Winnicott, D. (1963c). The mentally ill in your caseload. In D. Winnicott (Ed.), *The maturational processes and the facilitating environment* (pp. 217–229). New York: International Universities Press.

Winnicott, D. (1965). *The family and individual development*. London, UK: Tavistock Publishers.

Winnicott, D. (1971). *Playing and reality*. New York: Basic Books.

Chapter 2

# Relational, Self, and Physical Intimacy Needs: A Review

## Introduction

Prior to the 1960s, the concept of needs played a relatively important role in the theories of personality, social psychology, and motivational psychology. With the shift toward cognitive theories in the 1960s, the concept of need was repudiated and replaced by the concept of goal-directed behavior as the dominant motivational concept. Yet to fully understand goal-directed behaviors, psychological development, and well-being, it is necessary to address needs that give the goals their psychological potency and influence which regulatory processes impact the goals being pursued (Deci & Ryan, 2000).

This shift toward viewing motivation in terms of goal-directed behaviors rather than in terms of needs as an explanatory concept has affected psychotherapy theory, practice, and research. Although many of the contemporary theories of psychotherapy have moved beyond a behavioral and cognitive-behavioral approach, yet theories of psychotherapy tend to be built around one or more core concepts such as feelings (Greenberg et al., 1993), cognitive processes (Beck, 1976), and sensations and/or behaviors (Skinner, 1953; Wolpe, 1990) but fail to include needs as instrumental to change (Norcross, 1992). For example, in a recent book by Gurman (2008) on couple therapy, the concept of emotions received about 50 pages of coverage, cognitions 44 pages, intimacy 17 pages and needs received zero pages of coverage. These facts point to the lack of attention that is given to the significance of addressing needs in psychotherapy theory, practice, and research.

It is apparent, then, that contemporary theories of psychotherapy fail to take into account the whole of human experience by neglecting to address the significance of relational, self, and physical intimacy needs. Few empirical studies have investigated the role of this dimension in the change process. Yet personality theorists over the past four decades have pointed out the importance of considering needs in theory building and in clinical practice.

DOI: 10.4324/9781003272502-3

The central concept for Self-in-Relationship Psychotherapy (SIRP), in its theory, assessment and treatment, is core needs (Meier & Boivin, 2011). Where experiential and cognitive-oriented approaches considered emotions and cognitions to be the motivating forces in both adaptive and maladaptive behaviors, SIRP argues that needs, met or unmet, are the motivating forces in adaptive and maladaptive behaviors and in interpersonal interactions. SIRP identifies relational, self, and physical intimacy needs and strongly advocates for their inclusion in a theory of psychotherapy. It assumes that the satisfaction of these needs leads to healthy personality development and to meaningful relationships. It also assumes that when these needs go unmet for an extended period of time, the individual is prone to develop emotional and relational problems (Meier & Boivin, 2006). The goal of therapy is to help individuals and couples to recognize and accept their needs and to orient their individual and couple lives accordingly. It is crucial then that in addition to "cognition and affect" that a theory of psychotherapy integrate needs (DeLamater & Hyde, 2004, p. 15).

SIRP's emphasis on relational, self, and physical intimacy does not preclude the importance of physical (e.g., clothes, shelter), physiological (e.g., hunger, thirst), and higher-order needs such as universal values and belief systems. There are situations, such as trauma, abuse, and death, where one reaches beyond the confines of psychology and turns to the higher-order needs for solace, to gain a perspective and draw strength (Frankl, 1967; Maslow, 1968; May, 1953; Miller, 1999). Needs such as the need to become fully human (e.g., self-actualize) is a higher-order need that presumably embraces the relational, self, and physical intimacy needs.

Very little has been written about the role of relational, self, and physical intimacy needs in psychotherapy theory and practice. Since there is no publication that brings together in a single article the role that core relational, self, and physical intimacy needs play in psychotherapy theory and practice, this entire chapter is dedicated to this topic. The chapter is divided in two parts. The first part presents material related to relational and self needs, and the second part presents material related to physical intimacy needs. This chapter ends with a summary that provides the theoretical foundation for SIRP.

## Part I: Relational and Self Needs

This section begins by presenting definitions of needs and a rationale to include needs in psychotherapy theory and practice. This is followed by a discussion of methods to classify needs. This section ends with a presentation of the research that supports the inclusion of needs in psychotherapy theory and practice.

### *Definition of Relational and Self Needs*

Writers do not agree on the definition of a need and they often use it interchangeably with wishes, desires, yearnings, and wants. As well, they do not agree as to whether needs are innate and biologically based and are required for survival or whether one can survive without having them satisfied (Kasser, 2002).

In terms of dictionary definitions, a wish is a longing or strong inclination for something. A desire is a strong craving. A yearning is a persistent, often wistful melancholy desire or longing. To want is to desire greatly and to seek with intent to capture. Wants spring from desires or wishes. A need, on the other hand, is a motivating force that compels action for its satisfaction. Needs range from basic survival needs to cultural, intellectual, and social needs. Needs are finite but in contrast to wants, are boundless (Collins English Dictionary – Complete and Unabridged, 2003; the American Heritage Dictionary of the English Language, 2000). It can be seen from these definitions that needs are more fundamental, in a sense more primary than a wish, desire, yearning, and want.

Erskine (1998) conceives of needs, particularly relational needs, as being unique to a given situation. They are not the basic needs of life but they are the essential elements that enhance the quality of life. He adds that relational needs are the component parts of a universal human desire for relationship. Nevertheless, when needs, particularly relational needs, are not satisfied, the need becomes more intense and is "phenomenologically experienced as longing, emptiness, a nagging loneliness, or an intense urge often accompanied by nervousness" (p. 4). When needs go unmet, the needs take on a compulsive quality and become insatiable. The continued absence of the satisfaction of needs may be manifested as frustration, anger, and aggression.

Deci and Ryan (2000) define needs as innate, organismic necessities rather than acquired motives and define needs at the psychological rather than at the physiological level. More specifically, Deci and Ryan define needs as "innate nutriments that are essential for ongoing psychological growth, integrity and well-being" (p. 229). They identified three innate needs, namely, the need for competence, relatedness, and autonomy.

Kasser (2002) defines a need not just as something that a person desires or wants, but as "something that is necessary to his or her survival, growth, and optimal functioning" (p. 24). Just as a plant must have air, water, and soil to survive and thrive, so too all people require certain "psychological nutrients" for their health and growth (p. 24). Kasser adds that needs direct an individual to behave in ways that increase the likelihood that they will be satisfied. Kasser's position is that people have needs that must be satisfied for them "to have a high quality of life" (p. 28).

### *Rationale for Including Relational and Self Needs in a Theory of Psychotherapy*

Psychodynamic oriented theorists and psychotherapists and personality psychologists have for decades advocated for the inclusion of needs or their equivalent in a theory of psychotherapy and personality development. Current models of psychotherapy, in general, neglect to pay attention to needs. SIRP gives needs a central role in its approach.

Freud (1918, 1923, 1938) gave impulses and drives a central place in his psychoanalytic theory. It is to be noted that Freud did not use the term instinct to describe human behavior. He used the words drives/impulses (i.e., *Trieb*) to refer to human behavior and instincts to refer to animal behavior. In English, the terms drives/impulses have come to be translated as instincts (Bettleheim, 1984).

Freud's (1938) theory rests on two innate instincts, the life instincts (Eros) and the death instincts (Thanatos). Eros represents the life instinct sourcing from the libido, which stands for creativity and the sexual and life-preserving drives. Thanatos signals a desire to give up the struggle for life and return to quiescence and the grave. Expressing this more in relational terms, Freud (1938) stated that the aim of Eros is "to establish ever greater unities and to preserve them thus – in short, to bind together" and the aim of Thanatos is to "undo connections and so to destroy things" (p. 148). In relational terms, Eros refers to bonding, emotional connection, companionship, and romantic love and Thanatos to dispelling that which inhibits the acquisition of that which is pleasurable and moving toward separateness (p. 148).

Perls (1969) stated that needs are primary for without them, there would be no human motivation. He added that one attends to the most pressing need. According to Wallen (1970), the phenomenal world is organized by the needs of the individual. He states that "needs energize behavior and organize it on the subjective-perceptual level and on the objective-motor level. The individual then carries out the necessary activities in order to satisfy the needs" (p. 9). Wallen adds that we have a hierarchy of needs that continually develop and organize the figures of experience and then disappear.

Polster and Polster (1973) gave wants a significant role in therapy and stated that "people who have no wants – have no future" (p. 227). According to Polster and Polster, wants is an orienting function, it directs, mobilizes, channels, and focuses. A want integrates present experiences with the future where its gratification lies and also with the past which it culminates.

Korb et al. (1989) described how different human needs dominate and then recede into the background when fulfilled. They state that "needs arise, come to the foreground, and recede progressively as they receive attention and are satisfied ... Once fulfilled, a need recedes from prominence and others emerge to be fulfilled; they, in turn recede from prominence when fulfilled" (p. 6).

Yalom (1989), based on his clinical experience with groups, observed that people, regardless of their emotional state, are driven (pulled) by their need (want) to matter, to be important, to be remembered, and to be loved. He also observed that when people are wish-blocked, knowing neither what they feel nor what they want and are without impulses and inclinations, they "become parasites on the desires of others" (p. 9). He adds that an individual's deepest wants will never be fulfilled and it is when these unattainable wants dominate an individual's life, that he or she turns outward for answers.

Erskine (2011) stated that "we are motivated by our biological need ... to be in a relationship. Relationship is a biological imperative that exists throughout our lives" (p. 10). He added that when our relational needs are met, we have the "capacity to be expansive, creative, and intimate. When relational needs are repeatedly not met, we experience a sense of insecurity and emotional disturbance" (p. 11). He differentiated between meeting archaic or old needs and needs of the here-and-now. He stated that "often the intensity of old unmet relational-needs overshadows and distorts the relational-needs of the here-and-now therapeutic relationship. A major task of the psychotherapist is to help the client differentiate between current needs and archaic needs" (p. 11).

Stumpf suggests that the mind does not just consist of intellectual representations (cognitions) and raw feelings, but also desires and wishes of all kinds (cited by Reisenzein & Schnpflug, 1992, p. 43). Murray (1938) postulated the central role of needs in normal development and presented a taxonomy of needs. Maslow (1954) gave a place for needs and wants in normal development and offered a hierarchy of needs beginning with physiological needs (e.g., food) and extending to the need for self-actualization.

Max-Neuf et al. (1991) maintained that needs are finite, few, and classifiable. They add that "fundamental human needs are the same in all cultures and in all historical periods" (p. 18). Cultures do not determine the needs, rather they, might determine how the needs are met, that is, the satisfiers of those needs. Deci and Ryan (2000) maintain that to fully understand goal-directed behaviors and psychological development and well-being, it is necessary to address needs that give goals their psychological potency and influence which regulatory processes direct the goals being pursued.

### *Classification of Needs*

Personality and social psychologists were among the first to provide a theory-based classification of human needs and suggested that human needs are keys for understanding who we are. Researchers attempted to provide empirical support for the classifications by operationalizing the constructs and testing them out for their stability and validity. Results from these studies also added to the classification and/or rendered them more precise. This section begins by providing theory and practice-based classification of needs and terminates by providing the results from an empirical investigation of these needs.

#### *Needs derived from theory and practice*

Working from a motivation theory based on needs and press, Murray (1938) developed a list of 12 primary physiological needs and 28 secondary psychological needs. Four of the primary needs are water, sex, urination, and harm avoidance and four of the secondary needs are abasement, affiliation, dominance, and play. In understanding personality, the behavior of the individual must be understood in terms of the needs of the individual and the demands (press) from reality as interpreted by the individual. With the exception of the need for achievement, there have been very few studies to validate Murray's hypotheses (Corsini, 1977, p. 409) and therefore his list of psychological needs does not yet meet the criteria for scientific validity (Reiss, 2012).

A popular classification of needs is Maslow's (1954, 1971) five-stage hierarchy or pyramid of psychological needs. This hierarchy of needs stems from his work with Harlow on animal studies and from his time with Thorndike where he studied human sexuality (Boeree, 2006). Maslow gave needs a significant place in normal development. According to Maslow, this hierarchy of needs is "universal" and has an "instinctual character" and displays a "uniform sequence of emergence in development, some being more primary and fundamental than others" (Corsini, 1977, p. 309). At the base of this hierarchy lie the physiological, survival-oriented needs (e.g., hunger, thirst, and elimination), next are the safety and security needs. On the third level are the sexual and love needs. This is followed by the needs for esteem from self and others. At the peak of the hierarchy are the needs for self-actualization, that is, the need to reach one's fullest potential. The need for self-actualization "involves a kind of transformation or reorganization of the whole personality, a totally new way of thinking" (Corsini, 1977, p. 309). Although very popular in growth centers and in personal development and greater awareness, Maslow's hierarchy of needs is based on observations and wishes. The hierarchy has not yet received scientific validation.

Glasser (1999) postulated four basic needs, which are fun, freedom, power, and belonging. Fun refers to the need for pleasure, to play and to laugh. Freedom is the need for autonomy, independence, for control over one's life and for choice. Power is the need for empowerment, to achieve, to be recognized for achievement and skills, to have a sense of worth, and to contribute. Belonging is the need for love, for relationships, social connection, and to be part of a group. Glasser (1999) believes that the four basic needs are universal, innate, over lapping, conflict with other needs, and are satisfied from moment to moment.

Kohut (1977) classifies self needs, also called narcissistic needs, into three categories, namely, the need for mirroring, idealization, and twinship. The need for mirroring is a need for affirmation, admiration and echoing of an individual's sense of competence which feeds her sense of grandiosity. The need for idealization refers to the need to be with someone who is strong, perfect, and wonderful – omnipotent – and being with the other vicariously feeds the individual sense of lovability, self-worth, and goodness. The need for twinship refers to a yearning to feel an essential likeness with other people be it peer groups, rock groups and so on. It could be said that the three Kohutian needs are for competency, lovability, and equality.

Mahler et al. (1975) did not directly offer a set of psychological needs, but one can infer two primary needs from the separation-individuation process. From their concept of symbiosis one can infer the need for emotional bonding and connectedness. Symbiosis refers to a state of being undifferentiated in which the "I" is not yet differentiated from the "not-I" and to the state of being fused with the caregiver. As the child physically and psychologically separates from the caregiver it still has the need to maintain connection and will return to the caregiver for "emotional re-fueling." From Mahler and associates' concept of individuation one can infer the need for autonomy and mastery of one's life. Individuation denotes the evolution of intrapsychic autonomy, that is, to the development of psychic structure and personality characteristics. It denotes as well, assuming one's own individual characteristics, being one's own person. The child, teenager, and adult, it is assumed, assert their need for autonomy and mastery of their lives.

Based on the Three-Dimensional Theory of Interpersonal Behavior, Schutz (1966) construed three interpersonal needs that are inclusion, control, and affection. These needs were considered on two levels, that is, wanted and expressed needs (e.g., wants to be included; includes others).

### *Empirical support for needs*

Based on his review of psychological research and theory, Kasser (2002) concludes that at least four sets of needs are basic to an individual's motivation, functioning, and well-being. The four sets of needs are (a) need for safety, security, and sustenance; (b) need for competence, efficacy, and self-esteem; (c) need to be connected and related to other people; and (d) need to feel autonomous and authentically engaged in our behavior. Kasser concludes in saying that

> substantial research and theory suggest that people are highly motivated to feel safe and secure, competent, connected to others, and autonomous and authentically engaged in their behaviors … [and] … that well-being and quality of life increase when these four sets of needs are satisfied and decrease when they are not (p. 25).

Epstein and Baucom (2002) report empirically supported motives relevant to couples' relationships. They group these needs into two classes, namely, communally oriented motives and individually oriented motives. The communally oriented motives include affiliation, intimacy, altruism, and succorance. The individual-oriented motives include autonomy, power, and achievement.

From a study of transference and a qualitative investigation of the crucial factors in significant relationships, Erskine (1998) derived eight relational needs. Relational needs are "the component parts of a universal human desire for intimate relationship and secure attachment" (Erskine, 2011, p. 14). The eight relational needs inferred from the analysis are need for security; need to feel validated, affirmed and significant with a relationship; acceptance by a stable, dependable, and protective other person; confirmation of personal experience; need for self-definition; a need to have an impact on others; the need to have the other initiate; and the need to express love (Erskine, 1998).

Reiss (2012) produced an empirically derived list of 16 psychological needs. The 16 needs are acceptance (the need for approval), curiosity (the need to understand), eating (strength of interest in food), family (the need to spend time with family), honor (the need for character), idealism (the need to improve society), independence (the need for personal freedom), order (the need for structure), physical activity (the need for exercise), romance (the need for sex), power (the need for influence of will), saving (the need to collect), social contact (the need for friends), status (the need for prestige), tranquility (the need for safety), and vengeance (the need to fight back).

Bekker and van Assen (2006) studied the concept of autonomy particularly as defined by Mahler and associates (1975). Through their factorial studies, they identified three subscales of autonomy, namely, Self-Awareness, Sensitivity to Others, and Capacity to Manage New Situations.

The above authors do not organize needs according to a higher order, but basically present a number and/or a range of needs that can be characterized as being psychological and social needs. Some of the authors fail to differentiate between a need and a need satisfier. For example, Kohut (1977) speaks of the need for mirroring, idealization, and twinship. The basic needs are the need for competency (grandiosity), lovable (omnipotent), and being equal. Mirroring, idealization, and twinship are the manner in which the needs are satisfied. SIRP theoretically groups psychological needs according to self needs and relational needs.

### *Research and the Implication of Unmet Needs*

Theorists and practitioners have pointed out the negative effects in not having the relational and self needs met. Erskine (1998) states that when needs, particularly relational needs, are not satisfied, the need becomes more intense and is "phenomenologically experienced as longing, emptiness, a nagging loneliness, or an intense urge often accompanied by nervousness" (p. 4). When needs go unmet, the needs take on a compulsive quality and become insatiable. The continued absence of the satisfaction of needs may be manifested as frustration, anger, and aggression. When childhood needs go unmet, the individual might expect to receive them in adulthood (e.g., affection longed for in childhood but not received). Kasser (2002) maintains that people have needs that must be satisfied for them "to have a high quality of life" (p. 28). Erskine (2011) postulates that we are motivated by our biological need to be in a relationship and when our needs are met, we have the capacity to be expansive, creative, and intimate and when relational-needs are repeatedly not met, we "experience a sense of insecurity and emotional disturbance" (p. 11).

Studies that focused on the effects of core needs not being met in relationships are rare. Meier and Boivin (2006) investigated the resolution of intrapsychic conflicts from the perspective of client statements about feelings, thought processes, and social and affectional needs. The intervention was the Gestalt two-chair technique. The Gestalt two-chair segment of the session was divided into three parts using the length of the segment in time. They observed that the resolution of the conflict began by both parts (Topdog and Underdog) engaged in the expression of negative affective, judgmental, and critical statements. These feelings gave way to the expression of positive affective responses and the expression of needs. During the last stage of the process in resolving the conflict, the two parts expressed their unmet needs in their relationship and agreed to be responsive to each other's needs.

## Part II: Physical Intimacy Needs

This part of the chapter focuses on physical intimacy needs from a developmental, health, integrative, and holistic perspective. The former Surgeon General David Satcher, in his *Call to Action to Promote Sexual Health and Responsible Sexual Behavior*, stated that sexuality encompasses more than sexual behavior and it includes as well the "mental and spiritual." He added that "sexuality is the core component of personality … [and] … is a fundamental part of human life" (Office of the Surgeon General, 2001, p. ii) (cited by DeLamater & Hyde, 2004, p. 8). Robinson et al. (2002) state that "sexual health involves the ability to be intimate with a partner, to communicate explicitly about sexual needs and desires, to be sexually functional, to act intentionally and responsibly, and to set appropriate sexual boundaries" (p. 45). Thus, sexuality includes intimacy, communication, sexual behavior, self-regulation, and sexual self-esteem.

Although there are studies that support the inclusion of physical intimacy in a theory and practice of psychotherapy, this has not happened in a significant way for several reasons. First, much of the research on sexuality has focused on sexual dysfunctions rather than on healthy sexuality in close relationships (Harvey et al., 2004). Second, there is a cultural taboo in the expression of physical intimacy such as touching, cuddling, and kissing except for parent-infant and pair-bond relationships. This is particularly noticed in Canadian, American, German, and English cultures (Davis, 1999). In subcultures where extra-relationship contact is permitted, such as in prostitution, efforts to "avoid emotional involvement are common" (Zeifman & Hazan, 2008, p. 440). Davis (1999, p. 79) laments the fact that children are not given enough loving touch for them to distinguish between loving and sexual touch. Third, all families develop complex rules and attitudes about people touching each other. The rules are a mix of each adult's ancestral values and traditions about hugging, kissing, and caressing and can vary according to age, gender, and social roles. For example, sisters can kiss each other but brothers shouldn't. There might also be family rules about initiating touch, inviting touch, and how, and when to react to it. Families can also vary from being "very touchy-freely" to being "very cold … formal, polite, and reserved" (Gerlach, 2013, p. 1).

SIRP (Meier & Boivin, 2011) advocates, from a developmental and health perspective, for the inclusion of physical intimacy needs together with relational and self needs. It is assumed that these sets of needs are an inherent aspect of the human person. When these sets of needs are met, the individual proceeds to healthy development and establishes meaningful, rewarding, and fulfilling relationships. However, when these sets of needs go unmet, the individual is vulnerable to develop emotional problems and unsatisfying relationships. By not including intimacy needs, particularly emotional and physical intimacy needs, psychotherapy theory and practice is left incomplete and with a void.

This section begins by presenting definitions of physical intimacy needs and providing a rationale to include them in the theory and practice of psychotherapy. The section ends by providing research that supports the effects of having physical intimacy needs met or not met.

### *Definition of Physical Intimacy Needs*

Intimacy is a broad term that refers to an intense feeling of closeness that exists between two people. Intimacy provides the setting where people are able to share their deepest feelings, thoughts, needs, worries, and concerns and at the same time feel accepted for having these experiences. Intimacy can be manifested in different modalities such as intellectual intimacy, spiritual intimacy, emotional intimacy, and physical intimacy (Sawin, 2012). Although physical intimacy is the topic of this section, yet it is helpful to situate it within the context of emotional intimacy as often they are intertwined.

Emotional intimacy is the most meaningful kind of intimacy that can exist between two individuals. To achieve intimacy, one must (a) be oriented to value and seek closeness, (b) be able to tolerate, and even embrace, the intense emotions that are inextricably part of close relationships and to be able to share emotional experiences freely, and (c) be capable of self-disclosure, mutual reciprocity, sensitivity to the feelings of the other, and concern for the other's well-being (Collins & Sroufe, 1999). In intimacy, there is a sense of uninhibited trust, communication, respect, concern, self-disclosure, and understanding (Scharf & Mayseless, 2001). Gordon (2012) speaks of intimacy in terms of four Cs: communication, caring, commitment, and common values.

Mature intimacy simultaneously involves the capacity for autonomy, individuality, and separateness within relationships. An individual needs a coherent sense of self to be able to achieve closeness and sharing with others without fear of losing one's unique identity (Erikson, 1968). Mature and genuine intimacy involves a balance between emotional closeness (connectedness) and separateness (Mahler et al., 1975; Shulman & Knafo, 1997).

Physical intimacy involves being physically close to another person through a sensual proximity and/or physical affection such as hugging, kissing, touching, or sexual contact. It is an act/reaction or an expression of feelings such as close friendship, love, or sexual attraction, which people have for one another (Miller, 2011). To be physically intimate is intimacy with the body in such a way that "all one's sensitive spots, pleasurable or not pleasurable are known or being identified ... Physical intimacy is about being able to feel and sense with each part of one's body" (Ferlic, 2009, p. 1).

Physical intimacy can be thought of in terms sexual intimacy and of sensual intimacy. Sexual intimacy includes behaviors which include touching, hugging, caressing, and kissing with the intent of sexual expression. Sensual intimacy (i.e., sensual contact) can be thought of that which includes touch such as holding hands and hugging without the intent of sexual expression. Physical intimacy can exist without emotional intimacy and emotional intimacy can exist without being sexually intimate.

### *Rationale for Including Physical Intimacy Needs in Psychotherapy*

Gordon and Gordon (2012) assert that the experience of physical intimacy is a basic need for every individual and that it is a prerequisite for every healthy individual. In their view, touch relieves stress, makes us happier and healthier, provides an easy avenue to give and receive affection, and strengthens relationship. Within the context of families, a handshake, putting an arm-around-the shoulder and reaching out to touch an arm while conversing, promotes closeness between families. Within the context of marriage, sensual contacts, such as touch, keeps the emotional doors open between partners and helps them through arguments, conflicts, and financial pressures and thereby minimizes the effects of isolation and loneliness.

Gerlach (2013) states that every individual has a primal human need for physical contact with each other, starting in infancy. He continues, "most child development experts agree that newborns and infants need frequent soothing human skin-on-skin contact to thrive" (p. 1). He maintains that a young child's evolving personality and identity (e.g., "I am lovable") can be affected by whether she gets enough spontaneous hugs, caresses, and kisses. Touching is one of the many factors "that determine whether a growing child's developmental needs are well-enough and often enough" (p. 1). In spontaneous physical contact between two people, there is an exchange of an implied or assumed message such as "I like and care about you now" (p. 1).

The child or adult's psychological and relational experiences will affect the (a) primal needs for physical contact, (b) asserting or not asserting her needs, and (c) responding to touch. Individuals who are significantly wounded can have little or no need for touching, an exaggerated need for touching, and/or have trouble initiating, reacting to and decoding touching. For example, an individual can ignore her need for touching because she feels unlovable, feels that her need for and enjoyment of touching is wrong and selfish, and/or be inhibited from initiation touch for fear that she is intruding or will be rejected. The wounded individual might be unaware of her childhood-family's rules about touching and might not know what she is missing (Gerlach, 2013).

Depending on the amount of touch received during the formative years, one either has strong aversion or fondness for touch. Abusive touch could lead to physically and sexually violent relationships as where loving touch leads to nurturing close relationships. Given the impact it has on the quality of the relationships, touch plays a crucial role in the development of the emotional and physical health of individuals. Furthermore, attitudes toward touch are a result of social conditioning, influencing people's actions from birth to death. Individuals never outgrow their primal need for nourishing physical contact.

### *Development of Physical Intimacy and Sexual Needs*

Every individual has an innate need and capacity to express themselves fully as a sexual being. Freud, long ago, stated that we are sexual beings from the very beginning of our life and that we begin to learn about sexuality at the mother's breast. Freud's view has been confirmed by recent research (Haroian, 2000). Infants/children learn about sexuality by the way that their primary caregivers touch, caress, cuddle, and care for them. Later, they learn about sexuality by exploring and learning how their bodies feel to themselves and by exploring the bodies of children and adults. They continue to learn about sexuality in becoming attached to the parent of the opposite gender and by observing how members of the family express affection and care for one another. As well, infants/children learn about sexuality by the words that family members use to refer to body parts and in learning what constitutes sexually appropriate behavior (Pike, 2000).

The infant/child's sexual maturation parallels the orderly, logical, and self-regulation pattern of development in similar ways as observed in other aspects of human behavior such as from dependency on family of origin, to the development of the sense of an autonomous self and to the confidence and desire to form an intimate relationship and begin a family of one's own. The erotic response in infancy is global and undifferentiated and in childhood it shifts toward genital focus that is expressed in autoeroticism. The genital focus is intensified in pubescence and sexual experience in itself becomes the paramount goal. In adolescence sexuality becomes a powerful force that manifests itself in sexual reciprocity and mutual sharing (Haroian, 2000; Webber & Delvin, 2005).

Meier and Boivin (2011) state that

> the acknowledgement and affirmation of an infant/child's relational, self and physical intimacy needs and the extent to which they are realized, integrated and moderated by interactions with caregiver, others and reality (e.g., culture), affects all aspects of her personality including how she perceives the other, self and the world, the organization and structuring of experiences, relational patterns and quality of intimacy, and coping strategies used to deal with the frustrations of unmet needs. (p. 156)

### *Research and the Impact of Physical Intimacy*

Much of the research on the impact of physical intimacy has focused on touch which has been found to influence bodily functions and to affect an individual's health and well-being. Tiffany Field established the Touch Research Institute (TRI) in 1992 at the University of Miami School of Medicine. The goal of the TRI was to study the effect of touch therapy on health and well-being. The institute has produced hundreds of studies that showed that touch therapy has beneficial effects on health and well-being. In two of her books, Field (2000, 2006) shows how touch therapy has alleviated depression and anxiety, increased attentiveness, enhanced immune function, and reduced pain during medical procedures.

Fowler (2000) in reviewing the literature found that human touch has many beneficial effects such as improved immune function, decreased cortisol levels, and coherence of heart-generated magnetic fields (Ironson et al., 1996). Human touch was also observed to lower anxiety and lessen depression (Field et al., 1992; Field et al., 1997; Field et al., 1998).

Holt-Lunstad et al. (2008) studied the effect of "warm touch" (the non-sexual, supportive kind) on blood pressure, salivary oxytocin, alpha amylase, and cortisol. The subjects for the research were couples who gave each other a 30-minute massage three times a week for four weeks to promote emotional and physical closeness. The control group consisted of couples who were tested but did not provide massages. The authors found that massages and other supportive and caring touch lowered stress hormones and blood pressure among men, enhanced salivary oxytocin both early and late in the intervention group and alpha amylase was reduced at post treatment in intervention group husbands and wives relative to controls. Husbands in the intervention group had significantly lower post treatment 24-hour systolic blood pressure than the control group. They concluded that increasing warm touch among couples has a beneficial influence on multiple stress-sensitive systems.

## Summary and Conclusion

The review of the current theoretical, clinical, and research literature strongly supports the thought that self, relational, and physical intimacy needs be included in a theory of psychotherapy. The support comes from many different orientations including self-psychology, cognitive therapy, gestalt therapy, and psychodynamic theory and from a vast number of research studies. Research has demonstrated that needs can be defined and classified and that the construct of needs can be operationalized and reliably and validly measured. The relevant findings from the review of the literature regarding self, relational, and physical intimacy needs are the following:

1 Needs are considered to be innate, organismic necessities, nutriments that are essential for ongoing psychological growth, integrity, well-being, survival, and optimal functioning (Deci & Ryan, 2000, p. 229; Kasser, 2002, p. 24). Needs are the essential elements that enhance the quality of life and a sense of self; relational needs are the component parts of a universal human desire for relationship (Erskine, 1998). Individuals are driven by their biological need to be in a relationship (Erskine, 2011).
2 Needs are considered to be the primary motivators for all of the behaviors and interactions, give them focus and direction and mobilize and channel them; people are pulled by their needs (Kasser, 2002; Perls, 1969, p. 22; Polster & Polster, 1973, p. 228; Wallen, 1970, p. 9; Yalom, 1989).

3 Relational needs are universal and fundamental human needs are finite, few, and classifiable and are the same in all cultures and in all historical periods. Cultures do not determine the needs, but determine how needs are met (Max-Neuf et al., 1991). Relational needs are the component parts of a universal human desire for relationship (Erskine, 1998).
4 Innate needs can be classified on different parameters such as the need for competence, relatedness, autonomy (Deci & Ryan, 2000, p. 229); communal-oriented needs (affiliation, intimacy, altruism, succorance) and individual-oriented needs (autonomy, power, achievement) (Epstein & Baucom, 2002, p. 116); for competency and lovability (Kohut, 1977) and the need for emotional bonding (connectedness) and autonomy (separateness) (Mahler et al., 1975).
5 Needs are to be differentiated from that which satisfies the needs, that is, from their satisfiers such as a hug or a cuddle (Max-Neuf et al., 1991).
6 The satisfaction or lack of satisfaction of needs can be viewed on different parameters such as expressed needs and wanted needs (Schutz, 1966) and as unmet needs and met needs (Meier & Boivin, 2006).
7 Unmet needs lead to emotional disturbance and sense of insecurity (Erskine, 2011) and take on a compulsive quality and become insatiable (Erskine, 1998); the continued absence of satisfaction of needs may be manifested as frustration, anger, aggression, longing, emptiness, and loneliness (Erskine, 1998, Kasser, 2002); individuals who do not know their needs might become parasites on the needs of others (Yalom, 1989, p. 9).
8 Not all needs press for satisfaction at the same time, rather one or more human need dominates and then recedes into the background when fulfilled (Korb et al., 1989, p. 6; Wallen, 1970).
9 The primary needs can be operationalized and reliably and validly measured.
10 The experience of physical intimacy is a basic or primal human need for every individual and is a prerequisite for every healthy individual (Gerlach, 2013; Gordon & Gordon, 2012).
11 Physical intimacy is highly correlated with both psychological and physical health and well-being.
12 Sensual physical intimacy needs can be differentiated from sexual physical intimacy needs.

In conclusion, needs are considered to be the primary motivators of all behaviors and interactions. As well, needs can be broadly classified as relational needs (need for connection, need for autonomy), self needs (competency, lovability), and physical intimacy needs (sensual contact and sexual expression). Further, needs can be operationalized and validly and reliably measured. These ideas form the foundation for the development of SIRP to be presented in the next chapter.

## References


American Heritage Dictionary of the English Language, 4th Edition (2000). Boston, MA: Houghton Mifflin.

Beck, A. T. (1976). *Cognitive therapy and the emotional disorders.* New York: International Universities Press.

Bekker, M. H., & van Assen, M. H. L. M. (2006). A short form of the autonomy scale: Properties of the autonomy-connectedness scale (ACS-30). *Journal of Personality Assessment, 86*(1), 51–60.

Bettleheim, B. (1984). *Freud and man's soul.* New York: Vintage Books.

Boeree, C. G. (2006). *Abraham Maslow, 1908–1970.* Retrieved December 2012 from http://webspace.ship.edu/cgboer/maslow.html

Collins English Dictionary – Complete and Unabridged (2003). Scarborough, Canada: Harper Collins.

Collins, W. A., & Sroufe, L. A. (1999). Capacity for intimate relationships: A developmental construction. In W. Furman, Brown, B. B., & Feiring, C. (Eds.), *The development of romantic relationships in adolescence* (pp. 125–147). Cambridge, UK: Cambridge University Press.

Corsini, R. J. (1977). A medley of current personality theories. In R. J. Corsini (Ed.), *Current personality theories* (pp. 399–439). Itasca, IL: F. E. Peacock Publishers.

Davis, P. (1999). *The power of touch.* California: Hay House, Inc.

Deci, E. L., & Ryan, R. M. (2000). The "what" and "why" of goal pursuits: Human needs and the self-determination of behavior. *Psychological Inquiry, 11*, 227–268.

DeLamater, J., & Hyde, J. S. (2004). Conceptual and theoretical issues in studying sexuality in close relationships. In J. H. Harvey, A. Wenzel, & S. Sprecher (Eds.), *The handbook of sexuality in close relationships* (pp. 7–30). New Jersey: Lawrence Erlbaum Associates.

Epstein, N. B., & Baucom, D. H. (2002). *Enhanced cognitive-behavioral therapy for couples.* Washington, DC: American Psychological Association.

Erikson, E. H. (1968). *Identity: Youth and crisis.* New York: Norton.

Erskine, R. G. (1998). Attunement and involvement: Therapeutic responses to relational needs. *International Journal of Psychotherapy, 3*(3), 235–244.

Erskine, R. G. (2011). Attachment, relational-needs, and psychotherapeutic presence. *International Journal of Integrative Psychotherapy, 2*(1), 10–18.

Ferlic, K. (2009). *The need for physical intimacy.* Retrieved December 2012 from http://ryuc.info/creativesexuality/need_for_physical_intimacy.htm

Field, T. (2000). *Touch therapy.* Sydney, Australia: Churchill Livingstone; Harcourt Brace.

Field, T. (2006). *Massage therapy research.* Toronto, Ontario: Elsevier Health Sciences.

Field, T., Hernandez-Reif, M., Quintino, O., Schanberg, S., & Kuhn, C. (1998). Elderly retired volunteers benefit from giving massage therapy to infants. *Journal of Applied Gerontology, 17*, 229–239.

Field, T., Morrow, C., Faldeon, C., Larson, S., Kuhn, C., & Schansberg, S. (1992). Massage reduces anxiety in child and adolescent psychiatry patients. *Journal of the American Academy of child and Adolescent Psychiatry, 31*, 125–131.

Field, T., Sunshine, W., Hernandez-Reif, M., Quintino, O., Schanberg, S., Kuhn, C., & Burman, I. (1997). Chronic fatigue syndrome: Massage therapy effects on depression and somatic symptoms in chronic fatigue syndrome. *Journal of Chronic Fatigue Syndrome*, *3*, 43–51.

Fowler, R. (2000). *The effects of human touch on healing: A literature review.* Retrieved January 2013 from http://www.logan.edu/mm/files/LRC/Senior-Research/2000-Dec-25.pdf

Frankl, V. E. (1967). *Psychotherapy and existentialism: Selected papers on logotherapy by Viktor E. Frankl.* New York: Simon Schuster.

Freud, S. (1918). Lines of advance in psycho-analytic therapy. *Standard Edition*, *17*, 159–168.

Freud, S. (1923). The ego and the id. *Standard Edition*, *19*, 12–63.

Freud, S. (1938). An outline of psycho-analysis. *Standard Edition*, *23*, 144–1207.

Gerlach, P. K. (2013). *Are you getting enough healthy physical contact? A basic human need.* Retrieved January 2013 from http://sfhelp.org/touch.htm

Glasser, W. (1999). *Choice theory: A new psychology of personal freedom.* New York: Harper Collins.

Gordon, J. (2012). *The four C's of emotional intimacy.* Retrieved December 2012 from http://www.selfgrowth.com/articles/Emotional_Intimacy.html

Gordon, J., & Gordon, C. (2012). *Touch promotes physical intimacy.* Retrieved from http://www.the-intimate-couple.com/physical-intimacy.html

Greenberg, L., Rice, L., & Elliot, R. (1993). *Facilitating emotional change: The moment-by-moment process.* New York: Guilford Press.

Gurman, A. S. (2008). *Clinical handbook of couple therapy*, 4th ed. New York: Guilford Press.

Haroian, L. (2000). Child sexual development. *Electronic Journal of Human Sexuality*, *3*, 1–45.

Harvey, J. H., Wenzel, A., & Sprecher, S. (Eds.). (2004). *The handbook of sexuality in close relationships.* New Jersey: Lawrence Erlbaum Associates.

Holt-Lunstad, J., Birmingham, W. A., & Light, K. C. (2008). Influence of a "warm touch" support enhancement intervention among married couples on ambulatory blood pressure, oxytocin, alpha amylase, and cortisol. *Psychosomatic Medicine*, *70*(9), 976–985.

Ironson, G., Field, T., Scafidi, F., Hashimoto, M., Kumar, M., Kumar, A., Price, A., Goncalves, A., Burman, I., Tetenman, C., Patarca, R., & Fletcher, M. A. (1996). Massage therapy is associated with enhancement of the immune system's cytotoxic capacity. *International Journal of Neuroscience*, *84*, 205–217.

Kasser, T. (2002). *The high price of materialism.* London: Bradford Book.

Kohut, H. (1977). *The restoration of the self.* New York: International Universities Press.

Korb, M. P., Gorrel, J., & Van de Riet, V. (1989). *Gestalt therapy: Practice and theory.* New York: Pergamon Press.

Mahler, M. S., Pine, F., & Bergman, A. (1975). *Psychological birth of the human infant.* New York: Basic Books.

Maslow, A. H. (1954). *Motivation and personality.* New York: Harper.

Maslow, A. H. (1968). *Toward a psychology of being*, 2nd ed. New York: Van Nostrand.

Maslow, A. H. (1971). *The further reaches of human nature.*New York: Penguin.
Max-Neuf, M., Elizalde, A., & Hopenhayn, M. (1991). Development of human needs. In M. A. Max-Neuf (Ed.), Human *scale development: Conception, application and further reflections* (pp. 12–54). New York: The Apex Press.
May, R. (1953). *Man's search for himself.* New York: The New American Library.
Meier, A., & Boivin, M. (2006). Intrapsychic conflicts, their formation, underlying dynamics and resolution: An object relations perspective. In A. Meier & M. Rovers (Eds.), *Through conflict to reconciliation* (pp. 295–328). Ottawa, Ontario: Novalis.
Meier, A., & Boivin, M. (2011). *Counselling and therapy techniques: Theory and practice*. London, England: SAGE.
Miller, R. (2011). *Intimate relationships*. New York: McGraw-Hill.
Miller, W. R. (Ed.) (1999). *Integrating spirituality into treatment*. Washington, DC: American Psychological Association.
Murray, H. A. (1938). *Explorations in Personality*. New York: Oxford Press.
Norcross, J. C. (1992). Introduction to special Issue: The future of psychotherapy. *Psychotherapy*, *29*(1), 2–3.
Office of the Surgeon General. (2001). *The surgeon general's call to action to promote sexual health and responsible sexual behavior*. Rockville, MD: Public Health Service.
Perls, F. S. (1969). *Gestalt therapy verbatim*. Toronto, Ontario: Bantam Books.
Pike, L. B. (2000). *Sexuality and your child: For children ages 0 to 3*. Columbia, Missouri: University of Missouri-Columbia.
Polster, E., & Polster, M. (1973). *Gestalt therapy integrated*. New York: Brunner/Mazel Publishers.
Reisenzein, R., & Schnpflug, W. (1992). Stumpf's cognitive-evaluative theory of emotion. *American Psychologist*, *47*(1), 34–45.
Reiss, S. (2012). *Psychology of human needs. New ways of thinking about people. Who We Are*. Retrieved November 2012 from http://www.psychologytoday.com/blog/who-we-are/201205/psychology-human-needs
Robinson, B. E., Bockting, W. O., Rosser, B., Miner, M., & Coleman, E. (2002). The sexual health model: Application of a sexological approach to HIV prevention. *Health Education Research*, *17*, 43–57.
Sawin, D. (2012). *Intimacy: What is it and how do I find it?* Retrieved December 2012 from http://www.lstionline.com/article2.php
Scharf, M., & Mayseless, O. (2001). The capacity for romantic intimacy: Exploring the contribution of best friend and marital and parental relationships. *Journal of Adolescence*, *24*, 379–399.
Schutz, W. (1966). *The interpersonal underworld*. Palo Alto, CA: Science and Behavior Books.
Shulman, S., & Knafo, D. (1997). Balancing closeness and individuality in adolescent close relationships. *International Journal of Behavioral Development*, *21*, 687–702.
Skinner, B. F. (1953). *Science and human behavior*. New York: Free Press.
Wallen, R. (1970). Gestalt therapy and Gestalt psychology. In J. Fagan & I. L. Shepperd (Eds.), *Gestalt therapy now* (pp. 8–13). New York: Harper & Row.

Webber, C., & Delvin, D. (2005). *Sexuality throughout life*. http://www.netdoctor.co.uk/sex

Wolpe, J. (1990). *The practice of behavior therapy* (4th ed.). New York: Pergamon.

Yalom, I. D. (1989). *Love's executioner and other tales of psychotherapy*. New York: Harper Perennial.

Zeifman, D., & Hazan, C. (2008). Pair bonds as attachments: Reevaluating the evidence. In J. Cassidy & P. R. Shaver (Eds.), *Handbook of attachment: Theory, research, and clinical applications* (pp. 436–455). New York: Guilford Press.

Chapter 3

# Self-in-Relationship Psychotherapy

In recent years there has been a noticeable shift from unidimensional to integrated approaches in the formulation of psychotherapy theories. The attempts toward integration have taken place under the rubrics of technical ecclecticism, common factors approach, theoretical integration, and assimilative integration (Arkowitz, 1992; Messer, 1992; Norcross, 2005; Stricker & Gold, 2005). In addition to a shift toward integrative theories, there is also a movement from an individualistic to a relational paradigm in the way emotional problems and behaviors are understood and treated (Barrett-Lennard, 2013).

Self-in-Relationship Psychotherapy (SIRP) is an integrated therapeutic approach that focuses on relational and self issues in the understanding, assessment and treatment of emotional problems and behaviors. The SIRP approach includes both explanatory constructs and interventions (mechanisms) of change. The SIRP approach integrates explanatory constructs from psychodynamic-oriented therapies (i.e. psychoanalysis, ego psychology, object relations theory, self psychology, and intersubjectivity theory) and interventions from action-oriented therapies (i.e. person-centered therapy, Gestalt therapy, behavioral therapy, and cognitive-behavioral Therapy).

This chapter presents the basic principles and major constructs of SIRP. The first part provides an overview of SIRP in the form of a narrative that connects its constructs in a meaningful way. The second part presents more clearly the fundamental principles of the SIRP approach. The third part presents, defines, and illustrates SIRP's major explanatory constructs.

## An Overview of SIRP

The overarching concept that embraces and integrates SIRP constructs and processes and informs the shaping of personality is the concept of the psychological separation and individuation process which describes how an infant/child begins extrauterine life by becoming emotionally bonded with a significant caregiver (e.g., mother) and then emerges from this state to

DOI: 10.4324/9781003272502-4

achieve psychological separation, autonomy and individuation (Mahler et al., 1975). For the duration of his life, the infant/child, as he moves into the toddler, adolescence, and adult stages, strives to maintain connection with significant others and at the same time pursues and maintains his own sense of autonomy and individuality.

A major concept of SIRP is that the core relational, self, and physical intimacy needs propel the separation and individuation process. It is assumed that these needs, which emerge largely in the social interactions in infancy and childhood, propel all of human behaviors and interactions and remain present throughout one's entire life. The infant is born with the innate relational "need for emotional bonding" and with the innate relational "need to psychologically separate/individuate" and become his own person (Mahler et al., 1975). As the infant/child gradually grows away from emotional bonding and moves toward psychological separation/individuation, the self needs for "competency" and "lovability" emerge. The infant/child requires the parents' admiration and validation for his budding competencies (i.e., sense of omnipotence) and their affirmation for being loved and liked for moving away from emotional bonding toward autonomy and interdependence (Kohut, 1977). The infant/child also has the need for physical intimacy (e.g., touch), to connect bodily with the caregiver which serves to help the infant/child to connect bodily with himself which is the basis to build a core psychological self (Krueger, 1989; Mahler et al., 1975). That is, it is important for the infant to become physiologically, emotionally, and psychologically "anchored" in order to move toward becoming an individual. Later, this anchoring serves as a base or a "psychological home" (e.g., object constancy) from which to take direction for one's life.

In the movement from emotional bonding to psychological separation/individuation, the infant/child encounters a host of experiences about their self, others, and the world and stores these experiences bodily, perceptually, and conceptually as representation of self and other. These singular and initially isolated experiences and representations become organized to form internal structures and organizations (e.g., psychic organization) that represent internal (e.g., feelings, urges) and external realities (e.g., demands, expectations) and at the same time serve as a lens to process and interpret incoming information and shape the patterns of relating with others (Freud, 1923).

In his pursuit of separating and individuating, the infant/child acquires skills pertaining to how to relate to others and to the world, handle frustrations and anxieties, deal with emotions, internalize the demands and expectations of others, and realize his relational, self, and physical intimacy needs. All of the infant/child, toddler, adolescent, and adult's behaviors, interactions, and relational patterns are driven by attempts to satisfy his core relational, self, and physical intimacy needs. An infant/child that is brought up with "good enough" parents (Winnicott, 1965) will develop the necessary relational and coping skills to actualize his relational, self, and physical intimacy needs. On the contrary, an infant/child not brought up with "good enough" parenting might develop inadequate or dysfunctional relational and coping skills to actualize his needs.

SIRP views emotional problems and disorders in terms of developmental injuries and failures to develop adequate coping and relational skills (Mahler et al., 1975). More precisely, SIRP assumes that the majority of emotional and interpersonal problems (with the exception of those emanating from abuse and trauma and neurological deficits and biochemical imbalances) have their origin in failures in the developmental process of emotional bonding and psychological separation/individuation. It assumes, as well, that these problems stem from unmet relational, self, and physical intimacy needs and from unsatisfactory ways to compensate for their deprivation. To compensate for the disruption of healthy childhood relations, the individual develops relational patterns, defensive (protective) mechanisms, and self structures and psychic organizations that provide a semblance of security, protection, safety, and emotional connection, but in reality they become ineffective in adolescence and adulthood.

Since emotional problems began in a relationship, it is assumed that emotional problems are healed in a relationship. The goal of therapy is to help clients become aware of their unmet core needs, orient their lives around these, become agents of their own lives, establish meaningful relationships and acquire effective coping and relational skills and thereby free themselves from their symptoms and gradually change the organization of their internal structures and personality. The means to help a person change maladaptive psychic organizations, relational patterns, and address emotional problems is for the therapist to offer the client opportunities to experience other, self, and the world differently so as to allow new realities to come forward, rework developmental injuries and work with the client's transferences. The therapist's use of self (Lum, 2002) aids the intuitive understanding of the client, an understanding that complements a more formal and conceptual understanding of the client.

## Fundamental Principles

SIRP rests on a set of fundamental principles. The principles are presented and briefly explained.

1 SIRP assumes that core needs are the primary motivating force in human behaviors and interactions; that needs are innate, organismic necessities, an integral aspect of human nature and are potentially present when life begins (Deci & Ryan, 2000; Kasser, 2002).
2 The needs are construed in terms of relational, self, and physical intimacy needs. Relational needs include the "need for emotional bonding" and the

"need for psychological separateness/individuation/autonomy," self needs include the "need for competency" and the "need for lovability/significance," and physical intimacy needs include the "need for sensual contact" and the need for "sexual intimacy" (Meier & Boivin, 2011).

3 A child's specific relational, self, and physical intimacy needs evolve and change as he moves from being intimately bonded with his caregiver to becoming a separate and an individuated person and forming intimate relationships with others (Mahler et al., 1975). The core relational and self needs are reworked each time the person goes through a major phase in life, such as the initial separation from the caregiver, and later leaving his parents and home during adolescence to attend university (Meier et al., 2006).
4 The manner in which the caregiver responds to the infant's core needs will influence the quality of the physiological and psychological emotional bonding (i.e., safe anchorage), the separating/individuating processes, the formation of internal object and self-representations, the development of the psychic organization, self-structure, and relational patterns.
5 The infant/child has to experience an optimum level of challenges (i.e., frustration) in order to develop the ego and self resources to move through the separation and individuation process and achieve individuality and autonomy (Mahler et al., 1975).
6 Needs, together with affects and cognitions, form three parallel but interdependent systems (Benesh & Weiner, 1982; Lazarus, 1982; Reisenzein & Schonpflug, 1992; Zajonc, 1980). Within this triad, core needs are conceived to be the prime directional motivators of behavior, feelings are thought to be responses to either the satisfaction or the frustration of needs, and thoughts pertain to the stylistic ways of perceiving reality, to solving problems, managing reality, and to evaluating experiences and beliefs (Meier & Boivin, 2001).
7 The infant/child's innate needs interact with the social (e.g., good enough parenting) and physical milieu in shaping the individual's personality and the formation of new behaviors and attitudes including the formation of the superego (Meier & Boivin, 1983).
8 Identifying the unmet core needs is a crucial aspect of the SIRP approach. Needs may be expressively stated or inferred from the individual's style of communication and relating, his intrapsychic struggles and dominant emotional state.
9 The term, unmet core needs refers primarily to those needs not adequately responded to during infancy/childhood and continue to linger and push for fulfillment in adolescence and adulthood. The unmet childhood core needs are to be differentiated from unmet growth needs which are the age appropriate needs of adolescent and adult relationships.
10 When needs go unmet they may lead to emotional, behavioral, and relationship problems. The unmet core needs become the principle around which the person maladaptively organizes his life.

11 SIRP assumes that the majority of psychological, emotional, and relational problems begin in a relationship and therefore need to be healed in a relationship. The goal of therapy is to help clients become aware of their unmet core needs, orient their lives around these and thereby gradually transform the organization of their personality, become agents of their own lives, and free themselves of their symptoms.
12 SIRP focuses on an individual's subjective experience and psychic organizations assuming that in transforming the organization one will at the same time change an individual's overt behaviors and symptoms.
13 The primary means to bring about change, both intrapsychically and behaviorally, is for the therapist to offer opportunities for the client to experience self differently so as to allow new realities to come forward, to address the intersubjective therapeutic reality and work with the client's transferences.
14 SIRP assumes that the client has the inner resources to bring about the desired changes and to become the agent of his own change, within the context of a safe, secure, caring, and supportive therapeutic setting. The therapist is responsible for the therapy process and the client is responsible for the therapy work.
15 Psychotherapy evolves across space and time according to a pattern marked by phases (Meier & Boivin, 1983, 1998).

## Major Constructs

The major explanatory constructs that constitute the SIRP approach are incorporated from psychodynamic theory including psychoanalysis, ego psychology, object relations theory and self-psychology. The names of the original constructs, to a large extent, are kept but are modified and interwoven in the SIRP narrative. These constructs are presented, defined, and illustrated. For the purpose of simplicity, the illustrations will refer to the role that parents play in the origin of an individual's problem although more often than not other factors (e.g., trauma, losses, failures) play significant roles. Also, when speaking about father and mother, it is important to remember that the statements represent the individual's perception of his parents and do not necessarily correspond to who and how they truly were or are. The major constructs of the SIRP approach are presented in the following sections and are summarized in Figure 3.1.

### *Core Relational, Self, and Physical Intimacy Needs*

Core needs is a foundational concept of SIRP in the same way that thoughts and feelings are primary concepts of cognitive and experiential-oriented therapies, respectively. The authors arrived at the significance of human core needs from their clinical work with children, adolescents, and adults in the

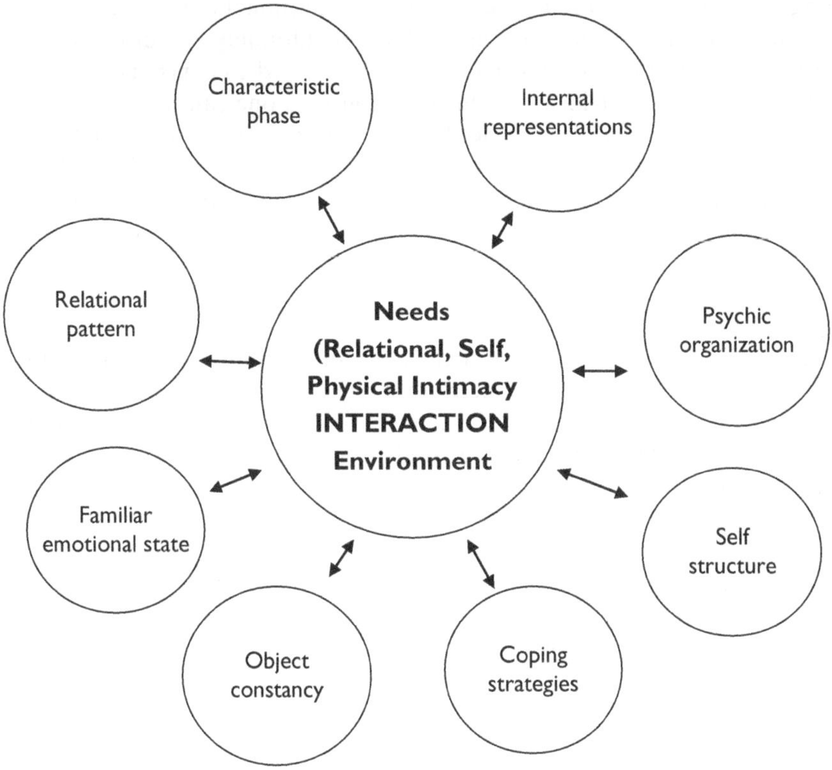


*Figure 3.1* Visual presentation of the core SIRP constructs.

context of individual, couple, and family therapy. They observed that children crave the love and affection of their parents and want to be included with their peers. They observed that teenagers want to have a voice in matters that relate to their lives, they want the freedom and autonomy and choose and make decisions. They observed in adults, particularly in couples, how one partner wants to spend more time with their partner while their partner wants more time for him/herself.

SIRP groups core needs according to relational, self, and physical intimacy needs. This grouping of needs is based in part, on the writings of Epstein and Baucom (2002), Deci and Ryan (2000), Reeves (2014), Mahler, et al. (1975), and Kohut (1977). Epstein and Baucom (2002) classify needs into two classes: communally oriented motives (e.g., affiliation, intimacy, altruism, and succorance) and individual orientated motives (e.g., autonomy, power, and achievement). Deci and Ryan (2000) and Reeves (2014) identified three innate needs, namely, autonomy, competency, and relatedness. Mahler et al. (1975) indirectly referred to needs when discussing the developmental process of separation and individuation. The two needs, referred to as relational needs, are the need for emotional bonding/connection and the need for separateness/individuation/autonomy. In discussing the structure of the cohesive self, Kohut (1977) referred to concepts of nuclear ambition and nuclear ideal. From these concepts one can infer two needs, referred to as self needs, the need for competency and the need for significance, respectively. To the two groups of relational and self needs, the authors added physical intimacy needs, which include the need for sensual contact and sexual intimacy.

### *Core relational needs*

The core relational needs comprise the need for emotional connection with a significant caregiver and the need to psychologically separate from the caregiver, to individuate and to become autonomous (Mahler et al., 1975). These two relational needs are referred to as the need for emotional connection and the need for autonomy.

*Need for emotional connection:* This refers to a need for a mutual emotional and psychological closeness that is characterized by affection and trust between people. Although one can develop emotional connections with pets, objects, and associations, the term, in this chapter, is reserved for emotional connection between people.

*Need for autonomy:* The need for autonomy implies the needs for psychological separateness and for individuation. The need for separateness refers to the need to psychologically separate from a person, that is, to experience oneself as different from the other. The need for individuation refers to the need to be autonomous, that is, the origin of one's own behaviors (Deci & Ryan, 2002), develop one's own interests, values, and goals in life and have the freedom to make choices and decisions. In terms of relationships, the need for autonomy is often expressed in terms of wanting one's psychological space and the freedom to be one's own person, to make decisions and choices and to have a voice in matters that concern him. The need to become one's own person and to be agent of one's own life is propelled by the inborn sense of "narcissistic omnipotence," that is, the illusion of omnipotent creativity and control (Winnicott, 1948, p. 163).

The quality of the core needs for emotional connection and for autonomy is dependent upon the age and stage of development of the infant/child. In the early stage of development, the infant/child has not developed a sense of "me" and "not me," that is, the boundary between self and other is tenuous. As well, the need for autonomy is merged with dependency needs at the early stage of development. Thus the definition of the need for emotional connection and the need for autonomy varies according to the developmental stage achieved (Mahler et al., 1975).

When the needs for emotional connection and for autonomy are not fully met in infancy/childhood, they will continue to push for satiation in adolescence and adulthood and may result in relational and self dysfunctions. The consequences of not having the needs for emotional connection and for autonomy met are illustrated by the following two examples.

***Illustration 1.*** Unmet need for emotional connection: Kami and Mario had been dating for two years and Kami always dreaded when Mario's travels kept him away from home. When he was away, Kami would become angry at him, feel that he was abandoning her, and was ready to terminate the relationship rather than to go through the pain of reconciling his absence. For her, when he was out of sight, he was out of mind. She could not comfort herself in thinking about the good times that they had together and to anticipate the moment when they would be together again. In exploring these feelings in therapy, Kami reported that as a child she craved the love and affection from her emotionally distraught, cold, and distant mother. Today she continues to incessantly crave for emotional connection with Mario, but she does not know what is a reasonable request and her need is only temporarily satisfied when they are together.

***Illustration 2.*** Unmet need for autonomy: Sofía and Enrique were married for seven years. Sofía worked outside of the home and after work took care of the children and the domestic tasks. Enrique was a life insurance salesperson and often spent the evenings with customers. Even when he was not meeting with customers, he continued to find excuses for not coming home early. In therapy he stated that Sofía begrudged him for being away from home and when he was home she always found something for him to do. He felt that he was being imposed upon when he was home and had no life of his own. In the course of the therapy he became aware that, as a child, he often felt imposed upon by his parents and he found relief by signing up for all school sports so as to stay away from home as much as possible. As a child, Enrique did not learn how to integrate his need for autonomy with his need for emotional closeness, thus he overly asserted this need even if it was unreasonable to do so.

### *Core self needs*

The core self needs include the striving to being competent and the striving to being significant. The child needs the caregiver's admiration and affirmations to foster his sense of omnipotence, empowerment, and competency and to experience that he is a good, significant, and lovable person for just being who he is and also for his movement out of the emotionally bonded relationship. These self needs are referred to as the need for competency and the need for significance. These two needs are inferred from Kohut's (1977, 1979) concepts of mirroring transference and idealizing transference and from the concepts of nuclear ambition and nuclear ideals.

Kohut (1977, 1984) did not differentiate between a need and the satisfier of a need. His focus was on the satisfier of the need. Thus the need for competency is satisfied by admiration (mirroring transference) received from others for being a competent worker, good father, good mother, to name a few. The need for significance is satisfied by receiving affirmation (idealizing transference) for being a worthwhile, significant, and lovable person that one likes to be with and cherishes.

Whereas the relational needs are about being connected to others and being one's own person in the presence of others, the self needs are about the subjective experience that one has of oneself, that is, a sense of being competent and a sense of being significant. The need for competency is nourished by the sense of grandiosity and the need for significance is nourished by the sense of merger, that is, to be like someone who is admired and with whom one identifies.

*The need for competency:* This refers to the need to experience oneself as effective in one's ongoing interactions with others (relational competency) and to experience opportunities to exercise and express one's capacities (self competency in relation to oneself) (Deci & Ryan, 2002).

*The need for significance:* This refers to the need to experience oneself as significant, lovable, worthwhile, and likeable, and as being a good person and attractive in relation to others.

The development of the self needs begins in early childhood with affirmations and validations from caregivers. With consistent positive validations, the child gradually develops a sense of competency and significance and requires less feedback from others regarding the two self needs. The self needs then become self-evaluative needs and therefore are less dependent on the positive and negative judgments of others. That is, a person who has a good sense of competency and feels significant (i.e., lovable), is able to maintain these despite negative responses from others. Equally, for a person who has a negative sense of his competency and significance, it is difficult to change these perceptions of self. The need for competency and the need for significance are illustrated by the two following examples.

***Illustration 1.*** Unmet need for competency: Rudi and Selma requested couple therapy because the former felt that his wife had become cold toward him, withdrew sexual favors, and showed no interest in his work and in his accomplishments. Despite being a highly successful and wealthy businessman in the community, Rudi never felt that it was enough; he had to prove himself over and over again. He craved for admiration and affirmation from Selma for having developed a successful business, but she could not give it to him in the way he wanted it. In an individual session, he reported that, as a child, his father constantly put him down, called him stupid and indicated that he would not make it in life. To this day, he continues to crave for the admiration and affirmation that he never received for being intelligent and competent. His unmet need for competency continues to push for satiation and the admiration and validations that he receives only provide temporary relief as he is not able to internalize them to bring about a sense of competency.

***Illustration 2.*** Unmet need for significance: Dodi and Adi, both in their late 20s, had been living together for 18 months and Adi was very unhappy in the relationship. She constantly nagged Dodi to do his part of the domestic tasks such as to put away dirty dishes and to take out the garbage but he always forgot to do so. Adi began to feel frustrated, felt what she said did not matter and was insignificant; she felt unlovable. When she described her childhood experiences, it became apparent that the feeling of being unloved and didn't matter was a familiar feeling that had its origins in her relationships with her parents who did not validate her feelings, needs, and thoughts. She began to feel that there was something wrong with her, that she was bad and flawed and began to think that she was unlovable. She has struggled since childhood to have her need for significance satisfied and has constantly failed in achieving it.

### *Core physical intimacy needs*

The core physical intimacy needs include the need for sensual contact and the need for sexual intimacy. The need for sensual contact is associated with an infant's need, as part of the emotional bonding, for bonding through the senses. Thus the need for sensual contact refers to the need for physical contact such as hugs and being cuddled.

Sensuality broadens to include sexual intimacy when the infant/child begins to experience pleasure in making physical contact with self by touching different parts of his body with the ultimate physical pleasure, in later years, by sexual intimacy. The need for sexual intimacy, therefore, refers to the need for physical contact with the intention of a sexual contact. This includes hugging, kissing, and fondling that find their mutual satisfaction and completion in genital expression.

Freud (1905) mentions that an infant/child learns about sexuality at the breast of the mother in terms of how the breast, that is, the mother relates to the infant. Freud's views have been given support by the research of Haroian (2000), Pike (2000), and Webber and Devlin (2005).

The need for sexual intimacy rarely, if ever, has its beginnings in childhood. When it has its beginnings in childhood, it is often related to sexual abuse and manifests itself as sexualized language and behaviors. In other cases, the child or pre-teenager might confuse the need for love and affection with sexual pleasure and sexual behavior or he might seek to have his need for emotional connection satisfied sexually. This is often observed in children who have been emotionally neglected and not validated, affirmed, and admired for their competencies and goodness as persons. Some children and pre-teenagers may have learned that in order to attract the attention of the other and to form a relationship with them, they have to be sexual even though at a deeper layer, they crave for an emotional relationship and a sensual contact. When this behavior extends into adulthood, the individual might feel compelled to engage sexually to attract the attention of the other in order to have a relationship but to discover later that his own need for emotional intimacy is being compromised and thus the relationship fades.

It is to be noted that age, gender, and culture often affect how the need for sensual contact and the need for sexual intimacy are expressed and satiated. These two needs are illustrated in terms of unmet needs by the following examples.

***Illustration 1.*** *Unmet need for sensual contact:* Crista, in her mid-20s, left home for a position as a computer analyst in city a few hundred miles away. She found being away from home extremely difficult and would return home once every two to three weeks despite the fact that she was not emotionally close to either of her parents. The mother was depressed most of her life and abused alcohol, and the father was often out at sea fishing. Crista craved for both emotional connection and sensual and physical closeness with her mother. She pictured her mother holding her in her arms, comforting and rocking her. To receive verbally expressed gestures of emotional connection did not satisfy Crista's need for closeness; she also had a need for sensual contact something that she rarely experienced as an infant and child. The unmet need for sensual contact impacted all of Crista's relationships including those with her mother and her male friends.

***Illustration 2.*** *Unmet need for sexual intimacy:* Klara and Klaus, married for 25 years, sought psychotherapy to work through the aftereffects of two affairs on part of Klaus. The first affair was brief and took place many years ago. The last affair, more recent, lasted three years. During the past five years, Klara and Klaus did not have sexual intimacy. Klaus explains his lack of sexual interest to being tired and on antidepressants, being sexually abused as a young boy, not trusting anyone including Klara, feeling not wanted, not belonging, being pushed out, and feeling abandoned. He is remorseful for his transgressionism, feels as if he does not measure up, and that he has messed up his life. He finds sex to be gross although he had two affairs. Klara did not believe his explanation for his lack of interest in having sexual intimacy with her. Klara is troubled by the fact that he was able to have sex with the two women, but he cannot have sexual intimacy with her. She finds that he is not sexually attracted to her; she often feels like a second class citizen in their relationship. Klara craves that their sexual intimacy will come back. For her to have sexual intimacy is an ultimate expression of being desired. Klara's craving for sexual intimacy represents an unmet growth need.

In summary, the relational, self, and physical intimacy needs play out together and impact each other. The manner in which caregivers acknowledge and affirm them and how they are realized and integrated affects all aspects of the personality. When these needs go unmet, problems are apt to occur. However, it is important to remember that unmet needs do not inevitably lead to the problems described above. One cannot make predictions about the outcome when needs go unmet, one can only trace a problem back to its roots. Even at that, one requires strong clinical evidence to support a hypothetical connection between the problem and unmet needs.

### *Internal Representations and their Linking Affects*

In the process of psychologically separating from his parents and moving on to individuation, the child/infant develops impressions and ideas about them and about himself. The impressions that a child develops of himself are based on how he perceives that he is percieved by his parents and significant others. These impressions, feelings, sensations, and ideas are referred to as internal representations of the other and of the self (Klein, 1946, 1959).

In addition to the formation of representations of others and self, the child and the parent develop feelings for each other. Masterson (1976) spoke about these mutual feelings in terms of affects that link the internalized representations of the other and the self. Another aspect of the relationship is how the child felt being in the presence of or living with the parents and other members of the family.

An individual's representations of his parents and of himself and the feelings that members of the family have for each other provides very useful information regarding the home environment in which he was raised. These perceptions and experiences greatly shaped the individual's formation of his psychic and self-organizations. SIRP pays particular attention to an individual's subjective experiences and inner world and how they impact his behaviors and his relationships.

#### *Internal representation of self and other*

In his early experiences with others, the child forms cognitive-affective representations of other and self. The representation of the other (e.g., caregiver) is a consequence of how he experiences them responding to his feelings, needs, and behaviors. An infant/child's first representations of self are through the eyes of the caregivers, that is, he sees himself as they see him. The representations can bear a positive, negative, or a mixed positive/negative valence and continue to persist into adolescence and adulthood and impact the quality and nature of future relationships.

The representations that an infant/child formed of himself and of the parents, provides information about the home climate and the quality of parenting. It also provides information that is helpful to understand how client's subjective experiences influenced the development of his psychic organization, self-structure, and coping strategies to secure his self and relational needs.

A client's internal representations of his childhood's caregivers can also give a clue as to which needs were met or unmet. For example, if an individual, as a child, experienced his mother as cold and rejecting, this might give a clue as to the client's need to emotionally bond and feel significant. If on the other hand, the client, as a child, experienced his father as being critical and demeaning, this might give a clue as to the client's need to be validated for being a competent person. Therefore, both a client's representations of others and self, can provide clues as to his unmet needs. In the same vein, a client's perception of self as seen through the eyes of a childhood caregiver can give a clue which needs were met or unmet. In terms of psychotherapy, one assesses whether the internal representations need to be transformed before one can expect behavioral and relationship changes.

### INTERNAL REPRESENTATIONS OF OTHER

This refers to the cognitive-affective image that a person has of the other which might be that they are seen as being strong, weak, domineering, cruel, compassionate, and responsible. The internal representation is a cognitive-affective image, not a feeling, that one has of the other. The representation of a person may correspond to how the person is in real life or it may deviate from it in some dramatic fashion.

*Examples:*

1 My father was self-centered, controlling; it was always about him. (Negative internal representation of other).
2 My mother was caring, did crafts with us, took us to the park, she was fair with us (positive internal representation of other).

### INTERNAL REPRESENTATIONS OF SELF

The internal representation of self is a cognitive-affective image of self formed from the infant/child's interactions with significant caregivers. The mental representation is influenced by the quality and nature of the caregiver's responses to the infant/child's needs, feelings, and behaviors. If the responses are positive the infant/child thinks of himself as a good person and as having caused the caregiver's positive responses. His self-representations might include seeing one as lovable, competent, and intelligent. The reverse happens when the caregiver's responses are negative, then he sees himself in negative images. Self representations are also formed from the comments and feedback from others. The mental representation that an individual has of himself is an image or picture and not a feeling about himself.

*Examples:*

1 With my father, I was never good enough, was not smart enough, I was the dumb and the clumsy one in the family (negative internal representation of self).
2 My mom helped me to realize that I was good at drawing, painting, doing crafts (positive internal representation of self).

### *Affect linking internalized other and self representations*

Masterson (1976) pointed out the importance to consider the mutual feelings that the parent and child have for each other. He described this relationship in terms of the affect that links the internalized representations of the other and the self. This affective linkage refers to the feelings that an infant/child had for a parent and the feeling that the parent had for the infant/child. This is seen through the eyes of the child and reflects his reality but not necessarily objective reality. This information regarding the affective linkages is useful as it may help to understand an individual's emotional responses to figures in position of authority. However, it is important to differentiate old (familiar) feelings related to past experiences from new feelings that are associated with current and real experiences with others.

#### AFFECT LINKING INTERNALIZED REPRESENTATION OF OTHER TO SELF

This refers to the client's perceived feeling that the parents had toward him when he was an infant or child. The feeling is from the perspective of the client which might or might not correspond to the way things were in reality. For example, the client might have felt that his parents felt frustrated, sad, and angry toward him but they might not have felt that way.

*Examples:*

1 My dad was constantly criticizing me, was impatient with me. He did not like me because I was not as smart as my older brother (father has negative feelings toward child).

2 My mother was affectionate, loving, caring. She would at times become angry with us, but we always knew that she loved us (mother has positive feelings toward her child).

### AFFECT LINKING INTERNALIZED REPRESENTATION OF SELF TO OTHER

This refers to the feelings that the client, as an infant or child, had toward a parent and might still have today but may not be aware of the feeling. For example, the client might have been angry toward his parents or frustrated with them. Or he might have been happy, content, joyful, and cheerful when with them. The client might experience the same feelings toward his parents today. Again, this is based on the perception of the client.

*Examples:*

1 My father's criticisms hurt me so much that I hated him and I am angry at him and I have no feelings for him (child's negative feelings toward his/her father).
2 I love my mother; she has always tried to be helpful and to make things pleasant for the family and for me (child's positive feelings toward his/her mother).

### THE FEELING WHEN IN THE PRESENCE OF OR LIVING WITH THE OTHER

This dimension describes how the person, as a child and teenager, felt when in the presence of or living with his parents and with the other members of the family. He might have felt safe, secure, and protected or he might have felt anxious, fearful, and resentful. The person, as an infant and child, might have felt lovable, significant, important, competent, nurturing and proud or tense, afraid, unaccepted, a nuisance, stupid, humiliated, and shamed. The person might have found it to be fun and exciting in living with the family members. These early experiences in being with significant others may continue to influence how the person feels in being with others and how others accept him socially.

*Examples:*

1 When I was with my father I felt very tense and anxious because I didn't know what he was going to criticize me about next. I walked on egg shells when around him (negative feeling in presence of father).
2 I felt safe and secure and protected when I was with my mother; she felt proud of me and I also felt proud of myself (positive feeling in presence of mother).

### *Psychic Organization*

The growing child's experiences with significant others and the representations that were formed gradually become organized and take on the quality of a structure. This structure together with the innate biological strivings and the innate adaptive capacities form what has come to be called the psychic organization. The psychic organization is dynamic and impacts all aspects of life and more often than not it operates outside of awareness. Psychodynamic-oriented theorists refer to this tripartite organization by terms such as psychic structure (Freud, 1923) and as ego states (Berne, 1961, 1964; Fairbairn, 1944).

According to Freud (1923), the psychic structure comprises three parts: the innate energy system (i.e., the id which embraces the instincts), the acquired social heritage (i.e., superego) which comprise acceptable behaviors and values by which to live and the adaptive and creative capacity to think, plan, and act (i.e., ego). The ego sees to it that the needs of the id and the demands and expectations of the superego and of reality work together for the benefit of the person. It is the encounter between an infant/child's innate needs and the societal demands and expectations that leads to their encoding and to the development of internal structures (i.e., superego) that are an amalgam of an infant/child's core needs, the expectation significant others, and the demands of reality.

SIRP has modified Freud's (1923) tripartite organization of the psychic structure in the following ways. With regards to the two instincts of the id, the *life instinct* has been replaced by the relational need for emotional bonding and by the physical intimacy needs for sensual contact and sexual intimacy and the *death instinct*, that is aggression, has been replaced by the need for autonomy. SIRP does not consider aggression to be innate but as an emotional reaction to interference in the pursuit of one's innate needs. However, the striving for autonomy is considered to be an innate need; it is an innate need to move away from the emotional bond, to psychologically separate, become autonomous and to individuate and to become one's own person. These needs are considered to be the prime motivators of much of human behavior and interactions. This modification of the two instincts is consistent with Freud's (1938) reformulation of the instincts where he wrote "The aim of the first of these basic instincts [Eros] is to establish ever greater unities and to preserve them thus - in short, to together; the aim of the second is, on the contrary, to undo connections (and so to destroy things)" (p. 148).

The SIRP approach embraces Freud's (1923) concept of the ego which is innate and potentially present at birth and is described as a "coherent organization of mental processes" (p. 17). The ego's innate characteristics are the capacity for perception, memory, and motility. The ego is an active agent and its functions, briefly, include thinking, planning, and action. The functions of the ego can be thought of in terms of adaptive functions and defensive functions. An adaptive ego is flexible, resourceful, and resilient and is capable to manage the challenges of daily living and the life problems that it faces in a creative, realistic, and rewarding manner. The ego in its defensive mode responds to intrapsychic conflicts and attempts to mediate between the needs of the id, the prohibitions of the superego, and the demands of reality. In its defensive mode, it protects the person from dangers and threats to one's psychological well-being.

SIRP adopts Freud's concepts of superego which comprises all of that which is socially inherited in terms of acceptable behaviors and conduct and in terms of values and ideals to live by. These behaviors and values become part of a person's life through the processes of identifications with significant others which begin at an early age and before the resolution of the Oedipus complex (Jacobson, 1964). Freud (1923) used the term "conscience" when referring to the socially acceptable and unacceptable behaviors and the term "ego ideal" to refer to the values and ideals to live by. The conscience is the part of the person that prohibits the behaviors that are unacceptable and upholds those that are desirable and acceptable. The ego ideal is the part of the person that has internalized, through identifications with loving persons, the values and ideals that rise above behaviors and are worth living for such as cleanliness, punctuality, and kindness. The superego can be considered as being moderate, severe, or harsh in its function (Jacobson, 1964). A moderate superego is able to integrate the prohibitions without compromising his innate needs and preferences. A severe superego is demanding of self and of others, tends to be perfectionist, feels obligated (rather than responsible), and has a need to be in control. A harsh superego is punitive, guilt ridden, and may self-harm and entertain suicidal thoughts.

### *Self-Organization and Sense of Self*

In the early days, weeks, and months of its life, the infant develops an emotional and physical bond with its mother. This bond is the foundation for the development of the self. The sense of self is believed to begin as a bodily sense of self (Allport, 1967) that emerges through the way the infant is physically handled (Mahler et al., 1975; Winnicott, 1965). The child's sense of self is further developed through the interactions and identifications with the primary caregivers and their feedback. These experiences are internalized as representations of self.

The idea of self has been the topic of many authors. Some have offered a definition of the self (Gergen, 1971; Masterson, 1985; Mead, 1977; Rogers, 1966; Symonds, 1951). Others focused on the emergence of the self (Stern, 1985). Postmodernists, on the other hand, believe that there is nothing of "essence" regarding the self and that the self is socially constructed (Butler, 2002; Detmer, 2003). Lichtenstein (1961), however, attests to the existence of the self by showing how individuals have the capacity to "remain the same in the midst of change" and how they are "conscious of such continuity of sameness" (p. 193).

Kohut (1977), the founder of self-psychology, was particularly interested in the components of the self and how the sense of self developed. He observed that an infant/child develops a sense of self from his interactions with caregivers as he goes through the process of psychological separating from them and moving toward individuation. Human infants, generally, are born with a self already in place, that is, a biologically determined psychological entity (Brinich & Shelley, 2002). Kohut (1977) states that the baby's self is a "virtual self" (p. 101). This potential for a self, interacts with caregiver's sense of what is self and from this interaction emerges the infant/child's organization of a cohesive self which is cognitive and affective in nature and is stored as an internal representation of self (Kohut, 1971). At the beginning of an infant's life, the ego is dominant but with the development of a self, the "living self" becomes the "organizing center of the ego's activities" (Kohut, 1971, p. 120).

In his study of narcissistically wounded clients, Kohut (1977) observed that the self structurally comprised three components which he named Nuclear Ambitions, Nuclear Ideals, and Nuclear Talents. Nuclear Ambitions comprise the grandiose and exhibitionistic self-images that are the result of interchanges with caregivers who confirm the child's innate vigor, greatness, and expanding states of mind. Nuclear Ideals are made up of idealized images of self and world and develop from the child's involvement with powerful others to whom the "child can look up and with whom he can merge as an image of calmness, infallibility, and omnipotence" (Kohut & Wolfe, 1978, p. 414). Nuclear talents and skills connect nuclear ambitions and nuclear ideals and enable the ambitions to turn into achieved goals (Baker & Baker, 1987). SIRP interprets nuclear ambitions as referring to the experience of competency and ability to pursue goals, nuclear ideals to the experience of being significant and lovable, and nuclear talents as referring to the capacity to moderate the needs for competency and self-esteem and to keep them in balance.

SIRP has incorporated Kohut's (1971) components of the self, that is, the need for competency and the need for significance. With regards to SIRP's taxonomy of core needs, the self needs for competency and significance are included under the construct of the self. The core self needs are not considered to be of the same order as the relational and physical intimacy needs which are more inherently relational and psychophysiological in nature. The impact on a relationship when the need for competency and significance are not validated is illustrated in the following case.

*Illustration* Stella and Radu, married for about 15 years, complained that they were drifting apart and that there was no intimacy between them. Radu was brought up in a family of four boys and being the youngest, he constantly felt inadequate, socially awkward, and incompetent. These experiences were reinforced by the constant criticisms from his parents and brothers. Stella was the youngest of five girls. She felt that she had no place in the family; she felt that what she wanted and what she said did not matter; she had no voice and felt unloved. Although the first years of their marriage were relatively harmonious, the next 10 years have been conflicted and highly troubled. Both felt unsupported by their partner. Radu had an enormous need to be affirmed and admired for his professional successes and achievements and Stella had an intense need to be a significant and meaningful partner. Stella felt that it was all about Radu and his needs and that her own needs were not responded to. Both Radu and Stella struggled with their unmet childhood self needs, the former with the experience of being incompetent and the latter with the experience of being insignificant and unlovable. Neither partner was ready to provide what the other needed to feel a complete and wholesome person.

### *Defense Mechanisms and Coping Strategies*

The infant/child inevitably meets frustrations, setbacks, and disappointments as no parents are able to consistently be attuned to the infant/child's feelings and needs. It is also possible that the infant/child may experience hurts and emotional injuries due to emotional neglect, abuse, and/or trauma. The infant/child develops coping strategies to deal with the realities of frustrations, disappointments, setbacks, hurts, and emotional injuries. The earliest of these strategies (e.g., dissociation), referred to as primary defense mechanisms, operate at an unconscious and instinctual level whereas the later coping strategies (e.g., displacement), referred to as secondary defense mechanisms, are more learned and cognitive in nature and, in a sense, less unconscious (Kaplan & Sadock, 1991; Sadock et al., 2014; White & Watt, 1981). Each individual develops a unique system of coping and protective strategies, which act as a coat of armor, based on the nature of issues dealt with and the age at which these were developed. With respect to the SIRP approach, the significant defense mechanisms include splitting, idealization, projection, introjection, and regression with splitting being the most significant.

Splitting is a developmental and defensive process of keeping incompatible feelings apart and separate. It refers to dividing external objects into "all good" and "all bad" accompanied by the "abrupt shifting of an object from one extreme category to the other" with possible "sudden and complete reversal of feelings and conceptualization about a person" (Kaplan & Sadock, 1991, p. 183). Splitting is a normal process for a young child as he does not have the capacity to reconcile and synthesize a caregiver's opposite behaviors (e.g., pleasurable, unpleasurable), a capacity that is acquired by the age of two to three (Mahler et al., 1975). Failure to synthesize opposites can lead to emotional problems.

Idealization and devaluation are characteristic of splitting, whether it be by an infant/child, teenager, or adult. Idealization refers to seeing external objects as "all good" and "endowing them with great power," whereas devaluation refers to seeing a person as "all bad" (Kaplan & Sadock, 1991, p. 183). Most often the "all good" object is seen as omnipotent, or ideal, while the "all bad" object is seen as completely flawed and worthless and is devalued.

Projection refers to "perceiving and reacting to unacceptable inner impulses and their derivatives as though they were outside the self" (Kaplan & Sadock, 1991, p. 183). That is, it is an unconscious tendency to attribute one's own unacceptable feelings, thoughts, and impulses to other persons or objects in the external world.

Introjection has both developmental and defensive functions. Developmentally, introjection is the process of incorporating the characteristics of a person (e.g., a favorite aunt) unconsciously into one's own psyche with the "goal of establishing closeness to and constant presence of the object" (Kaplan & Sadock, 1991, p. 183). Defensively, introjection can serve the purpose of coping with the anxiety with regards to a lost object or a feared object and in coping with a sense of guilt. For example, with regards to a lost object, an individual deals with the grief by internalizing the characteristics of the lost object thereby nullifying or negating the loss (Kaplan & Sadock, 1991, p. 183).

Regression refers to returning to a previous stage of development or functioning to avoid the anxieties or hostilities involved in later stages (Kaplan & Sadock, 1991, p. 183). That is, it refers to behavior where the individual reverts to a behavior more appropriate to an earlier stage of development or to reaction patterns long since outgrown.

*Illustration* Belinda, single, in her late 20s, experienced childhood physical, emotional, and sexual abuse by her caregivers and by her stepfather's male friends. In her early teens she was placed in an institution because of her acting out, raging, and destructive behaviors. In her late teens she became addicted to drugs and alcohol and took up burlesque dancing. To cope with the stressors of her life and her emotional states, Belinda developed an armor of protective strategies that included dissociation, splitting, projection, idealization, and regression. Belinda often tried to reconcile with her parents. On one Christmas Day, Belinda visited her parents. She attempted to suppress the negative experiences that she had toward her parents and to see them (*idealize*) as caring and kind (*projection*). After greeting her mother, who ignored her and walked away, Belinda became enraged (e.g., *split*) and assaulted her mother who charged Belinda for assault with bodily harm. During the court proceedings, as she listened to the psychologist explain the impact of abuse on personality formation and the phenomenon of uncontrollable rage, Belinda became distraught, left the room, *dissociated,* dropped to the floor and then *regressed* to an infantile state uttering "Papa, get off from me." At first she allowed no one to approach her. When she became sufficiently grounded with the help of the psychologist, she was helped to safely find her way home. This case illustrates the unique pattern of coping and protective strategies that Belinda developed as a child and which continued into adolescence and adulthood.

### *Quality of the Emotional Bond*

This construct refers to the quality of an infant/child's emotional bond and investment of energy in the caregiver on whom the infant/child would normally depend for safety, security, nurturance, stability, and comfort (Mahler et al., 1975). It refers to the degree to which an infant/child feels emotionally and physically bonded and anchored. The quality of an infant/child's emotional bonding reflects the extent to which the caregiver spontaneously responded to the infant/child's feelings and needs.

The two essential components of an emotional bond are that the person's needs are satisfied ("confident expectation") and that the person feels comfortable, safe and secure in being with the other ("safe anchorage") (Mahler & Furer, 1968). Thus the degree of satisfaction of needs and the nature of the feelings define the quality of an emotional bond. The failure to develop a secure emotional bond could be experienced as a longing, emptiness, and a nagging loneliness and take on a compulsive quality and become insatiable (Erskine, 1998).

The quality of the emotional bond can be considered according to four categories: emotionally connected, striving for emotional connection, avoiding emotional connection, and emotionally disconnected. To be emotionally connected means that the infant/child (later an adolescent, adult) has developed a satisfying, secure, and comfortable connection with the significant other. The other types of emotional bonding are explained and illustrated.

#### *Seeking emotional connection*

To seek emotional connection refers to eagerly search for a meaningful, satisfying, and comfortable emotional relationship with a significant other. This form of connection might manifest itself in the fear of abandonment, emotional enmeshment, and emotional entanglement with the expression of negative emotions.

*Illustration* Emotional connection seeking behavior is manifested by an individual pursuing a significant other. In the case of a child, he follows the mother from place to place with the hope of emotionally and physically connecting. Mahler et al. (1975) refer to this as shadowing behavior. Something similar can happen with adults. For example, Pedro and Priscilla, married for 15 years, had a conflicted relationship with the former feeling very insecure and the latter being dominant and controlling. Following an argument and feeling rejected by his wife, Pedro typically followed his wife from room to room in their house with the wish to talk to her and to be reassured about her love for him and that she would not leave him. The more he pursued her, the more she avoided him and the more she avoided him the more he pursued her.

### *Avoiding emotional connection*

Avoiding emotional connection refers to keeping emotionally distant from significant others. This might happen when the significant other is imposing, overbearing and demanding and does not allow the individual space to be himself, or when being emotionally close is too painful and the individual avoids getting emotionally close to another.

*Illustration* Rory and Sileas, married for about 10 years, sought therapy because Rory was very frustrated with the lack of sexual and emotional intimacy in their relationship. Sileas was brought up in a home where she could not rely on her parents to respond to her feelings and needs and she prematurely became independent and autonomous and took care of herself. She trusted that no one would be there for her. Rory was brought up in a home where he was belittled, demeaned, and called names such as being stupid and an idiot. Rory's unmet childhood need was to be affirmed and validated for being competent. He constantly sought validation from Sileas for his accomplishments and successes. In the process Sileas felt that her own needs and feelings were being dismissed. She became resentful and refused to respond to Rory's need for validation as she felt used. Given their current situation, Sileas avoided any form of emotional and physical connection for fear of being emotionally hurt.

### *Emotionally disconnected*

To be emotionally disconnected refers to having limited feelings of affection and empathy for the other and to being emotionally cut off from the other. Or, the person may be connected to the other in different ways such as in travelling, partaking in sports and dining out but not emotionally. This may occur when the infant/child, after many attempts to emotionally connect, experiences continued rejections and hostilities which bring about feelings of hurt and emotional disconnection.

*Illustration* Jenö and Lányka were married for about 15 years and enjoyed each other's company but were emotionally disconnected. Lányka described their relationship in terms of boxes arranged similar to a wheel with a hub and a rim. The boxes on the rim included the love of travelling, playing sports, fine dining, intellectual discussions, and going to movies and the box in the middle represented emotional connection. Lányka stated that they were connected on each of the outer boxes, but they were disconnected at the level of emotions. Both were brought up in oppressive homes where there was little if any emotional expressions. Both sets of parents were cold toward each other. Although both Jenö and Lányka wanted emotional connection, both feared this for different reasons. They did not know how to be emotionally close to each other.

### Characteristic Emotional State

A characteristic emotional state is one that is familiar, was first intensely experienced in the past (e.g., childhood) and is carried into the present. A characteristic emotional state is typically brought about by a persistent dissatisfaction in not having a core relational, self, and physical intimacy need met in childhood. The telling sign of a characteristic emotional state is that it is familiar and its expression is disproportionate to a given event or response from another. The emotional state, when carried into adulthood might, manifests itself as a constant underlying emotion (e.g., anger, depression, anxiety), which can become intense when triggered by experiences resembling those of childhood.

An individual's characteristic emotional state provides information regarding his unmet childhood needs. Emotions indicate the satisfaction or the unfulfillment of core needs. In exploring and processing the characteristic emotion one can uncover the early unmet childhood needs which are still pushing for response in adulthood but are being frustrated.

*Illustration* Aileen, single, in her mid-30s, presented for therapy because of her life-long intense fear to assert herself in her relationships. She was brought up in a home with domineering and critical parents who did not validate and affirm her feelings, thoughts, and needs, but rather, they were dismissed as not being important. The consequence was that Aileen was out of touch with her needs and did not know how to express them. Moreover, she feared to express them lest she be treated by her boyfriend in the same way that she was treated by her parents. Aileen's characteristic emotion was fear, that is, fear to assert her needs.

### Object Constancy

One of the significant achievements of the growing child is the development of object constancy. Object constancy can be defined as the ability to remain libidinally (i.e., love and pleasure) connected to a loved person whether the person is present or absent. A child's development of object constancy is a significant moment as it represents the formation of an internal "psychological place" to which he can turn to gain a perspective in troubled times, to comfort himself and to psychologically lift himself up. In developing object constancy, the individual feels anchored within himself and is not at the mercy of the negative reactions from others. Mahler and associates (1975) describe object constancy as a mental representation of a positive libidinally connected person to whom an individual can consistently and reliably turn internally for safety, security, protection, nurturance, love, and self-soothing.

The development of object constancy begins in infancy/childhood and is associated with consistent and reliable positive behavior on part of the caregiver to whom the child is emotionally connected and turns for comfort and protection. Object constancy conjures up pleasant feelings, sensations, and memories of the significant person; it conjures up the feeling of "safe anchorage" and "confident expectations" that its needs will be responded to (Mahler & Furer, 1968). It also gives the sense of being known and being wanted. Object constancy is a feeling of where I am there you are.

A significant aspect in developing object constancy is that the infant/child gradually internalizes the characteristics of the parents, that is, their functions, ideals, and behaviors, to comfort self and others. Object constancy permits the infant/child to function separately in familiar surroundings despite moderate degrees of tension and discomfort and acts as an agent to self comfort (Edward et al., 1981). This implies maintaining the positive mental representation regardless of the presence or absence of the love object and despite internal stress or need. Having an internalized positive object is essential to good emotional health as it provides a resource to which an individual can turn for comfort, regulate emotions, and gain perspective on situations. An individual who lacks object constancy, feels adrift, disconnected from self and others, and struggles to regulate his emotions as he has nowhere to turn to gain perspective on life's problems.

*Examples:*

1 When my boyfriend goes out with the guys to watch the Superbowl and if he does not come home before midnight, I feel lonely, get enraged, want to end the relationship; and I hope that he does not come home on time so that I can rightfully be angry at him (object constancy mostly absent).
2 Even though I cannot see her as often as I would like to because she is busy with school work and family, I know that she cares for me and loves me and that is reassuring and comforting (object constancy fully present).

### *Social Self*

An infant/child in his interactions with his caregivers and significant others learns how to be socially with others; he develops a social self. He might organize his life according to his values, interests, ambitions, and dreams that are congruent with his sense of self and self-identity, or he might organize his life around the expectations, values, wishes, and demands of others. The former is referred to as living from the *true self* and the latter is referred to as living from the *false self* (Winnicott, 1960, pp. 145–146). The false self begins to emerge during childhood as compliance due to an inability to live from the true self because of the lack of inner resources to balance the demands from significant others and his own relational, self, and physical intimacy needs. The purpose of the false self is to protect the true self from the criticisms and judgments of others and from one's own unacceptable needs and demands.

The false self can readily be recognized in an individual who compromises the true self to maintain relationships for fear that if he asserts himself he might be rejected. It can also be recognized in an individual who has very little sense of who he is, what he wants to do in life, and is without ambitions and goals. Enmeshed relationships and being extremely pleasant are other signs of living from a false self.

*Illustration* Anselm, middle-age, married, but childless, sought professional help because of a major depression (Meier et al., 2006, p. 116). It was his fourth episode with depression during the past 15 years. His father, a college professor, was emotionally absent from the family. His mother, anxious, insecure, and demanding, rewarded him for compliance to her wishes but withdrew her affection and love and became critical of him when he asserted his autonomy and independence. Anselm felt angry, worthless, and guilty when he asserted his autonomy and he felt intruded upon and violated when he complied. To maintain the love and affection of his parents, and later of his wife and supervisors at work, Anselm shaped his life according to their wishes and expectations and suppressed his own. He lived not according to his true self but according to his false self. Anselm's depression lifted when he became more authentic and genuine and developed the courage and competency to live from his true self and to re-orient his life according to his core relational and self needs and became master of his life.

### Communication Pattern

In his interactions with caregivers and significant others, a child learns from them, how to communicate with them, how to express and assert his thoughts, feelings, needs, and preferences and how to manage disagreements and conflicts. He learns how to verbally and non-verbally "convey information, make meaning with one another, and respond – internally and externally" (Satir et al., 1991, p. 31). This includes the "words, tone, and quality of expression" (Luthman, 1974, p. 59).

The child develops a pattern of communication that is influenced by the person communicated with. When communication with others is very difficult and troublesome, the child might learn indirect and dysfunctional ways of communicating. Satir (1972) and Satir and associates (1991) point to four dysfunctional stances that a person may take in his communication with others. These include placating (i.e., disregarding his own feelings and worth and hands it over to someone else) and blaming (i.e., finds faults in others, is the boss), being super reasonable (e.g., focus on facts, not feelings; logical) and irrelevant (e.g., distracts from real issue).

Communication can also be carried on as an internal dialogue, that is, as "self-talk (Meichenbaum, 1977). The internal dialogue often takes place between what the person would like to do (i.e., id), what he thinks he is expected to do (i.e., superego), and what is the best action to take (i.e., ego). Each of these constituents has its own unique voice. The id represents the voice of the inner child (e.g., is needy, angry), the superego is the voice of the parent (e.g., demanding, authoritative), and the ego represents the voice of reason and adaptive capacities.

The pattern of internal communication can be externalized in his communication with real people. In his communication with others, he could take the stance of the critical and demanding parent or he could take the stance of the oppositional and/or the needy and whining inner child. An individual's pattern of communication can reveal many aspects of his personality including his psychic organization, unmet needs, and coping strategies.

The following is an example how a couples' unresolved internal dialogues manifested themselves in their communication. Stefan and Carina, in their mid-30s, married, sought psychotherapy because of communication problems. Stefan was brought up in a chaotic family with a domineering father who constantly demeaned and criticized his children. In order to avoid the wrath of his hypercritical father, Stefan identified with his father's criticism of his siblings. In the process, Stefan became an internal critical parent who demeaned the needs and feelings of his own inner child (e.g., id). He could not tolerate his neediness nor the needs of others. On the other hand, Carina was brought up in a large family where communication among family members was congenial. Stefan and Carina's communication problem was due to Stefan externalizing his own internal dialogue on to Carina by constantly making demands on her and finding something about her which to criticize such as her indulgent parent style, not being punctual and not following his rules. Carina, on her part, opposed Stefan's demands and criticisms. She often found him to be attacking and she defending.

### *Relational Patterns*

An infant/child is born with the innate capacities to form meaningful, satisfying, and enduring interpersonal relationships. The core relational, self, and physical intimacy needs propel the person to develop meaningful relations and the child's expression of these needs together with the responses from others shapes the quality and nature of these relationships.

In a "good enough" (Winnicott, 1965) home environment, the infant/child and adolescent acquire the attitude and skills to form meaningful intimate relationships. They learn to problem solve, to negotiate, compromise, reconcile conflict, forgive, repair broken relationships and to be empathic toward others. When the infant/child is exposed to an environment that is not good enough, he might acquire relational skills and patterns that are helpful at that age, but become problematic in adolescence and adulthood. That is, they might acquire repetitive, compulsive, and ineffective relational patterns that are driven by unmet core needs which unrelentlessly push for a positive response from others. The individuals have as their purpose to establish and maintain relationships and to control (e.g., orchestrate) the nature of these relationships. The manner in which the individuals perceive themselves (e.g., helpless, unlovable) and how they perceive others (e.g., powerful, lovable) influences the nature and quality of the relationship.

These repetitive and compulsive interpersonal patterns have been called "maladaptive cyclical patterns" (Strupp & Binder, 1985) and "projective identifications" (Cashdan, 1988; Klein, 1959).

The common forms of projective identification are (a) dependency – the need to be taken care of, feeling helpless and dependent on the other; (b) power – portraying oneself as being more competent than his partner and wanting to be in charge; (c) ingratiation – laying on guilt trips to get the needed response from the other; and (d) sexuality – using one's sexuality (e.g., flirting, dress) to create sexual arousal in the other so as to get his/her attention (Cashdan, 1988). Projective identifications are driven by unmet childhood needs. In projective identifications, an individual takes a specific stance (e.g., sense of helplessness) which draws forth from his/her partner a specific responses (e.g., a caretaking response). Individuals enter into a relationship with the hope that the partner will respond to their unmet childhood needs.

Although these are initially responded to, nevertheless, as the relationship shifts from the honeymoon stage to the real love stage (Hendrix, 2008), one or both partners may no longer want to respond to their partner's unmet childhood needs either because they are frustrated that their own unmet childhood needs are not being responded to or because they have outgrown the relationship.

*Illustration* Remi and Simone, middle age couple, were married for three years; it was Simone's second marriage and Remi's third. Simone was brought up in an uncaring home where she learned to fend for herself although she constantly craved the love and affection from her parents. Remi, the youngest of three boys, was brought up in a home where he was often criticized by his brothers and parents for being poor in school work and athletics and socially shy and awkward. He craved affirmation for being as talented as his brothers. Simone and Remi, in the first year of marriage, responded positively to each other's unmet childhood needs. Remi craved affirmation for his competencies as a lawyer and legal successes. Simone wanted Remi to treasure her and take care of her as she was tired of taking care of others. After one year of marriage, both began to experience that their partner no longer was willing to respond to his/her relational and self needs. This led to arguments, tension between the two of them, and threats to separate. In the course of therapy, both became aware of their own and of their partner's unmet childhood needs and their projective identifications. Simone's projective identification was that of power (e.g., to take charge of her relationships) as she could not trust that others had her best interest at heart and Remi's projective identification was that of dependency (e.g., to be affirmed for being competent).

### *Developmental Processes and Phases*

A significant aspect of SIRP is viewing the origin of emotional problems and their treatment within the context of human development and its phases. Although interested in all of the developmental phase that span the life cycle (Erikson, 1950, 1968), SIRP is particularly interested in the early phases of development, referred to as the pre-oedipal phases, since an individual's personality begins to be formed in these earlier phases. Failure to negotiate the tasks of the pre-oedipal phases can lead to serious emotional problems in childhood, adolescence, and adulthood. SIRP has incorporated the phases that Mahler and associates (1968, 1975) identified based on their research and clinical observations. The phases that have significant relevance for SIRP are symbiosis, differentiation, practicing, and rapprochement. The developmental tasks for these phases are presented in Figure 3.2.

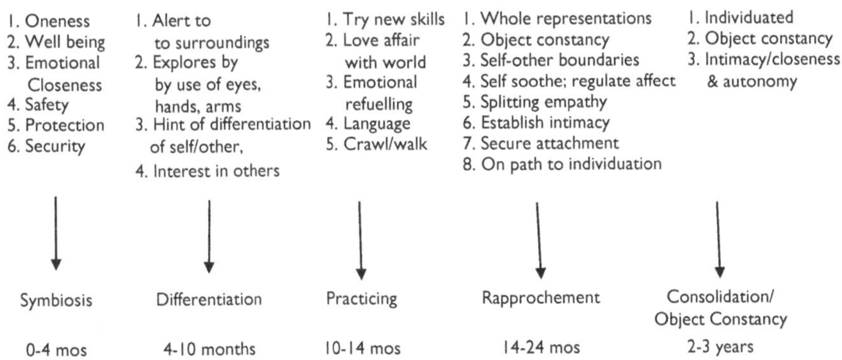


*Figure 3.2* Separation-individuation process: developmental tasks.

### *Symbiotic phase*

Symbiosis represents a state of intermittent fusion with the mother, a state of undifferentiation in which the "I" is not yet differentiated from the "not I" and the inside and outsides are only gradually coming to be sensed as different (Mahler et al., 1975, p. 8). This is not to say that the infant is fused with the mother at all hours. Rather, the mother and infant are separate entities from the beginning (Bergman, 1975) and there are moments in the infant's day when merger or fusion is close to the reality of the infant's experience (Pine, 1975). An example is when the infant, crying ravenously, begins suckling at the breast, achieves satisfaction and melts drowsily "into the mother's body" (Pine, 1975, p. ix) – this represents fusion. Thus the infant's merger with mother represents, more accurately, "moments of merger" (Bergman, 1975, p. xvi).

The major tasks of this phase are the achievement of "safe-anchorage" with the caregiver, the development of "confident expectation" that its needs will be met, the formation of an inner core and bodily self, and formation of representations of other and self (Mahler & Furer, 1968, p. 17). The infant's inner body experiences contribute to the development of the body ego and body self and form the very core of the self. These experiences are the crystallization point around which a sense of identity will become established (p. 11). The failure to adequately achieve the capacity to merge and to develop a bodily self, can lead to problems such as a lifelong yearning for emotional connection, a disconnection from self and other, and inability to invest energy externally and find his path in life.

The effects of failed "safe-anchorage" is illustrated by Ektor, in his late 20s, whose parents divorced when he was two years of age. His mother grieved the loss of the relationship with her husband, was constantly depressed, and emotionally not available to her son. As a young child, preteen and teenager, Ektor spent most of his time alone in solitary activities. His one pleasure was to go into the woods with his dog. Ektor left his country in search for the love that he did not have as an infant and child and to find his place in life. He was in a series of short-term relationships but all of them left him emotionally empty as he could not allow himself to become emotionally intimate and bonded. At the core of his being he felt empty, disconnected from himself and from others. He continued to search for a soul mate with whom he could become fused so as to repair the early childhood deprivation.

### *Differentiation and body image subphase*

Differentiation refers to the process of emerging from the "symbiotic state of oneness with the mother, in the intrapsychic sense" (Mahler et al., 1975, p. 290). It is outward and goal directed (p. 54). One of the main characteristics of this subphase is the formation of identity. This refers to the earliest awareness of a sense of being; it is a feeling that includes in part the investment of the body with libidinal energy. Identity is not "a sense of who I am" but a sense "that I am" (p. 8).

A major task of this subphase is for the child to psychologically separate from the love object (i.e., the caregiver) and to develop a sense of identity. To help the child differentiate in a timely fashion, it is important that the caregiver be emotionally available and to support and to validate the child's efforts to move toward psychological separation and to be available when the child returns for emotional closeness. It is also important not to prematurely burden the child with adult responsibilities and problems and to place the child in the position of being a caregiver to the parent or to take on responsibility for his own life and thereby become self-sufficient and independent. The caregiver provides a balancing act between nurturing the child when needed and nudging the child when ready.

The most serious developmental dangers occur at this phase when the child fails to differentiate or differentiates prematurely. The former may lead to psychoses and the latter is apt to lead to borderline and narcissistic disorders (Mahler et al., 1975). Some of the dangers or disturbances that might occur in this subphase are the following: (a) delayed differentiation which refers to the failure to intrapsychically separate from the symbiotic object and to establish the "I" and the "not I" (p. 58); (b) premature differentiation which means that the infant moved out of the "safe anchorage" before it was ready (pp. 59–60); (c) premature ego development that implies that the infant took over functions from his mother or started to do so (Mahler & Furer, 1968, p. 16); (d) development of a false self which refers to the "as if" personality (p. 16); and (e) narcissistic compensation that refers to the infant or toddler taking over a function that is not being provided by the mother (Edward et al., 1981, p. 219).

An example of a person who did not successfully complete the differentiation subphase is illustrated in Angelina's continued enmeshed relationship with her mother. Angelina had not spoken to her mother in three years. She is married, has two young children and wanted to repair her relationship with her mother so that her children could have a relationship with their grandmother. Angelina described her mother as being intrusive and imposing her demands and not respecting those of Angelina. Beginning in Angelina's early teenage years, the mother shared with Angelina her relational difficulties with her husband. Without being conscious of it, Angelina became a confidant of her mother which served as a barrier for Angelina to emotionally and psychologically separate from her mother and to invest energies in her own growth toward individuation and to a sense of identity. In the course of couple therapy, Angelina informed her mother the type of mother that she needed in the past and wants today. The mother, who was totally unaware of the dynamics of their relationship, painfully listened to her daughter's complaints, and agreed to mend her ways knowing that it would be a new, difficult, and painful journey. With continued couple therapy, Angelina and her mother worked through their emotional enmeshment and achieved a greater sense of their personhood and began to relate to each other as two differentiated persons.

### *Practicing subphase*

The practicing subphase represents the child's movement from the "maternal nest" to exploring the expanding world that lies beyond the relationship with the caregiver; he begins a "love-affair" with the world (Mahler et al., 1975, p. 70). The child exercises his developing motor capacities (e.g., crawl, walk) and cognitive capacities (e.g., manipulate objects, language), and reality tests his sense of omnipotence. The child feels elated and exhilarated with his own faculties, with the greatness of his own world and in using his body to explore and master the "other-than-mother" environment and to "escape from fusion with, from engulfment by, mother" (Mahler et al., 1975, p. 71). In being away from the mother for a significant period of time, the toddler develops anxiety. He acquires the capacity to self soothe, first by internalizing the maternal functions that originally served to soothe, calm, and regulate affect, and later by creating a transitional object (e.g., blanket) that is invested with the mother's tension-relieving and soothing functions. The transitional object loses its importance when the child begins to perform soothing operations for himself without the need for the external soother (Edward et al., 1981). This subphase leads to the toddler asserting his individuality and to identify formation.

To negotiate this subphase, it is important that the caregiver validate the toddler's efforts toward separation and his strivings toward mastery of his world and be emotionally available when the toddler feels anxious in his separation experiences. Failures to negotiate this subphase could be brought about by the caregiver pushing the toddler too early to psychologically separate and by being critical, rather than validating, of the toddler's efforts to master his environment resulting in feeling inadequacy and low self-esteem, and fear to risk and venture out. Also, the toddler who has failed to become emotionally bonded in the symbiotic phase, might indeed be more preoccupied in being with the caregiver rather than to venture out and explore his expanding world. The toddler may carry these failures into adolescence and adulthood.

The effect of the failure to negotiate this subphase is illustrated by Percy, married, in his late 30s, and the youngest of three boys. He sought therapy because he felt inadequate in his job despite having received many awards for his performance. As a child and pre-teen he was criticized by both his siblings and his father for being the dumb one, not good in school, and athletically awkward. He was left feeling inadequate, a loner, and an outsider. He sought the company of women for comfort and validation of his competency and lovability. His preoccupation about wanting to feel lovable and emotionally bonded, impeded the exploration of his "other than mother" world and thereby he failed to develop the experience of being competent and adequate.

### *Rapprochement subphase*

This subphase marks a pivotal developmental point in the child's struggle toward establishing his individuality. During the rapprochement subphase, the child continues to strive to (a) become securely emotionally connected, (b) establish a comfort zone between the "need to be emotionally connected" and the "need to be separate/individuated"; (c) establish physical and psychological boundaries between himself and others (e.g., establishes "what is mine" from "what is yours"); (d) internalize representation of good persons (e.g., object constancy) to whom he can turn mentally to gain perspective on issues, comfort self, and regulate affect; (e) relate to others empathically and in their own right (e.g., whole-objects); (f) replace splitting with repression; and (g) and move toward individuality (Mahler et al., 1975). The two main achievements of this subphase are the establishment of object constancy and individuality.

To help a child to achieve these goals, it is important for the caregivers to be sensitive to the child's emotional needs and to validate self-directed movements toward individuality. Whereas in the previous months, the child was rather oblivious of the caregiver's absence, now being in her presence is vital. The child manifests this by bringing toys and books to the caregiver and invites her to participate in his activities. It is also important for the caregivers to provide a structure to help the child to contain his feelings and behaviors and to provide the child with explanations for the limits that are being imposed.

Failure to complete the developmental tasks of this subphase as listed above can lead to serious emotional problems that are carried into adolescence and adulthood such as borderline personality disorder. The core unmet need is for emotional bonding which might be accompanied or triggered by the feeling of abandonment. The goal of therapy is to undo the developmental disturbances by the therapist meeting the child (client) at the level at which the injury occurred.

The consequence in failing to negotiate this subphase is illustrated by Belinda (mentioned earlier) who was court-ordered to consult a psychologist to deal with her anger and rage as she was charged with physically assaulting her mother. Belinda was brought up in an emotional depriving and dysfunctional home. As an infant she did not experience physical/emotional closeness and bonding with her caregiver as the latter was emotionally cold toward her daughter. Belinda entered the practicing stage preoccupied with establishing an emotional bond and relationship with her mother rather than with leaving the nest and exploring the other than mother world. She moved into the rapprochement subphase without having established a secure emotional bond with the caregiver and without having freely explored the other-than-mother world. During the same period she suffered from emotional, physical, and sexual abuse on part of both her father and mother. These combined experiences, prevented Belinda from (a) leaving the nest to become her own person; (b) establishing appropriate boundaries between she and her parents; (c) establishing object constancy; (d) learning how to regulate affect; and (e) developing empathy toward her caregivers and, thereby, failing to reverse the defense of splitting.

Belinda carried the failure to negotiate the rapprochement subphase into adolescence and adulthood. Her adult behaviors continue to be characterized by (a) splitting, idealizing, fear of abandonment, and rage; (b) an inability to regulate affect; (c) feeling unlovable; and (d) a difficulty to form intimate and meaningful relationships. When she felt unloved, pushed aside, and/or criticized by her mother, she felt abandoned, engaged the defence mechanism of splitting, and became enraged, which resulted in assaulting her mother.

## *Etiology and Classification of Emotional Problems*

### *Etiology of emotional disorders*

The SIRP approach differs from both the Millon and Kernberg systems that focus on undoing defenses. SIRP focuses on how unmet core childhood relational, self, and physical intimacy needs underlie emotional problems and how these unmet needs lead to an individual's skewed perceptions of self, other, and the world, to the failure to establish object constancy and regulate affect, to the development of dysfunctional relational patterns and communication styles, to the failure to establish a comfortable zone between being connected without losing sense of self and being separate without losing sense of connection, to mention a few. SIRP views emotional problems in terms of developmental deficits and in terms of relational and self issues. Rather than focusing on the defenses and on the troubled behaviors, SIRP focuses on the person's subjective experience and helps the individual to uncover the unmet core needs that drive the behaviors, help the person to bring them to consciousness, and to reorient his life according to these needs. This means living from a true self rather than from a compromised self.

An example is that of Anselm (mentioned above) who was struggling with bouts of clinical depression. The root of his depression was that he compromised himself for the sake of others rather than to live from his "true self" (Winnicott, 1960). When he became aware of his unmet needs and of the manner in which he wants to live his life, he developed the courage and skills to shift the orientation of his life and his depression lifted. In summary, the SIRP approach is characterized by its focus on unmet needs, helping individuals to uncover these, and redirect their lives according to them.

The position that unmet core needs are related to emotional problems and disorders is consistent with Schmdit and Harnandez' (2007) observation that when an individual's unmet needs were addressed in treatment, his emotional problems diminished. The position is consistent with Hendrix's (2008) assumption that unmet childhood needs and with Johnson's (2004) assumption that unmet attachment needs underlie couple problems. The position that unmet needs can lead to emotional problems is supported by Spitz's (1945) observation that children of incarcerated mothers, who are not touched, held, and cuddled, become depressed and shut down physiologically. The position is also supported by two empirical research projects. In the first study, Meier and Boivin (2006) investigated the process of resolving intrapsychic conflicts. They observed that in identifying and responding to their unmet needs, the individuals resolved their intrapsychic conflicts. In a second study, Briscoe-Dimock (2013) studied the relationship between unmet relational and self needs and couple distress. The author found that the unmet "need for lovability" and the unmet "need for autonomy" were related to couple distress.

### *Classification of emotional disorders*

SIRP does not view emotional problems and maladaptive functioning in terms of diagnostic classification systems such as the *Diagnostic and Statistical Manual of Mental Disorders* (DSM-5; American Psychiatric Association, 2013) and the International Classification of Diseases (ICD-10; World Health Organization). The DSM-5 and the ICD-10, that classify mental disorders primarily according to symptoms and behaviors, are useful for their division of mental disorders according to major groupings such as mood, anxiety, somatoform, and personality disorders. These constructs provide a context within which to understand a specific emotional problem; however, they are limited in describing the unique way in which an individual came to struggle with an anxiety, mood, somatoform, and personality disorders.

SIRP is more inclined to adopt an approach to understanding mental problems similar to Millon's "biosocial approach" (Millon, 1969; Millon et al., 2004) and Kernberg's (1984) object relations approach. The Millon and Kernberg psychological approaches are explanatory in nature and indicate how a mental disorder is constituted by a group of psychological processes. For example, Kernberg views emotional problems in terms of the level of personality organization, such as higher, intermediate, and lower levels and the psychological processes that constitute them. He describes these levels in terms of the quality and/or nature of instinctual development, superego development, nature of defenses, and quality of object relations. Representative emotional problems for the higher, intermediate, and lower levels are, respectively, hysterical, narcissistic, and borderline personality disorders.

SIRP views emotional problems in terms of psychological and psychosocial bipolar themes, that is, of the self and relationship issues that constitute them. For example, the bipolar themes that underlie depression might include being non-assertive versus being assertive, feeling obligated versus being responsible and being compliant versus being autonomous. The underlying unmet needs are to live from the true self and the need to connect. In treating depression, therefore, one does not treat depression as such, but one addresses and treats the bipolar themes underlying it particularly the need to connect and live authentically.

This chapter presented the basics of SIRP, outlined its fundamental principles, and presented, defined, and illustrated its major theoretical constructs. The constructs are interrelated and interwoven by the more encompassing concept of the separation and individuation process. All of the constructs take shape within the separation and individuation process. The following three chapters indicate how to apply the SIRP constructs to conceptualize and assess clinical cases using an assessment instrument specifically designed for SIRP.

## References

Allport, G. W. (1967). *Becoming: Basic considerations for a psychology of personality*. New Haven: Yale University Press.

American Psychiatric Association. (2013). *Diagnostic and statistical manual of mental disorders (DSM-5)*. Washington, DC: Author.

Arkowitz, H. (1992). A common factors therapy for depression. In J. C. Norcross & M. R. Goldfried (Eds.), *Handbook of psychotherapy integration* (pp. 402–432). New York: Oxford Press.

Baker, H. W., & Baker, M. N. (1987). Heinz Kohut's self psychology: An overview. *The American Journal of Psychiatry*, *144*(1), 1–9.

Barrett-Lennard, G. (2013). *The relationship paradigm: Human being beyond individualism*. United Kingdom: Palgrave MacMillan.

Benesh, M., & Weiner, B. (1982). On emotion and motivation: From the notebooks of Fritz Heider.*American Psychologist*, *35*(8), 887–895.

Bergman, A. (1975). Preface by Anni Bergman. In M. Mahler, F. Pine, & A. Bergman (Eds.), *The psychological birth of the human infant* (pp. xv–xix). New York: Basic Books.

Berne, E. (1961). *Transactional analysis in psychotherapy*. New York: Gove Press.

Berne, E. (1964). *Games people play*. New York: Grove Press.

Brinich, P., & Shelley, C. (2002). *The self and personality structure: Core concepts in therapy*. Buckingham, England: Open University Press.

Briscoe-Dimock, S. (2013). *Unmet self, relational, and spiritual needs in distressed couple relationships* [Unpublished doctoral thesis]. Ottawa, Ontario: Saint Paul University.

Butler, C. (2002). *Postmodernism: A very short introduction*. Oxford: Oxford University Press.

Cashdan, S. (1988). *Object relations therapy: Using the relationship*. New York: W. W. Norton.

Deci, E. L., & Ryan, R. M. (2000). The "what" and "why" of goal pursuits: Human needs and the self-determination of behavior. *Psychological Inquiry*, *11*, 227–268.

Deci, E. L., & Ryan, R. M. (2002). *Handbook of self-determination research*. Rochester, NY: University of Rochester Press.

Detmer, D. (2003). *Challenging postmodernism: Philosophy and the politics of truth*. New York: Humanity Books.

Edward, J., Ruskin, N., & Turrini, P. (1981). *Separation-individuation: Theory and application*. New York: Gardner Press.

Epstein, N. B., & Baucom, D. H. (2002). *Enhanced cognitive-behavioral therapy for couples*. Washington, DC: American Psychological Association.

Erikson, E. H. (1950). *Childhood and society*. New York: Norton.

Erikson, E. H. (1968). *Identity, youth, and crisis*. New York: W. W. Norton.

Erskine, R. G. (1998). Attunement and involvement: Therapeutic responses to relational needs. *International Journal of Psychotherapy*, *3*(3), 1–20.

Fairbairn, W. R. D. (1944). Endopsychic structure considered in terms of object relationships. In *An object-relations theory of the personality* (pp. 82–136). New York: Basic Books.

Freud, S. (1905). Three essays on the theory of sexuality. *Standard Edition*, *7*, 23–243.

Freud, S. (1923). The ego and the id. *Standard Edition*, *19*, 12–63.

Freud, S. (1938). An outline of psychoanalysis. *Standard Edition*, *23*, 144–207.

Gergen, K. J. (1971). *The concept of the self*. New York: Holt, Rinehart and Winston.

Haroian, L. (2000). Child sexual development. *Electronic Journal of Human Sexuality*, *3*, 1–45.

Hendrix, O. (2008). *Getting the love you want: A guide for couples*. New York: St. Martins Press.

Jacobson, E. (1964). *The self and the object world*. New York: International Universities press.

Johnson, S. (2004). *The practice of emotionally focused couple therapy: Creating connections*. New York: Brunner-Routledge.

Kaplan, H. I., & Sadock, B. J. (1991). *Synopsis of psychiatry: Behavioral sciences clinical psychiatry* (6th ed.). London: Williams & Wilkins.

Kasser, T. (2002). *The high price of materialism*. London: Bradford Book.

Kernberg, O. (1984). *Object relations theory and clinical psychoanalysis*. Northvale, NJ: Jason Aronson. (Original work published 1976)

Klein, M. (1946). Notes on some schizoid mechanisms. In *Envy and gratitude and other works 1946–1963* (pp. 1–24). New York: Delacorte Press/Seymour Lawrence.

Klein, M. (1959). Our adult world and its roots in infancy. In M. Klein (Ed.), *Envy and gratitude and other works 1946–1963* (pp. 247–263). New York: Delacorte Press/Seymour Lawrence.

Kohut, H. (1971). *The analysis of the self.* New York: International Universities Press.

Kohut, H. (1977). *The restoration of the self.* New York: International Universities Press.

Kohut, H. (1979). *Four basic definitions of self psychology.* Paper presented to the Workshop on Self Psychology, Chicago, IL.

Kohut, H. (1984). *How does analysis cure*? Chicago, IL: Chicago University Press.

Kohut, H., & Wolfe, E. S. (1978). The disorders of the self and their treatment: An outline. *International Journal of Psycho-Analysis, 59*, 413–425.

Krueger, D. W. (1989). *Body self and psychological self: A developmental and clinical integration of disorders of the self.* New York: Brunner/Mazel.

Lazarus, R. S. (1982). Thoughts on the relations between emotions and cognition. *American Psychologist, 37*, 1019–1027.

Lichtenstein, H. (1961). Identity and sexuality: A study of their interrelationships in man. *Journal of American Psychoanalytic Association, 9*, 179–260.

Lum, W. (2002). The use of self of the therapist. *Contemporary Family Therapy, 24*(1), 181–197.

Luthman, S. (1974). *The dynamic family.* Palo Alto, CA: Science and Behavior Books.

Mahler, M., & Furer, M. (1968). *On human symbiosis and the vicissitudes of individuation.* New York: International Universities Press.

Mahler, M. S., Pine, F., & Bergman, A. (1975). *Psychological birth of the human infant.* New York: Basic Books.

Masterson, J. F. (1976). *Psychotherapy of the borderline adult: A developmental approach.* New York: Brunner Mazel Publishers.

Masterson, J. F. (1985). *The real self: A developmental, self, and object relations approach.* New York: Brunner/Mazel Publishers.

Mead, G. H. (1977). The self and the organism. In A. Strauss (Ed.), *George Herbert Mead on social psychology* (pp. 199–246). Chicago: University of Chicago Press.

Meichenbaum, D. (1977). *Cognitive-behavior modification: An integrative approach.* New York: Plenum.

Meier, A., & Boivin, M. (1983). Towards a synthetic model of psychotherapy. *Pastoral Sciences, 2*, 137–176.

Meier, A., & Boivin, M. (1998). *The seven-phase model of the change process: Theoretical foundation, definitions, coding guidelines, training procedures and research data* [Unpublished manuscript]. Ottawa, Ontario: Saint Paul University.

Meier, A., & Boivin, M. (2001). Conflict resolution: The interplay of affects, cognitions and needs in the resolution of intrapersonal conflicts. *Pastoral Sciences, 20*(1), 93–119.

Meier, A., & Boivin, M. (2006). Intrapsychic conflicts, their formation, underlying dynamics and resolution: An object relations perspective. In A. Meier & M. Rovers (Eds.), *Through conflict to reconciliation* (pp. 295–328). Ottawa, Ontario: Novalis.

Meier, A., & Boivin, M. (2011). *Counselling and therapy techniques: Theory and practice*. London: SAGE.

Meier, A., Boivin, M., & Meier, M. (2006). The treatment of depression: A case study using theme-analysis. *Counselling and Psychotherapy Research*, *6*(2), 115–125.

Messer, S. (1992). A critical examination of belief structures in integrative and eclectic psychotherapy. In J. C. Norcross & M. R. Goldfried (Eds.), *Handbook of psychotherapy integration* (pp. 130–168). New York: Basic Books.

Millon, T. (1969). *Modern psychopathology: A biosocial approach to maladaptive learning and functioning*. London, UK: W. B. Saunders.

Millon, T., Millon, C. M., Meagher, S., Grossman, S., & Rammath, R. (2004). *Personality disorders in modern life*. New York: Wiley & Sons.

Norcross, J. C. (2005). A primer on psychotherapy integration. In J. C. Norcross & M. R. Goldfried (Eds.), *Handbook of psychotherapy integration* (2nd ed., pp. 3–23). New York: Oxford Press.

Pike, L. B. (2000). *Sexuality and your child: For children ages 0 to 3*. Columbia: University of Missouri.

Pine, F. (1975). Preface. In M. Mahler, F. Pine, & A. Bergman (Eds.), *The psychological birth of the human infant* (pp. vii–xiii). New York: Basic Books.

Reeves, J. (2014). *Understanding motivation and emotion* (6th Ed.). New Jersey: John Wiley & Sons.

Reisenzein, R., & Schonpflug, W. (1992). Stumpf's cognitive-evaluative theory of emotion. *American Psychologist*, *47*(1), 34–45.

Rogers, C. R. (1966). Client-centered therapy. In C. H. Patterson (Ed.), *Theories of counseling and psychotherapy* (pp. 403–439). New York: Harper & Row.

Sadock, B. J., Sadock, V. A., & Ruiz, P. (2014). *Kaplan and Sadock's synopsis of psychiatry behavioral sciences clinical psychiatry* (11th ed.). New York: Walter Kluwer.

Satir, V. (1972). *People making*. Palo Alto, CA: Science and Behavior Books.

Satir, V., Banmen, J., Gerber, J., & Gomori, M. (1991). *The Satir model: Family therapy and beyond*. Palo Alto, CA: Science and Behavior Books.

Schmidt, S. J., & Hernandez, A. (2007). The developmental needs meeting strategy: Eight case studies. *Traumotalogy*, *13*(1), 27–48.

Spitz, R. A. (1945). Hospitalism: An inquiry into the genesis of psychiatric conditions in early childhood. *Psychoanalytic Study of the Child*, *1*, 53–74.

Stern, D. S. (1985). *The interpersonal world of the infant: A view from psychoanalysis and developmental psychology*. New York: Basic Books.

Stricker, G., & Gold, J. (2005). Assimilative psychodynamic psychotherapy. In J. C. Norcross & M. R. Goldfried (Eds.), *Handbook of psychotherapy integration* (pp. 221–240). New York: Oxford.

Strupp, H. H., & Binder, J. L. (1985). *Psychotherapy in a new key: A guide to time-limited dynamic psychotherapy*. New York: Basic Books.

Symonds, P. M. (1951). *The ego and the self*. Westport, CT: Greenwood Press.

Webber, J. G., & Devlin, D. (2005). *Sexuality throughout life*. Retrieved from http://www.netdoctor.co.uk/sex

White, R., & Watt, N. F. (1981). *The abnormal personality*. Chichester, West Sussex, England: Whiley & Sons.

Winnicott, D. (1948). Pediatrics and psychiatry. In D. Winnicott (Ed.), *Through paediatrics to psychoanalysis* (pp. 157–173). New York: Basic Books.

Winnicott, D. (1960). Ego distortion in terms of true and false self. In D. Winnicott (Ed.), *The maturational processes and the facilitating environment* (pp. 140–152). New York: International Universities Press.

Winnicott, D. (1965). *The family and individual development.* London: Tavistock Publishers.

World Health Organization. (2010). *The international classification of diseases (ICD-10).* Geneva, Switzerland: Author.

Zajonc, R. B. (1980). Feeling and thinking: Preferences need no inferences. *American Psychologist*, *2*(35), 151–175.

# Part II

# Assessment and Conceptualization

Chapter 4

# Psychodynamic Case Formulation

Clinical case formulations are at the heart of psychotherapy as they bring understanding to the client's problems and inform an approach to treatment. A case formulation, in general, serves three objectives, namely, it provides a theoretical explanation of the client's problem, organizes a vast amount of assessment data and provides a guide for treatment. A psychodynamic formulation has been an explicit or implicit aspect of psychodynamic psychotherapy from the outset (Hinshelwood, 1991; Messer & Wolitzky, 2007).

The topic of this chapter is case formulation. It begins by providing a definition of psychodynamic formulation and outlines its procedures from the perspective of Self-in-Relationship Psychotherapy (SIRP). The chapter ends by illustrating a conceptualization for a client.

## Definition of Psychodynamic Case Formulation

There are varying definitions for case formulations. The definitions differ in terms of the nature of the behaviors that therapy should change, the important constructs in a case formulation, and the role of personal and social histories (Eells, 2007; Sturmey, 2009).

Case formulations have been defined as a "hypothesis of how an individual comes to present with a certain disorder or circumstance at a particular point in time" (Weerasekera, 1996, p. 5), "explains the nature of a client's problems and how he or she came to have them … [and] … organizes assessment data into meaningful outline, applying research and theory to make sense of a client's current presentation" (Porzelius, 2002, p. 3), and explains "who the client is like" … [and] … "why the client is like this" (Berman, 1997, p. xi). According to McWilliams (1999), a case formulation, from a psychodynamic perspective, puts "all the assessment information into a narrative that makes this human being and his or her psychopathology comprehensible to us, and we derive our recommendations and our way of relating to the client from that Narrative" (p. viii).

DOI: 10.4324/9781003272502-6

SIRP adopts a biopsychosocial model (Barker, 1995; Weerasekera, 1996) in formulating a case conceptualization with an emphasis on the psychological and social dimensions. The biological dimension may include medical conditions, prenatal exposure to alcohol, traumatic brain injury, temperament, and side effects from medications. The psychological dimension may include issues such as low self-esteem, rigid thinking, and difficulty to regulate affect. The social dimension may comprise poverty, racial discrimination, domestic violence, and loss of a significant person. In formulating a conceptualization, it is essential to determine the extent to which biological, psychological, and social dimensions are contributing to the person's symptoms and/or to the presenting problem and to rule out those dimensions that are not contributors.

When the biological, psychological, and social dimensions and their influences have been determined, the SIRP-oriented psychotherapist begins to formulate a conceptualization of the individual's symptoms and/or presenting problems. The therapist presents a conceptualization in terms of four factors, namely, predisposing, precipitating, perpetuating, and protective factors (Barker, 1995; Weerasekera, 1993).

*Predisposing factors* are areas of personal vulnerability that increase the risk to develop a particular symptom, emotional response, and/or psychological problem. In psychological terms, a predisposing factor is a thought, perception, and/or representation of self that a person has internalized (e.g., feeling unloved, unwanted). *Precipitating factors* are the specific events or circumstances that trigger the onset of the emotional responses and psychological problems (e.g., breakup of an intimate relationship). *Perpetuating factors* are circumstances or events that maintain the symptoms and the psychological problem over a period of time (e.g., failed dating experiences). *Protective factors* counteract the predisposing, precipitating, and perpetuating factors. They include an individual's own areas of talents, skill, competency, and interests (e.g., reading romantic novels), which reduce the intensity of the problems and promote healthy and adaptive functioning.

From the perspective of SIRP, a psychodynamic formulation pays particular attention to the client's unmet core relational, self, and physical intimacy needs and how they impact the presenting problems. With the exception of trauma and abuse, it is assumed that the client's unmet childhood core needs, such as the need for emotional connection and significance, push for a response and when it is not forthcoming, the client finds other means (e.g., compensatory strategies) to fulfill the need and/or protect herself from the anxiety and hurt associated with the failure to provide the needs. The unmet needs also shape how the person thinks about herself (e.g., unlovable) and others (e.g., depriving) and affects the development of the style of relating such as pursuing or avoiding a relationship.

## Procedures for Case Conceptualization

The procedures to conduct a psychodynamic case formulation include the statement of the client problem, obtaining relevant data, selecting theoretical constructs, conceptualizing the problem, planning treatment, formulating a prognosis, and writing a report. Each of these components is briefly described.

### *Statement of Client Problem*

The therapist sees the problem through the lens of the SIRP constructs with a special focus on unmet core relational, self, and physical intimacy needs. This perspective shapes the gathering of the information.

It is important to explore the problem as thoroughly as possible and to present clearly the difficulties, complaints, concerns, and impairments for which the client seeks help. The title of the problem should be clear, specific, descriptive, and expressed in the language of the client. It is imperative to determine the intensity and extensity of the problem and whether it interferes or has interfered with educational, occupational, and social functioning. One wants to know whether this is an old problem or a new problem, when did the individual first experience the problem and how did she manage it. Did she seek professional help and if so, how was it helpful?

It is important to differentiate between a "problem and a normal life difficulty" (Watzlawick et al., 1974). With a problem there is a discrepancy between how things are and how they are expected to be whereas with normal life difficulty, there is no such discrepancy. Life is normal, has its ups and downs, problems exist, bad things happen, and things change.

Psychiatric disorders are best understood in terms of their constituents. For example, a major depressive disorder might be viewed in terms of a sense of powerlessness, inauthenticity, need to please, feeling obligated, and lack of assertiveness (Meier et al., 2006). For some emotional problems such as depression, one tries to identify the path that led to depression. For some clients it might be a loss experience and for others it might be that they fail to live up to their own expectations.

### *Obtain Relevant Data*

SIRP uses a semi-structured interview that has been designed to obtain information to assess its constructs (Meier & Boivin, 2021a; see Appendix 4.1). The domains about which information is obtained include the presenting problem, family of origin, educational background, occupational experiences, social experiences, relational experiences (i.e., friends, dating, marriage), use of leisure time and hobbies, trauma and abuse, history of misuse of substances, and sources of strength. Questions about hobbies and leisure are helpful to assess for balance between living from one's needs and from a sense of duty and obligations. The questions about sources of strength open the door to a discussion about one's philosophy of life and how it helps to face the tasks of daily living and major crises in one's life. In obtaining information about these dimensions, SIRP pays particular attention to relational and self experiences.

In addition to obtaining information by the use of a semi-structured interview, SIRP also obtains information from the results of the SIRP Assessment Form (SIRP-AF) (Meier & Boivin, 2021b) that is applied to a client's psychosocial history. The SIRP-AF assesses the individual's functioning on the SIRP constructs such as relational, self, and physical intimacy needs; representations of self and other; emotional bonding; psychic organization; and so on. The SIRP-AF provides operational definitions for each of the constructs and criteria for assessing them. The results from the analysis using the SIRP-AF paint a picture of the client's strengths and weaknesses. (These constructs were presented in Chapter 3 and are defined and operationalized in Chapter 5.) The therapist's observations of the client's pattern of relating, style of communicating, openness to disclose private material about self, also are part of the information used for assessment.

In making an assessment using SIRP one obtains as much information as possible about the client's problem and her psychosocial history which serves as a context. One also tries to obtain developmental and subjective history (e.g., trauma, abuse) about the individual's experiences during early childhood, pre-adolescence, and adolescence since SIRP assumes that these internalized and structured early experiences influence future attitudes about self, other, and the world, and behaviors and interactions.

Assessment is ongoing which implies that as therapy progresses, the initial assessment might be modified, broadened, and enriched. This might be facilitated by two additional sources of information, namely, the therapist's intuitive and empathic understanding of the client's presenting problem and underlying dynamics and by the therapist's countertransference. To facilitate an empathic understanding of the client, the therapist might ask herself the following question: "What is like to be in the body of the client?" By using empathic immersion (Kohut, 1977) one tries to experience the client's feelings, thought processes, and needs and thereby gain an appreciation of the client's sense of self, organization of the psychic structure, coping strategies, and so on. To become aware of one's countertransference in therapy, the therapist can ask herself the following question: "What might it feel like to journey with the client?" That is, what relational problems might emerge in being with the client? Countertransference can provide insight into the client's typical way of relating and the problems that it might create. It is important to distinguish between one's own unresolved childhood experiences from the feelings that emerge in a current relationship. It is imperative that one reality test one's empathic understanding of the client.

### *Constructs for Assessment*

Unlike some of the other orientations such as cognitive-behavioral therapy (Beck et al., 2004) and rational-emotive therapy (Ellis & Dryden, 1987) that have few constructs to assess, the SIRP approach has many constructs that are assessed and form part of the conceptualization. The SIRP constructs that are assessed using the SIRP-AF include (a) unmet relational, self, and physical intimacy needs; (b) representations of other and self; (c) affect that links representations of self and other and vice versa; (d) ego organization; (e) self-structure; (f) coping mechanisms; (g) quality of emotional bond; (h) object constancy; (i) characteristic; (j) projective identifications; (k) characteristic phase (Mahler et al., 1975); and (l) characteristic position (Klein, 1961). The constructs overlap, are interrelated, and together present a whole picture of the client. For example, underlying projective identifications are unmet core self, relational, and/or physical intimacy needs that push for satiation. The results from the assessments of the constructs lead to a theoretical consistent and coherent formulation. By using a great number of constructs, the therapist is better able to grasp the uniqueness of each individual.

The constructs that are relevant for one client may differ from the constructs that are relevant for another client. For example, for a client that is driven and is a high achiever, the constructs that might stand out for her are the superego (e.g., feeling duty-bound), projective identification of power, need for affirmation for her competency, and a dominant feeling of anger. For a client struggling with depression, the constructs that might stand out are affirmations for being a lovable person, projective identification of dependency, craving for emotional connection, and be arrested at the differentiation and rapprochement subphases. The same constructs for different clients may also differ in terms of their intensity. For example, for one client the striving for emotional connection may be moderate and for another client it might be intense.

In assessing clients on the different constructs, the therapist assures herself that there is a consistency across the constructs and together, as a group, they make sense of the client's struggles. The therapist assesses the client for current level of functioning, that is, the therapist indicates where the client is at phenomenologically regarding the construct. This differs from assessing a client's capacity regarding a specific construct such as to regulate affect (PDM Task Force, 2006).

### *Constructing a Psychodynamic Conceptualization*

From the perspective of SIRP, one can consider five steps in constructing a psychodynamic conceptualization. The conceptualization seeks to explain the client's current symptoms by linking them to predispositions (i.e., vulnerabilities), precipitating stressors, situations that maintain the symptom and to compensatory behaviors to minimize the presenting problem. SIRP pays particular attention in the way unmet core needs are related to the presenting problem.

To illustrate each of the steps, reference will be made to Stefan who sought therapy because he was depressed. Stefan did not report any physical ailments and misuse of alcohol; he did not experience any trauma and sexual abuse. He stated that his relationship with his wife was stressful; he enjoyed playing with his young children. The formulation of a psychodynamic conceptualization can be described in the following steps. The manner in which the five steps are included in a formal conceptualization is illustrated in the case of Tim and Leanne at the end of this chapter.

### *Step 1: Identify and clearly describe the problems, symptoms, and concerns*

The first step in conceptualization is to identify the problems and to describe their intensity and extensity. The identified problems are concisely and clearly described and named and it is indicated whether they are new problems or whether they are reoccurring problems. If the latter, it is indicated when they were first experienced. Where possible, the constituents of the problem are pointed out. For example, the constituents of depression might be a sense of powerlessness, inauthenticity, need to please, feeling obligated, and lack of assertiveness (Meier et al., 2006).

***Illustration*** Stefan stated that he has been depressed for most of his life. He first felt depressed when he began school as he was not validated for his school work whereas his classmates were. The teacher consistently pointed out how he could improve his work but she did not do that for the other students. He felt that he was not as good as his classmates. He added that his father was very critical of him but not of the client's younger brothers.

### *Step 2: Indicate the factors that predispose him to depression*

Predisposing factors are areas of personal vulnerability that increase the risk to develop a particular symptom, emotional response, and/or psychological problem. In a few sentences mention how the individual's past experiences, particularly early childhood experiences predisposed her to be vulnerable to develop her current problems.

***Illustration*** Stefan was brought up in home where his father was critical of him but not of his brothers. Although his mother was loving and caring, she was not able to stop her husband from being critical toward Stefan. As a child, Stefan felt that he was not as good as his brothers and that his father was correct in being critical of him. In the process he became critical toward himself and developed an inner world dominated by a severe superego, a low sense of self, a craving for competency and significance and became prone to depression. The childhood experiences in being criticized predispose him to feeling depressed.

*Step 3: Determine the precipitating events and factors that triggered the symptoms*

Precipitating factors are the specific events or circumstances that trigger the onset of the emotional responses and psychological problems. Determine the events or factors in the person's current life that triggered the symptoms. Are these events and factors new in the person's life and if not for how long has the person been subjected to them?

***Illustration*** Stefan reported that he became depressed after receiving a performance evaluation at his workplace. He added that he was very sensitive to being evaluated and recalled his first such experience was when he was criticized by his grade one teacher and by his father who was very critical of him but not of his younger brothers.

*Step 4: Indicate factors in the person's current life that serve to perpetuate the symptoms*

Perpetuating factors are circumstances or events that maintain the symptoms and the psychological problem over a period of time.

***Illustration*** Stefan often finds himself in settings or in relationships wherein he feels less adequate and important than the others. The competitive environment in which he works tends to maintain his sense of being inadequate and insignificant which lead to depressive states. He is in a marriage where his wife constantly criticizes him for not being a good father and for being emotionally distant from her. These situations tend to maintain his feelings of inadequacy, insignificance, and depression.

*Step 5: Indicate the protective factors*

Protective factors minimize the potency of the predisposing, precipitating, and perpetuating factors. They include an individual's own areas of talents, skill, competency, and interests, which reduce the intensity of the problems and promote healthy and adaptive functioning.

***Illustration*** Stefan was a member of the executive of an athletic organization in his community. He received many expressions of appreciation for the excellent work he did for the organization. Stefan's sense of competency and self-esteem were fostered by his involvement with the organization and helped him to cope with his inclination to become depressed.

## Formulating a Conceptualization and a Treatment Plan

In the case of Stefan, there are several potential SIRP constructs that explain his feelings of inadequacy, insignificance, and his depressive state. Among these are a severe superego, low sense of self, inability to regulate affect (i.e., lacking object constancy), weakened coping strategies, unmet core self and relational needs, a false self, and projective identification of dependency. Undoubtedly, all of the phenomena associated with these constructs will be included in the conceptualization. But which of these constructs is more dominant? This is the question that a therapist is asked to consider.

### *Conceptualization – Stefan*

Stefan sought therapy because he was struggling with feelings of inadequacy, insignificance, and depression. These feelings were precipitated by an evaluation of his performance at work. He mentioned that he was sensitive and vulnerable to criticisms and to statements that sounded like a belittling. These are familiar feelings which he linked to his childhood experiences of being criticized and belittled by his father. Being a young child with limited resources, he believed the criticisms of his father to be true. He gradually internalized these criticisms, made them part of his inner world (i.e., severe and demanding superego) and tried to evaluate and guide his behavior by them. He learned to see himself less adequate and significant (i.e., low self-esteem) than others (i.e., his brothers). This feeling of being inadequate and insignificant became his life script (i.e., projective identification). He entered into relationships where he craved to feel adequate and significant (i.e., unmet core needs) but, deep within, he did not feel that way. He craved for their validations, but they were insufficient as he was not able to retain them (i.e., lacking object constancy); after they were spoken, they evaporated. His feelings of inadequacy, insignificance, and tendency toward a depressive state are maintained by his competitive co-workers and his wife (perpetuating factors) who is critical of his parenting and of his lack of emotional closeness. For all of his life, beginning in childhood, Stefan has been in a search to satisfy his unmet core needs for a sense of adequacy and significance.

### *Treatment Plan for Stefan*

In terms of treatment, the goal is for the therapist and Stefan to address his feelings of inadequacy, insignificance, and depressive state. These feeling states appear to be a function of his critical and demanding critic (i.e., severe superego), of his impoverished sense of self (i.e., low self-esteem), of his inability (i.e., impoverished ego) to evaluate his performance at work and the quality of his relationships with his children and wife, and of his difficulty to assert his psychological space with others (i.e., need for autonomy).

It appears that a therapeutic priority is to help Stefan to be less dependent on others and to become more autonomous. This includes taking distance (i.e., differentiating) from others, becoming his own person (i.e., individuating) and establishing his standards as an employee, father, and husband and becoming proud when they are achieved. Because of his strong dependency needs, it is important to validate them and to integrate them while at the same time for Stefan to pursue his sense of autonomy. Techniques and exercises that might be helpful to achieve these goals are experiential focusing and Task-Directed Imagery (Meier & Boivin, 2011). Experiential focusing can be used to help the client get in touch with his feelings in becoming less dependent and more autonomous. In helping Stefan to become more autonomous, a Task-Directed Imagery exercise could be designed for him to experience what it is like to be autonomous and free of dependency needs. These exercises might be helpful to tame his internal critic and give more power to his inner child and thereby lift his depressive mood and bring about a greater sense of competency and significance.

## Prognosis and Writing a Report

A prognosis is a prediction, based on the conceptualization, as to whether the person can benefit from psychological treatment given the client's internal and external resources. The assessment of two factors can be of help in predicting therapeutic success. Bellak et al. (1973) state that "the triad of synthetic functioning, autonomous functioning and thought processes is assumed to be most highly related to a good long-term prognosis, as subjects who are high in those areas are believed to have better-integrated premorbid personalities" (p. 403).

Synthetic functioning refers to the capacity to integrate potentially contradictory experiences, ideas, and feelings and to organize and unify other aspects of the personality. This means the capacity to be in the grey zone rather than in the black and white or all or nothing zone. Autonomous function refers to the ego's ability to function (e.g., concentrate, attend, learn, work) free from the influence of impulses, intense emotions, and conflicts. Thoughts processes refers to the ability to have logical, coherent, and abstract thoughts. The capacity to form relationships, particularly to be empathic, is a second factor that can be useful to determine good therapy outcome. The therapeutic relationship, which assumes a capacity to form a relationship, is the main vehicle to change as it is in the context of the client's new experiences in the relationship that she develops new representations of self and other, object constancy and the ability to regulate affect, self-esteem, and so on.

The communication of the conceptualization can take different forms dependent upon its purpose and writing style of the therapist. Berman (1997) presents six non-inclusive different writing styles: assumption-based style, symptom-based style, interpersonally based style, developmentally or historically based style, thematic or metaphorically based style, and diagnostic-based style. SIRP incorporates elements from several of these styles (e.g., assumption, symptom, interpersonally, and developmentally based) in presenting the conceptualization of a case.

The written report according to the SIRP approach includes the following information: (a) The report begins with a clear articulation of the emotional, behavioral, and/or relational problem that indicates its intensity and extensity and whether it is a new problem or an old problem. (b) This is followed by a description of the individual's vulnerability (predisposition) to experience the reported problem. The vulnerability is linked to the childhood experiences (e.g., being neglected) and how these led to the formation of the vulnerabilities such as low self-esteem. (c) Next there is a description of the actual experience that led to the onset of the presenting problem. This could include information about the persons current lived reality (e.g., relationships, work, health). (d) The report mentions the current situation that tends to perpetuate the problem and (e) indicates the individual's readiness to address her problems. And lastly, (f) the report specifies possible short-term and long-term therapy goals, suggests issues to be addressed, and indicates interventions that might be helpful to achieve the goals.

An example of a written report that includes the information just described is presented in the clinical case: Tim and Leanne. A more detailed report of a conceptualization following an assessment using a semi-structured interview and the SIRP-AF is presented in Chapter 6.

## Clinical Case – Tim and Leanne

### *Psychosocial History*

Tim, in his mid-30s, was married for ten years to Leanne and they have two pre-school age children. Tim comes from a farming family driven by the work ethic. There was limited communication in the family and the expression of feelings and needs was not acceptable. Both parents were very demanding of their children. Family meals took place in front of the TV. Although they related with each other on practical things, emotionally they were distant. His father was easily given to anger when something did not go his way. Leanne was brought up in the city and in a family with both of her parents being professionals and achievement and success oriented. There was little family time spent together.

When they were married, Tim was self-employed and Leanne worked with him in his business. At the same time, she continued with her education and gave birth to two children and raised them. After completing her education, Leanne took on full-time employment outside of the home. This situation marked the beginning of their couple problems. Tim missed her working next to him in his business. He felt that Leanne had no interest in him and in his work and that her priorities became her work and the children and that he was relegated to the bottom of the totem pole. He became embittered toward her for going to work and not making herself available to help him in his business. He felt betrayed and abandoned by her and became depressed and suicidal.

### *Conceptualization and Treatment*

Tim's current feelings of bitterness toward Leanne and his feeling of depression, betrayal, and worthlessness and suicidal thoughts were precipitated by Leanne graduating from university and accepting full-time employment. These feelings are perpetuated because Leanne continued to work outside the home, took delight in her work, and refused to work for Tim's business.

Tim was predisposed to his feelings because of his childhood experiences of having had critical parents, having been put down, made to feel worthless, and by the parents not adequately responding to his needs and feelings.

These experiences were internalized to form an internal critic which is hard on himself and dismissive (superego) of his affectional needs, a needy pattern of behavior to attempt to secure his affectional needs (projective identification of dependency), a perception of himself as being worthless (enfeebled nuclear self) and not deserving of love and affection, and an inability to regulate his affect (inadequate object constancy).

In terms of therapy, short-term goals could include the establishment of a solid, safe, secure, and accepting therapeutic relationship so as to help Tim to become aware of and articulate his feelings, thoughts, and needs regarding the current situation including his relationship with Leanne. Long-term goals could include working through and completing the separation-individuation process so that he can better tolerate Leanne's absence and feel more comfortable with emotional intimacy or closeness. Other goals could include the development of capacity to regulate affect (develop object constancy) and to relate as a whole person to a whole other (whole representations) and to develop ego resources to assertively and correctly articulate his needs and feelings and to harmonize demands he places on himself and his affectional needs (psychic organization).

The therapist could use experiential focusing to help Tim uncover his underlying needs and Task-Directed Imagery to develop object constancy and a sense of being worthwhile. To aid him to connect his current emotional state to earlier and childhood state, the therapist could engage the client in ego state therapy to heal the early wounds of rejection and emotional neglect. Task-Directed Imagery could be used to develop the capacity for intimacy (which means being connected to Leanne in her absence and maintaining his individuality when close) and the Gestalt two-chair technique to give the voice to and empower the child within and bring about greater intrapersonal harmony.

This chapter used the topics derived from the review of the literature on conceptualization to define psychodynamic conceptualization, from the perspective of SIRP, and to indicate the procedures to formulate a conceptualization that includes both a treatment plan and a prognosis.

It also suggested a model to communicate the conceptualization. The following chapter presents the SIRP Assessment Form designed to evaluate constructs inferred from a semi-structured interview.

## References


Barker, P. (1995). *The child and adolescent psychiatry evaluation: Basic child psychiatry*. Oxford, UK: Scientific, Inc.

Beck, A. T., Freeman, A., & Davis, D. (2004). *Cognitive therapy of personality disorders* (2nd ed.). New York: Guilford Press.

Bellak, L., Hurvich, M., & Gediman, H. K. (1973). *Ego functions in schizophrenics, neurotics and normals*. New York: John Wiley & Sons.

Berman, P. S. (1997). *Case conceptualization and treatment planning: Exercises for integrating theory with clinical practice*. California: SAGE.

Eells, T. D. (2007). History and current status of psychotherapy formulation. In T. D. Eells (Ed.), *Handbook of psychotherapy case formulation* (2nd ed., pp. 3–32). New York: Guilford Press.

Ellis, A., & Dryden, W. (1987). *The practice of rational-emotive the*rapy. New York: Springer.

Hinshelwood, R. D. (1991). Psychodynamic formulation in assessment for psychotherapy. *British Journal of Psychotherapy*, *8*, 166–174.

Klein, M. (1961). *Narrative of a child analysis*. London: Hogarth Press.

Kohut, H. (1977). *The restoration of the self*. New York: International Universities Press.

Mahler, M. S., Pine, F., & Bergman, A. (1975). *Psychological birth of the human infant*. New York: Basic Books.

McWilliams, N. (1999). *Psychoanalytic case formulation*. New York: Guildford.

Meier, A., & Boivin, M. (2011). *Counselling and therapy techniques: Theory and practice*. London, UK: SAGE.

Meier, A., & Boivin, M. (2021a). *Self-in-relationship psychotherapy semi-structured assessment interview (SSAI)*. Ottawa, Ontario. (Unpublished document).

Meier, A., & Boivin, M. (2021b). *Self-in-relationship psychotherapy assessment form (SIRP-AF)*. Ottawa, Ontario. (Unpublished document).

Meier, A., Boivin, M., & Meier, M. (2006). The treatment of depression: A case study using theme-analysis. *Counselling and Psychotherapy Research: Linking Research with Practice*, *6*(2), 115–125.

Messer, S., & Wolitzky, D. L. (2007). The traditional psychoanalytic approach to case formulation. In T. D. Eells (Ed.), *Handbook of psychotherapy case formulation* (pp. 67–104). New York: Guilford.

PDM Task Force. (2006). *Psychodynamic diagnostic manual*. Silver Spring, MD: Alliance of Psychoanalytic Organizations.

Porzelius, L. K. (2002). Overview. In M. Hersen & L. K. Porzelius (Eds.), *Diagnosis, conceptualization, and treatment planning for adults: A step-by-step guide* (pp. 3–12). Mahwah, NJ: Lawrence Erlbaum.

Sturmey, P. (2009). Case formulation: A review and overview of this volume. In P. Sturmey (Ed.), *Clinical case formulation: Varieties of approaches* (pp. 3–30). New Jersey: John Wiley & Sons.

Watzlawick, P., Weakland, J., & Fisch, R. (1974). *Change: Principles of problem formation and problem resolution.* New York: Norton.
Weerasekera, P. (1993). Formulation: A multiperspective model. *Canadian Journal of Psychiartry*, *38*(5) 351–358.
Weerasekera, P. (1996). *Multiperspective case formulation: Steps towards treatment integration.* Malabar, Florida: Krieger Publishing Co.

## Appendix 4.1: Self-in-Relationship Psychotherapy Semi-structured Assessment Interview (SIRP-SSAI)

**Augustine Meier, Ph.D. and Micheline Boivin, M.A. Ottawa, Ontario 2021**

The assessment interview used by Self-in-Relationship Psychotherapists does not differ that much from the assessment interview used by professionals of other orientations. The notable difference is that a Self-in-Relationship Psychotherapist focuses more on the development of the sense of self and the quality of relationships across time and persons beginning with the childhood experiences and extending to current relationships. The assumption is that many presenting problems are relational and self in nature. Special attention is paid to the nature and quality of relationships that the client has be it with parents, siblings, people at work, peers, etc. These relationships are explored with reference to how they were then and how they are now, repeated patterns, typical problems that emerge, how one sees the other and self in these relationships, how one feels about self with reference to these relationships, how one deals with relational problems, resources to turn to, etc.

Using the topics of a typical assessment interview, suggested questions are offered for each topic within the context of SIRP perspective. The questions that are keyed to each topic are to be considered only as guidelines. Often the client offers the information spontaneously and therefore there is no need to ask the questions. One must adapt oneself to the client and to the situation.



## Semi-Structured Assessment Interview (SIRP-SSAI)

1 *Reason for requesting counseling and the presenting problem:* The client contacting a therapist to seek help regarding a personal or interpersonal problem launches the therapeutic process. During the first 10 or 15 minutes, the therapist explores with the client the nature of the problem, its duration and intensity, its extensiveness, how it affects him/her, when the problem occurs and when it is more intensive, etc. Assuming that the client reports being *depressed*, one might ask the following exploratory and clarifying questions (for other problems replace depressed by that problem).

1a For how long have you felt this way?
1b When do you feel most depressed? How strongly do you experience this feeling?
1c Is there anything going on in your life now that might be related to you being depressed?
1d Have you felt depressed in the past? (If yes, explore the various episodes.)
1e Have you seen someone in the past because of your depression? (If yes, explore.)
1f Are you seeing anyone now for your depression? Who? How do you find this?
1g Have you ever thought it would be better not to be alive? Have you wished it? Have you thought of taking your life? (If yes, explore how it would be done, when and where. If no, inquire what it is that is keeping you going despite the difficulty.)
1h Are you on medication? (If yes, explore kind, dosage per day.)

2 *Appearance and behavioral observation:* The manner in which a person presents himself/herself and behaves in the therapy session can provide useful information regarding his/her mental state, coping strategies, relational style, and capacities. Typically, one asks questions about how the person presents himself/herself only when something stands out. How do you experience the client? What do you experience when with the client? What is the nature of the client's sharing of personal information? Is he or she open and forthright? Is the client retentive?
3 *Family background:* Information about one's family and childhood would include the relationship of the person to his/her father, mother, and siblings; the relationship of the parents to each other; the nature of the father and mother's work; the quality of the parents' relationship to their own families, their co-workers, friends, relatives, etc. The purpose is to gain an understanding as to how the person perceives his parents and himself and how the person feels about the parents and himself with reference to the parents. Having these goals in mind, one might ask the following questions (interspersed with empathic responding, etc.).

3a When you think of your childhood and teenage years with your family, what stands out most for you? Could you describe or say more.
3b What was it like for you to live in and be with your family?
3c How would you describe your relationship with your mother when you were a child? How is your relationship with your mother today? How would you describe your mother as a person?
3d Repeat question 3c for father, sibling, uncle, aunt, grandparent, and any other significant figure in the person's life.
3e (If there are siblings.) Where are you in the birth order? (Obtain

names and ages of sibling.) How do you get along with your sister (brother)? Say more.

3f How did your father (mother, sibling) feel about you? What did they think of you? How did you feel about the way they thought of you and felt about you?

3g As a child, who took care of you? If he/she was with a caregiver, inquire as to when this began, how often per week, and for how long. Where were the parents? Working? What was it like to be taken care of by others?

3h Have there been any deaths in your family? (If yes, could you say more, particularly how this affected you?) Any tragedies? Any serious illnesses? (Ask the person to say more about these and how he/she was affected by them.)

3i Have you experienced any abuse in your family? Mental abuse? Physical abuse? Sexual abuse? By whom? Say more about this.

3j Is there anything else about your family and your relationships with your father and mother that would be useful for me to know?

4 *Educational background:* In exploring a person's educational background pay attention to how well the person did in school, to his/her extracurricular activities, friends, peer groups, how well he/she related with the teacher, to his/her academic and career goals, etc. This information helps to understand how the person invested his/her energy, his/her enthusiasm and zest for life, academic aspirations and goals, etc. This information is helpful to understand the perceptions that he developed of others – peers, teachers – and of himself. The following questions may be helpful to obtain information for this domain.

4a How has school been for you? How well did you do in primary school? High school? College? University? How would you describe yourself as a student? Bright, average?

4b Did you take part in extracurricular activities? Which ones? How did you get started with this?

4c What were your favorite subjects?

4d Did you have friends at school? If yes, what did you do together? How did you get along with them? Do you still have friends from the school days?

4e How did you get along with your teachers? Tell me more.

4f Were there any drugs at school? Vaping? Where are you with that?

5 *Occupational background:* The level of the person's satisfaction with his/her work, the nature of his/her relationship with co-workers and supervisors, and quality of his/her work provides useful information regarding the person's sense of self, competency, adequacy, and quality of relationships. In obtaining information about this area, one might ask

the following questions. If the client is still going to school and has a part time job, adapt the questions to the situation.

5a What is the nature of your work? For how long have you done this kind of work? How are you enjoying your work?
5b For how long have you worked at your current place of employment? Have you worked at other places? Where? What made you change places of work?
5c How would you describe the working atmosphere of your current place of work?
5d How well do you get along with your co-workers? Do you prefer to work with men or with women? Alone? With others?
5e How would you describe your relationship with your supervisor?
5f Have you been promoted at your place of work? If yes, how is that for you? Do you have aspirations for the future? Could you say more about this?

6 *Social background:* A history of a person's social background provides information about his/her ability to relate to others, to get along, and to be in touch with reality. One might ask the following questions.

6a How is your social life? Do you have friends? What do you and your friends do when together? Do you like being with people? Are you able to be alone?
6b (If single) Do you have a boyfriend/girlfriend? Is this your first boy/girlfriend relationship? How is this like for you? Is this your first intimate relationship? When did you first date? What was that like for you?

7 *Marital and couple relations background:* Couple relationships are the most challenging of all relationships. Knowledge of this relationship provides information about a person's ability to be intimate, empathic and accepting; about his/her ability to integrate sexuality within the context of a set of values and one's own self-identity and self-acceptance; a person's ability to compromise, collaborate, resolve conflicts and to be altruistic. If the couple have children, how they relate with them, perceive, accept, and discipline them, etc., provide additional information about the parents. The following questions may be germane in securing information about this domain.

7a How are things between the two of you? (If they have problems, explore the duration, extent, intensity of the problems). Have you experienced these problems in the past? When? What has brought on the problems?
7b How would describe your relationship? How do you feel about that?

7c How do you go about resolving conflicts? Making compromises? Making decisions?
7d Are you able to count on each other? Are you there for each other?
7e How is your love life? Do you have difficulty in being intimate with each other? How? How often do you make love? Is there chemistry between the two of you? Do you want to be together?
7f (If they have children) How many children do you have? What are their gender and age? How would describe your relationship with your children? Their relationship with you?

8 *Health (physical and mental):* Inquire about the person's physical and mental health. If there have been ailments (physical and emotional) determine their duration, seriousness and what brought them on and ask if they have received treatment. If yes, what type of treatment and for how long. How satisfied were they with the treatment and with those providing the treatment? Has the person struggled with addictions: alcohol, medications, streets drugs, gambling, and so on.
9 *The experience of trauma:* Inquire whether the person has experienced traumas. If so, you can proceed with the following questions.

9a Tell me more about your experience.
9b How old were you when you experienced the trauma?
9c Was the traumatic event physical (e.g., car accident), relational, sexual?
9d Were you able to talk to someone about your traumatic experience?
9e Did you consult a professional regarding the trauma?
9f How is the traumatic experience affecting you today?

10 *The experience of abuse:* Inquire whether the person has experienced emotional, physical, and/or sexual abuse in the past. If so, follow up with these questions.

10a Tell me more about your abuse.
10b How old were you when the abuse occurred?
10c Who was (were) the offender(s) of the abuse?
10d Were you able to talk to someone about the abuse? Who?
10e How is the abuse affecting you today?
10f Have you consulted a professional to talk about the abuse? Who?

11 *Hobbies and leisure:* The ability to relax, play, have fun, and engage in creative projects and activities gives us information about how well the person has integrated external demands, internal pressures with the need to respond to one's wishes, desires, interests, etc. Leading questions to explore this topic may include:

11a How do you spend your free time? For how long have you been spending your free time this way? How do you feel using your time this way? (Notice whether or not he/she feels guilty and if so explore these.)

11b Are you able to sit down and merely do nothing? Do you have to do it for a purpose?

11c How does his hobby help you to take care of yourself, etc.?

12 *Sources of strength:* To assess a person's capacity to deal with current difficulties, that is, his or her resilience, it is helpful to obtain information concerning the place he/she turns to in time of difficulties (e.g., to another person, within, to a higher power, etc.). Questions that can be asked about this topic may include:

12a To where do you turn in times of difficulty for support and comfort? If the person states several sources, explore each as fully as possible. Be curious.

12b What is it about (this source) that helps you to feel better? (Explore fully.)

In concluding the interview ask the person whether there is anything else, that has not been covered, that would be good for the therapist to know to understand him/her better and be of assistance to him/her.

Chapter 5

# Self-in-Relationship Psychotherapy Assessment Form

This chapter presents the *Self-in-Relationship Psychotherapy Assessment Form (SIRP-AF)* to assess the constructs of Self-in-Relationship Psychotherapy and the *Operational Criteria and Coding Procedures and Guidelines* to code them (Meier & Boivin, 2013). The clinical material, in the form of a client's psychosocial history, to be coded is provided by the *Self-in-relationship psychotherapy semi-structured assessment interview (SSAI;* Meier & Boivin, 2011; Attachment 4.1, chapter 4). The use of the SIRP-AF assumes familiarity with The SIRP constructs.

The use of the Operational Criteria and Coding Procedures and Guidelines assures consistency in coding the SIRP constructs. The SIRP-AF has demonstrated very good interrater reliability the results of which are presented at the end of this chapter.

This chapter begins with a presentation of the SIRP-AF (Attachment 5.1, at end of chapter). This is followed by guidelines for using the SIRP-AF. The next part presents the operational criteria and coding procedures to be used when coding the SIRP constructs. For each of the constructs, there is a brief conceptual definition and description followed by procedures to code it. The last part provides the results from the interrater agreement studies.

## The SIRP Assessment Form

To use the SIRP-AF, it is important to carefully read and study it and become familiar with its structure and with the constructs to be coded. The SIRP constructs were presented in detail in chapter 3 and will only be briefly presented here.

On the first page of the SIRP-AF are to be entered biographical information including name, age, gender, and marital status. It also provides instructions for using the SIRP-AF. On the second page are constructs for which written information is to be provided. On the third page, the examiner codes the constructs according to a continuum or according to the degree to which they are present or operative. The last page provides space for a conceptualization and for treatment suggestions.

DOI: 10.4324/9781003272502-7

## Coding Guidelines

In using the SIRP-AF and the Operational Criteria and Coding Procedures to assess client material, the examiner is reminded to pay attention to the following guidelines:

1 Read the protocol to be coded from beginning to the end in order to get a sense of the whole before beginning to code the constructs.
2 Read the protocol for the second time and underline parts of the protocol that relate to different constructs and note these constructs in the margin of the protocol.
3 As you read the protocol, imagine being the client and ascertain what this might feel like. The goal of this exercise is to enhance the ability for empathic understanding.
4 As you read the protocol, imagine what it would feel like to be with the client. This is to access your countertransference and learn how to use it effectively to understand the client. The purpose of this and the previous guideline is to deepen your emotional (intuitive) understanding of the client. Typically, our emotional knowing of the client precedes our conceptual knowing of the client and provides a context for conceptual knowing. The intuitive understanding and the conceptual understanding work together to form a holistic understanding of the client. It is very important to recognize the difference between one's own unfinished business from the feelings that emerge because of being with this person.
5 In coding a construct, compare or contrast it to other constructs to assess for consistency of coding. For example, if one indicates that a dominant fear is abandonment, then it is logical that one might code for splitting, idealization, and devaluation as possible coping strategies.
6 When the information to code a construct is unavailable, make an inference from the available clinical material keeping in mind to assure consistency in coding and in conceptualization.
7 Using the SIRP-AF and the Operational Criteria, proceed to code the protocol for each of the SIRP theoretical constructs.
8 When the coding is completed, prepare the report which contains the conceptualization of the case and suggestions for therapy.

## Operational Criteria and Coding Procedures

Brief conceptual definitions are presented for each of the SIRP theoretical constructs. This is followed by operational definitions with examples and coding procedures for the theoretical constructs. It is to be noted that some constructs are coded on a 5-point scale continuum, other constructs are coded on a 5-point scale as to the degree of their striving quality, and the remainder constructs are checked off and/or rank ordered.

The Operational Criteria and Coding Procedures for the SIRP-AF (Meier & Boivin, 2013) have been modified for inclusion in this book. In using the Operational Criteria and the Coding Procedures, carefully read the psychosocial history of the client to get a sense of the client. The coding for the conceptual and operational definitions are presented in two parts, namely, one part for the descriptive data and a second part for the scaled data.

## Part I: Descriptive Data

The client's psychosocial history provides the clinical material for the analysis of his unmet needs, mental representations, and affect. These three classes of data are seen as comprising an interrelated cluster and are not seen in isolation from each other but as forming one entity. Although the "other" is often referred to as father or mother, "other" might refer to any significant person in the client's life such as uncle, aunt, and grandparent for example.

The descriptive data present the client's perception and feelings of himself and of the significant persons of his childhood. The data provide a picture of the atmosphere of the home environment in which the individual was raised and what it was like to have lived with others in the home of his childhood. These experiences also provide information how the child might have responded to them and tried to make sense of them, which is reflected in his perceptions of others and self. It is assumed that the manner in which these experiences were perceived and internalized continue to impact a person's relationships and day-to-day living. In this part, the examiner is asked to describe the unmet needs, mental representations of significant others and of self, the affects linking these representations, and the quality of his/her childhood interactions and experiences with his/her caregivers.

### *Organizing Unmet Core Relational, Self, and Physical Intimacy Needs*

**Definition and description:** The term unmet core needs refer primarily to those needs not adequately responded to during infancy/childhood and which continue to linger and push for fulfillment in adolescence and adulthood. The core needs are grouped according to core relational, self and physical intimacy needs (see Chapter 3). Relational needs refer to the need to be emotionally connected and the need to be autonomous (Mahler et al., 1975). Self needs refer to the need to be competent and the need to be significant (Kohut, 1977). Physical intimacy needs include the need for sensual contact and for sexual intimacy.

**Operational definition and coding procedure:** Operational definitions are given for each set of core needs taken separately. With regards to the unmet core needs, code these using, as much as possible, the names of the needs included in the Taxonomy of Needs, namely, connection (emotional bonding), autonomy (individuation), competency, significance, sensual contact, and sexual intimacy.

With reference to needs, one codes for the person's striving such as striving to be competent and striving to feel significant. One codes for the strength of this striving and not for its state or presence within an individual. Examples are provided for each set of needs.

The first set of unmet core needs are the two relational needs, that is, the need for emotional connection and the need for autonomy. The need for emotional bonding can be expressed in terms of words or in terms of a feeling or fear of being abandoned, rejected, cut-off, and not considered to be important. The need for autonomy can be expressed in terms of wanting to have a voice in matters that affect him.

*Examples:*

1 I want you to spend more time with me, I am lonely without you, I miss you, I need more quality time together (Need for emotional bonding)
2 I need to spend time alone, I need to have time to do my things, you are impinging upon my life and my freedom (Need for autonomy).

The second set of unmet needs are the two self needs, namely, for significance and competency which are manifested when a person seeks affirmations for them. Examples of these needs are the following.

*Examples:*

1 I just want to be told that I am okay, that you still care for me, that you accept me for who I am (Need for significance)
2 I do all of these things. I run a million-dollar business. I organize charities. I organize all of our vacations, and yet I do not hear a word of appreciation from you how well I am doing (Need for competency).

The third set of unmet core needs are the need for sensual contact and the need for sexual intimacy. The need for sensual contact includes those behaviors that involve touch (e.g., physical closeness, touch, hugging, kissing, and so on) but not with the intent of sexual intimacy. The need for sensual contact also includes those behaviors where there is no touch, but a wanted physical presence (e.g., to be in the same space but not engaged in touch).

*Examples:*

1 I need to be held, touched, and cuddled. We don't do enough of that anymore. We used to do a lot of that when we first dated, but we lost it (Need for sensual contact)

2 The last time that we had sex was three months ago. I need to have sex; a person needs to have sex (Need for sexual intimacy).

When the relational, self, and physical intimacy needs are not adequately satisfied in infancy and early childhood, the person may strive continuously to seek them in adolescence and adulthood. These needs become the organizing principle around which the person might live his life. It is important to differentiate unmet needs of the past from unmet needs appropriate to current relationships. These are referred to as unmet childhood needs and unmet growth needs, respectively.

### *Internal Representation of Other*

**Definition and description:** The internal representations of the other are cognitive and affective images formed from the infant/child's experience with significant caregivers (Klein, 1959). The representations can bear a positive, negative, or a mixed positive/negative valence. Representations are not to be confused with the feelings that one has for others. It is important to understand the nature and quality of the clients' representations of the significant other that were formed in childhood as these representations may persist into adult life. The representation that one has of others is intimately related to having or not having his early core childhood needs positively responded to.

**Operational definition and coding procedure:** A mental image that a person has of the other might be that he is weak, sad, and sensitive or the individual is domineering, cruel, strong and responsible. When identifying a person's internal representations of others, the focus is on the mental and affective image and not on how the person feels about the other or in the way the other is needed. The mental picture of a person may correspond to how the person is like in real life or it may deviate from it in some dramatic fashion.

*Examples:*

1 My father was self-centered, controlling; it was always about him and about no one else. He was heartless (Negative internal representation of father)
2 My mother was caring, did crafts with us, took us to the park, she was fair with us, and yet she expected that we participate in household chores (Positive internal representation of mother).

### *Internal Representation of Self Relative to Other*

**Definition and description:** The internal representation of self is a cognitive and affective image of self formed from the infant/child's interactions with significant caregivers (Klein, 1959). The mental representation formed about self is very much influenced by the quality and nature of the parents' responses to his needs, feelings and behaviors. These self-representations might include seeing one as lovable, competent, wanted, and intelligent or their opposites.

**Operational definition and coding procedure:** The focus when identifying the mental representation of self is on the image or picture that the child has of himself and not on how he feels about himself or on his needs.

*Examples:*

1 With my father, I was never good enough, was not smart enough, I was the dumb and the clumsy one in the family (Negative internal representation of self with regards to father)
2 My mom helped me to realize that I was good at drawing, painting, doing crafts (Positive internal representation of self with regards to mother).

### Affect Linking Representation of Other to Self

**Definition and description:** This refers to the feeling that the individual perceives the other (e.g., parents) to have had toward him when he was an infant/child (Kernberg, 1976; Masterson, 1976).

**Operational definition and coding procedure:** The linking affect represents the emotional response of the parents toward the client when he was an infant or child, but from the perspective of the client which might or might not correspond to the way things were in reality. For example, the client might have felt that his parents felt frustrated, sad and angry toward him but they might not have felt that way in reality.

*Examples:*

1 My dad was constantly criticizing me, was impatient with me. He did not like me because I was not as smart as my older brother (Father's negative feelings toward child)
2 My mother was affectionate, loving, and caring. She would at times become angry with us, but we always knew that she loved us (Mother's positive feelings toward her child).

### Affect Linking Representation of Self to Other

**Definition and description:** This construct describes the feelings that the client, as an infant or child, had toward a significant caregiver and which he might still have today (Kernberg, 1976). Again, this is the client's feeling of the situation.

**Operational definition and coding procedure:** The linking affect represents how he felt about the significant persons in his infancy/childhood. For example, the client might have been frustrated with and angry toward his parents or he might have been happy, content, and cheerful when with them. The client might experience the same feelings toward his parents today. It is important to differentiate old (familiar) feelings related to past experiences from new feelings that are associated with current experiences with others.

*Examples:*

1 My father's criticisms hurt me so much that I hated him and I am angry at him and I have no feelings for him (Child's negative feelings toward his/her father)
2 I love my mother; she has always tried to be helpful and to make things pleasant for the family and for me (Child's positive feelings toward his/her mother).

### How I Feel/Felt When in the Presence of the Other

**Definition and description:** This dimension assess how the person felt when in the presence of the significant other such as father and mother.

**Operational definition and coding procedure:** The person as an infant/child might have felt safe and secure or he might have felt tense, afraid and insecure when with a significant other such as father and mother. The person might still feel this way about being with the other today.

*Examples:*

1 When I am with my father, I felt very tense and anxious because I didn't know what he is going to criticize me for next. I walked on egg shells when around him (Negative feeling in presence of father)
2 I felt safe and secure and protected when I was with my mother; I also felt proud of myself (Positive feeling in presence of mother).

### Quality of Being Parented

**Definition and description:** This refers to the infant/child's experience of being parented and of being brought up by his parents (Winnicott, 1965).

**Operational definition and coding procedure:** This construct touches areas of concern in parenting such as: Was parenting consistent and free of conflict and violence? Was there structure in the home? Did the person feel encouraged to develop his abilities and potentialities? Was there sufficient freedom for the child to be himself and have time for fun and to play? Did the person feel that he was a significant part of the family and made a meaningful contribution to the family? Did the person feel safe, secure, and protected?

It is assumed that if these early relationships were satisfying and the infant/child blossomed within context of these relationships, the infant/child will have a positive view of himself and of others and acquire the skills to deal the day-to-day challenges of life. However, if the infant/child's experiences of others (i.e., caregivers) were more negative in that the caregivers might have been emotionally neglectful and cold and there was a lack of structure and lack of love, caring and support, the individual's experience would have been negative.

*Examples:*

1 My home life was chaotic; my mother was depressed; my father was on drugs and was unemployed; there was no food in the fridge; they shouted and screamed at each other; we were left to ourselves; my home was oppressive (Depriving and emotional neglecting parenting)
2 Living with my parents and older sister was okay; my parents were immigrants and worked hard to have money to buy their first house; we often celebrated with my relatives; there was music, singing, and a lot of food (Good enough parenting).

## Part II: Scaled Data

The results from the scaled data provide a picture of the person's inner world that was formed in large part through his interactions with significant others. The inner world is composed of memories, affects, motives, image, perceptions, and sensations that influence, to a great extent, how the person processes incoming information and shapes his interactions with others and with the world.

This part consists of the SIRP constructs that are assessed either on a five-point scale or are checked off as being present in the clinical material. The conceptual definitions of these constructs were presented earlier in detail and the operational definitions for these constructs are provided in the Operational Criteria presented later.

In general, when scoring the following dimensions in terms of the extent to which they describe the client's experience or the strength/extent to which they are present, consider whether the dimension lies to the left or right of the mid-point on the 5-point scale. You can also begin by eliminating categories or ratings that do not fit and then determine which of the remaining ratings or categories best describe the client's experience and behavior and/or your inference of these. Use as a point of reference clients with whom you have worked. The scores you assign to the various dimensions are based on your inference that is grounded on the material reported in the client's psychosocial history.

### *Manner of Relating to Significant Others*

**Definition and description:** This dimension address the manner in which an individual relates to others. When an individual relates to the other as the individual needs them (e.g., for advice, emotional support), the other is referred to as a part-object. When the individual relates to the other as someone who has needs, feelings, and thoughts and a life of his own, the other is referred to as a whole-object (Klein, 1952).

**Operational definition and coding procedure:** In rating the manner in which an individual relates to a significant other (caregiver) take into consideration how the individual generally related to her father, mother, or sibling. Does the person relate to the significant other as he or she is needed (i.e., part-object) or as a differentiated person (i.e., whole-object)? On the 5-point continuum, 1 = part-object, and 5 = whole-object, a score of 3 indicates that the person might at one time relate to the other as a part-object and at another time relate to the person as a whole-object.

*Examples:*

1 My mom and I always got along well; when I came home from kindergarten, she made lunch for us and asked about my day; today, we are like friends (Relates to her mother as whole-object)
2 My mother was an alcoholic; when I came home from kindergarten and grade school, she was lying on the floor drunk; I had to prepare the meals for her; today I still crave for the love that she never gave me and I also hate her for not having been a mother to me; I need a mother (Relates to her mother as a part-object).

### *Psychic Organization*

**Definition and description:** The construct, psychic organization, comprises the internalized demands and expectations of others and the world, his own innate needs, and an agent (reason) to negotiate these needs. Freud's (1923) concept of the psychic organization includes the concepts of the Id, Ego, and Superego. The id includes all of that which is inherited (e.g., instinct) and that which has been repressed because it was unacceptable. The superego comprises the conscience and the ego-ideal. The ego comprises defensive and adaptive functions.

The Freudian concept of the psychic organization has been slightly modified. Freud's concept of the id has been expanded. The two instincts, libido and aggression, have been replaced by four core needs, namely the needs for emotional bonding, sensual contact, autonomy, and sexual intimacy. These four needs are symbolized, respectively, as EB, SC, AU, and SI.

Freud's concept of the superego refers to both acceptable and unacceptable behaviors and to ideals and values to live by. Freud referred to these as the conscience and ego ideal, respectively. SIRP adopted Freud's notion of the superego, however, the coding is only for the conscience which is characterized by a sense of duty and obligation and includes acceptable and unacceptable social behaviors. A sense of duty and obligation are not to be confused with ideals and values to live by. There is a sense of freedom in choosing to live by one's ideals and values whereas in living by duty and obligation there is not the same sense of freedom. The superego can be severe and harsh, moderate, or non-existent.

Freud's concept of ego has been extended to include, in addition to a defensive function, also an adaptive function. The defensive function of the ego has the purpose to protect the person from anxieties and conflicts, particularly, internal conflicts, and to maintain self-esteem. The adaptive functions of the ego include the capacities to negotiate, compromise, accept, forgive, repair relationships, to mention a few. The energy of the ego's adaptive functioning is more creative than the energy used in defensive functioning. In coding the ego, one takes into consideration the ego's global capacity to mediate the person's core needs, the demands of the superego and of the external realities

The structures of the psychic organization are in constant interaction with each other but one structure (e.g., superego) might be dominant at one time and the others are latent. The configuration of the psychic organization affects the development of personality and relationships. For example, if in an individual the superego dominates, such a person might be demanding of self and might also be demanding and controlling of others.

**Operational definition and coding procedure:** The task of the coder is to assess the degree to which the client's psychic organization is in harmony, that is, the degree to which the ego has integrated the demands of the superego, the relational, self, and physical intimacy needs and demands of reality. Each part (e.g., superego) of the psychic organization is scored according to a 5-point scale where 1 means that the part (e.g., AU) is minimally striving for satiation and 5 means that it is actively striving for satiation. The score assigned to a specific aspect is meaningful only when it is considered in relationship to the scores assigned to the other parts.

In the case of an ego organization that is in harmony with itself, scores of 3–5 might be assigned to each of the parts depending upon the level of energy and passion. The greater the energy, striving and passion, the higher the assigned scores. For a psychic organization that is demanding, self-critical, self-punitive, oppressive, and moralistic and at the same time striving intensely for emotional connection, one might assign a value of 4.5 for superego, a 3.5 for EB, and a 2.5 for ego. In this case the person is characterized as having a domineering superego and need for emotional bonding that is suppressed but is pushing to be realized and an ego that is weakened. In the case of a psychic organization that results in aggressive, promiscuous and violent behavior, one might give a score of 4–5 for SC, a 1–2 for superego, and a 2–3 for ego depending on the ego's ability to regulate affect and impulses. For a psychic organization that is characterized by logical thinking and practical concerns, one might assign a score of 4 to the ego, 2–3 for EB, and a 2–3 to superego.

*Examples:*

1 I am in a constant state of conflict with an inner voice telling me to continue to do the right things and not to give into my craving to take another drink and at times I find both the voice and my craving overpowering and I want to go to bed (Possible coding: Superego = 4; EB = 4 and Ego = 2.5 since both the demanding voice and craving are strong and overpowering)
2 I don't give a darn what others think; I am not hurting anyone and I enjoy playing the slot machines; I have tried to stop and it didn't work, I just go back into it, I have given up trying (Possible coding: Superego = 3; AU = 4; ego = 3).
3 The one time that I can take time to play and try to relax is when I take the dog for a walk (because I should play with the dog); I find it a waste of time to watch TV; when I watch TV, I am reading for my work (Possible coding: Superego = 4; AU = 2; ego = 3 because the person is should, ought and performance driven).

### *Self-structure*

**Conceptual definition and description:** Human infants, generally, are born with a self already in place, that is, with a biologically determined psychological entity (Brinich & Shelley, 2002). The baby's self is a "virtual self" (Kohut, 1977, p. 101). The virtual or potential self is shaped by the child's interactions with his caregiver's sense of what self is and by the individual's reflections in context of the responses of others in his interactions with them. This evaluation is cognitive and affective in nature and is stored as an internal representation of self. According to Kohut (1977), these interactions lead to the organization of a self that comprises (a) a sense of competency and (b) a sense of self-esteem, and (c) a capacity to maintain a sense of competency and self-esteem at times of anxiety and stress. Thus, the self refers to both an embodied experience and the expression of oneself interpersonally in terms of one's storied (narrative) sense of self. Kohut's self-structure has been modified in that the sense of competency refers to a striving for competency and self-esteem refers to a striving for significance.

**Operational definition and coding procedure:** Each of the core self needs, need for competency and need for significance, is assessed on a 5-point scale as to the extent to which it is pressing to be responded to and is striving for satiation. A score of 5 means that the core need is greatly seeking to be responded to and a score of 1 means that it is minimally pressing to be responded to. The latter possibly means that it has been integrated and has already become an integral part of the person's sense of self. A score between 2.5 to 3.5 indicates that a person feels relatively competent and significant. With regards to the capacity to regulate competency and significance, which is similar to ego resources, a score of 1 indicates that the person lacks the capacity to maintain these two core needs, whereas a score of 5 indicates that the person has the capacity to maintain a sense of competency and significance.

*Examples:*

1 I feel so ashamed, I feel that I cannot do anything right, and when my partner treats me like a kid, I lose it (Possible coding: competency = 3.5, significance = 3.5 and capacity = 2 because the individual strives to feel competent and significance and has limited resources to maintain a sense of being competent and significance when he receives negative response from others)
2 I know myself and I try not to let what others think of me affect how I feel about myself and about my work and my importance to the company (Possible coding: significance = 3; competency = 3; capacity to maintain sense of competency and significance = 4, because the person's striving for competency and significance appears integrated, and he has the resources to maintain his sense of competency and significance despite the opinions of others).

### *Social Self*

**Definition and description:** This construct refers to the extent to which an individual organizes his life according to that which is integral, genuine and congruent with his sense of self and self-identity or whether the person lives from the expectations, values, wishes, and demands of others. The former is referred to as living from the True Self and the latter is referred to as living from the False Self (Winnicott, 1965).

**Operational definition and coding procedure:** To simplify coding on the True Self and False Self continuum, coding will only be for the True Self. From this code one can calculate the code for the False Self. In coding for True Self, use a 5-point scale where 1 indicates that the construct is minimally operative and 5 indicates that the construct is strongly operative.

*Examples:*

1 I just became a pleaser, I aimed to please the people around me, to impress people, and it was easier to do it that way than to speak for

myself. I don't like it, I want to get out of it and I keep slipping back into old patterns (Possible score, True Self = 1.5)
2 I just like to be me and not have to worry about what others think (Possible score, True Self = 4).

### *Defense Mechanisms and Coping Strategies*

**Definition and description:** Coping mechanisms serve the purpose to maintain and enhance an individual's self-esteem by managing conflicts, anxieties, and tensions (Freud, 1923). Every person uses a variety of defense mechanisms and the mechanism used depends on the issue dealt with. Persons who struggle with significant emotional problems tend to use a limited number of defenses repeatedly and rigidly.

Coping strategies can be thought of as being conscious such as negotiation, compromise, endearment, empathy, and problem solving and as being unconscious such as dissociation, splitting, denial, and repression. The pattern of coping strategies provides information regarding the nature of an individual's emotional problems and the age of their onset. The use of splitting and dissociation compared to the use of rationalization, indicates an earlier onset of the emotional problem. The brief definitions of the coping mechanisms are taken from White and Watt (1981), Kaplan and Sadock (1991), and Sadock et al. (2014).

1 Repression: the defense by which unwanted thoughts and feelings are kept out of awareness.
2 Dissociation: the inhibition or alteration of some aspect of consciousness or memory, such as observed in amnesias and fugue states.
3 Denial: the blocking out disagreeable realities or information by ignoring or refusing to acknowledge them.
4 Splitting: a developmental and defensive process of keeping incompatible feelings (e.g., love and hate) apart and separate as seen in idealization and devaluation.
5 Idealization: is the psychological process of coping with anxiety caused by ambivalent feelings by attributing overly positive and exaggerated qualities to another person or thing and negating negative qualities.
6 Devaluation: refers to the psychological process of coping with the anxiety caused by ambivalent feelings by attributing completely flawed, worthless exaggerated negative qualities to another person and discounting positive qualities.
7 Projection: is the unconscious tendency to attribute one's own unacceptable feelings, thoughts, and impulses to other persons or objects in the external world.
8 Introjection: the process of incorporating (without scrutiny) the characteristics of a person or object unconsciously into one's own psyche.

9 Displacement: is the conscious or unconscious substitution of an object (e.g., dog) for the appropriate object (e.g., person, place, thing) which is missing toward whom one expresses negative feelings.
10 Sublimation: entails the channeling of libidinal and aggressive energy into a socially approved mode of behavior.
11 Rationalization: means giving a probable reason for one's type of behavior.
12 Regression: refers to behavior where the individual reverts to a behavior more appropriate to an earlier stage of development or to reaction patterns long since outgrown.

**Operational definition and coding procedure:** Using the above definitions, select the pertinent mechanisms that constitute the person's defensive structure. The cluster of defenses will often comprise the more "primitive" defenses such as repression, dissociation, denial, splitting or the more advanced defenses (i.e., secondary defenses) such as rationalization, sublimation, reaction formation, displacement and so on.

Code the defense mechanisms that are repeatedly and rigidly used to deal with the same or similar issues. Indicate the defense mechanisms that are repeatedly and rigidly used by placing an X in the space preceding the defense mechanism. If one of the defense mechanisms stands out, indicate this by placing the number one ("1") in the space preceding the defense mechanism and place an X in the space preceding the other defense mechanisms. To assure yourself of the correct selection, determine whether your selection is supported by other concepts or structures such as the nature of the ego organization, self-structure, nature of object and self-representations and so on. If the client exhibits a defense mechanism not indicated on the form, add it as Other.

### *Quality of the Emotional Bond*

**Definition and description:** This construct refers to the quality of an infant/child's investment of psychic energy in another person on whom the individual would normally rely for safety, security, nurturance, stability, and comfort (Mahler et al., 1975). It refers to the degree to which an infant/child feels emotionally connected to and emotionally anchored in the significant other. The quality of an infant/child's emotional bonding reflects the extent to which the caregiver spontaneously responded to the infant/child's feelings and core relational, self, and physical intimacy needs.

The two essential components of an emotional bond are that the person's needs are satisfied and that the person is feeling comfortable, safe, and secure with that person. The former is referred to confident expectation and the latter as emotional anchorage (Mahler et al., 1975). Often the quality of the emotional bond manifests itself behaviorally, but the behavior does not define an emotional bond. The satisfaction of needs and positive feelings and living from them define an emotional bond. An emotional bond has more to do with the underlying dynamics that supports the behavior rather than with the behavioral manifestations as one can mimic a secure connection.

**Operational definition and coding procedure:** The quality of emotional bonding is assessed using the four categories – emotionally connected, striving for emotional connection, avoiding emotional connection, and emotionally disconnected.

1 To be *emotionally connected* means that the infant/child has developed a satisfying, secure, comfortable connection with the caregiver. This is due to the parent responding in a satisfying way to the infant/child's needs and feelings.
2 To *seek emotional connection* refers to eagerly searching for a meaningful, satisfying and comfortable emotional relationship with a significant other. This search for emotional connection often occurs when the caregiver is inconsistent in her responses or when the caregiver does not adequately respond to the infant/child's needs. This form of connection might manifest itself in emotional pursuit and entanglement with the expression of negative emotions when not achieved.
3 To *avoid emotional connection* refers to keeping emotionally distant from significant others. This might happen when the parent is overbearing and demanding and does not allow the infant/child space to be himself, or when being emotionally close is too painful and the infant/child avoids getting emotionally close to another.
4 *To be emotionally disconnected* refers to having no emotional feeling for the other and is emotionally cut off from them. This may the result when the infant/child, after many attempts to emotionally connect, experiences continued rejections and hostilities which bring about feelings of hurt, anger and cut-off.

In terms of coding, simply indicate which of the four categories describes the person's emotional bond with significant others. Place an X in the space preceding the category.

*Examples:*

1 I have no feeling for my mom, I hate her and I don't care if I ever see her again (Emotionally disconnected).
2 I remember when I was very young, I would follow mom around the house, I wanted her to talk to me, play me with, and hold me; I just

wanted to be with her but she did not have the time; I still seek her attention (Seeking emotional connection).

3 When I was very young, I did not want anyone to hold me, touch me, or get close to me; when they touched me, I felt violated (Avoiding emotional connection).

### Object Constancy

**Definition and description:** Object constancy refers to maintaining a libidinal (i.e., affectionate) connection with a significant other whether the person is present or absent. Object constancy refers to a mental representation of a positive libidinally cathected inner image of caregiver (Mahler et al., 1975).

From another perspective, object constancy is the "capacity to recognize and tolerate loving and hostile feelings toward the same object; the capacity to keep feelings centered on a specific object; and the capacity to value an object for attributes other than its function of satisfying needs" (Mahler et al., 1975). It implies that the good and bad object have been unified into one whole representation. The presence of object constancy permits the child to function separately in familiar surroundings despite moderate degrees of tension and discomfort and acts as an agent to self-comfort and self soothe.

Within the context of psychotherapy, one can see the formation of object constancy by the client saying to himself, when troubled, what would my therapist say about the situation. One can also observe this when a client writes down a therapist's saying be it about values or behaviors. These behaviors indicate the gradual formation of object constancy where the person internalizes the values, ideals and functions (i.e., skills and capacities) of the therapist.

**Operational definition and coding procedure:** Object constancy refers to the formation of an internal representation of a significant other formed from their positive interactions. The internal representation provides an emotional psychological home to which the person can turn to have a different perspective on an issue, to comfort and soothe oneself and find a way to uplift oneself when emotionally challenged or troubled. On the five-point scale, place in X in the space before the appropriate selection.

*Examples:*

1 When my boyfriend goes out with the guys to watch the Super-bowl and if he does not come home before midnight, I feel lonely, get enraged, want to end the relationship (Object constancy minimally developed and is mostly absent),

2 Even though I cannot see her as often as I would like to because she is busy with school work and family, I know that she loves me and that is reassuring and comforting (Object constancy fully developed and is present).

### *Characteristic Emotional State*

**Definition and description:** This refers to an individual's characteristic mood or emotional state which is typically brought about by a persistent dissatisfaction in not having one's primary relational, self and physical intimacy needs met when young. A characteristic emotional state might be that of anger, anxiety, sadness, and/or depression. The emotional state when carried into adulthood might manifest itself in periodic bouts with overwhelming emotions which can easily be triggered by experiences resembling those of childhood. The telling sign of a characteristic emotion is that it is a familiar emotion and has been part of the person's life since childhood and it is disproportionate to the event that precipitated it.

**Operational definition and coding procedure:** When coding for the characteristic emotional state, consider the emotion that a person has carried across time and across persons. Differentiate the characteristic emotion from an emotion triggered by a current event. For example, if a person easily becomes angered, consider whether the person is angry because of a current situation or whether the person has an underlying emotion such as anger. In such cases, one could identify anger as a characteristic emotion. Code only for one characteristic emotion.

*Examples:*

1 I have been depressed for the past month; I often felt depressed as a teenager; I think that I have been depressed all my life (Depression is the characteristic feeling).
2 When I play hockey and a guy slashes me on the shins, I become enraged and slash him back twice as hard; I felt the same way toward my dad, when as a child, he forced me and my brother to fight each other until we were hurt (Rage is the characteristic emotion).

### *Projective Identifications*

**Definition and description:** These are compulsive and repetitive relational patterns driven by underlying unmet core needs which have as their purpose to establish and maintain relationships and to influence the nature of these relationships (Klein, 1959). The manner in which clients perceive themselves (e.g., helpless; unlovable) and how they perceive others (e.g., powerful; admirable) influences the nature and quality of their relationship. The common forms of projective identification include playing the role of the helpless and dependent person (Dependency), portraying oneself as being more competent than the partner (Power), laying on guilt trips to get the needed response from the other (Ingratiation), and arousing a sexual experience in the other (Sexuality) (Cashdan, 1988).

**Operational definition and coding procedure:** Identify the dominant projective identification (PI) and place a check mark in the box next to it. If there are two or more PIs rank order them with 1 = most prominent, 2 = second most prominent, and so on.

*Examples:*

1 She just doesn't get it; the baby was crying for 20 minutes and then she asks me to bring the bottle of milk from the fridge; couldn't she figure it out that maybe the baby was hungry (Possible coding is PI of Power since he gives the impression that he knows more about child care than his partner)
2 My daughter is so selfish. When she needs to have something repaired, I do it right away. When I asked her to pick up something at the store – and she was next to it – she said that she had no time. I became angry at her and told her how I gave up my time to do things for her and that she could do something for me (Possible coding is PI of Ingratiation as the mother's behavior elicits the feeling that the daughter owes the mother something in return for her deeds)
3 My girlfriend gets angry at me when I ask her to take care of paying the bills because she is good at finance and budgets and I am not; I rely on her. In my home my mother took care of the finances (Possible coding is PI of Dependency because the guy seems to be looking for a caretaker).

### *Characteristic (Developmental) Phase*

**Definition and description:** The term phase refers to one of the pre-oedipal phases of which the Symbiosis, Practicing, Differentiation, Rapprochement and Consolidation/object constancy subphases are significant (Mahler et al., 1975). Each of the subphases has specific developmental tasks that need to be completed. The developmental task for each subphase is presented in the third chapter (Figure 3.2). The developmental task of the symbiosis phase, for example, is for the infant/child to emotionally bond with the mother. For the differentiation subphase it is for the child to psychologically separate and establish "me" and a "not-me." The developmental task of the practicing subphase is for the child to explore the non-mother world, to practice its new cognitive and motor skills, and to make choices as to the toys it likes and dislikes which is the foundation to making a commitment. The rapprochement subphase comprises many developmental tasks including the establishment of boundaries and object constancy, relating to people in their own right, regulating affect, and replacing the mechanism of splitting by repression, to mention a few. When the developmental tasks of a subphase are not adequately negotiated (i.e., completed), the person will push to complete them in adolescence and adulthood.

Failure to complete the developmental tasks of a specific subphase can have significant implications for development in adolescence and adulthood. The failure can begin at: (1) the Symbiotic phase if the infant does not become emotionally anchored; (2) the Differentiation subphase if the infant/child has not psychologically separated and individuated; (3) the Practicing subphase if the toddler does not have opportunity to try out his newly acquired cognitive and motor skills and explore his external world; (4) the Rapprochement subphase if intense fears of fusion and isolation (abandonment) interfere with leaving the nest and becoming one's own person; and at (5) the Consolidation and Object Constancy Phase if the individual failed to work out a balance between being connected to the love object and being his/her own person and having internalized good objects to whom to turn to self-comfort.

**Operational definition and coding procedure:** Identify the developmental tasks that the person has not completed or wishes to complete. Indications that an individual has not completed the developmental tasks specific to a subphase are: (1) Symbiotic subphase: the individual insatiably yearns for emotional connection, for closeness, for intimacy, is dependent upon the other, is not able to move toward psychological separation and autonomy and is in search of the unreachable; (2) Differentiation subphase: the person is enmeshed or seeks a dependent relationship and the ME and Not-ME are not clearly established; (3) Practicing subphase: the individual has no life of his own, does not know what he wants to do, is not committed, has no practical ambitions in life, fears taking risks, is not adventuresome, feels inadequate, has an insatiable need to prove himself as being competent; (4) Rapprochement subphase: the individual has great difficulty to negotiate and compromise, throws "adult" temper tantrums when things do not go his way, wants others to take part in his activity but is not ready to participate in the activities of others, is not able to wait, has low frustration tolerance, not able to establish boundaries, has not developed object constancy and capacity to self-soothe, and (5) Consolidation and Object Constancy: the individual has failed to establish boundaries between self and other, to replace splitting by repression, to achieve libidinal object constancy and the ability to regulate affect.

To determine the specific developmental tasks that an individual has not completed, ask the question: Is the person in constant pursuit of connection which means the symbiotic phase? Does the person resist psychologically separating from the caregiver which might indicate that the differentiation subphase characterizes his subjective experiences, behaviors, and relational interactions? Is the person in pursuit of proving himself or feels inadequate which is characteristic of functioning at the practicing sub-phase? Is the person in a power struggle, emotionally unregulated, and manifests mood swings and boundary issues which characterizes functioning from the rapprochement sub-phase?

In terms of coding, indicate the subphase or subphases for which the developmental tasks were not achieved or are pushing to be satiated. Use a scale of one to five to indicate the degree to which the developmental tasks of a specific phase failed to be completed. Failures to complete the developmental tasks are easily recognized by their push to be satiated. On the five-point scale 1 = minimally achieved and 5 = greatly achieved. It is possible that the developmental tasks of two or more subphases have not been completed and best describe the persons behaviors and relational patterns.

*Examples:*

1 I don't know what I want to do in life. I don't like my work. I am not too crazy about school. My girlfriend wants me to make up my mind about our relationship. She wants an answer in three months. I am not able to commit myself to anything (Possible coding is the Practicing Phase because the individual, as a child, did not have opportunity to adequately explore alternatives and to experiment).
2 At the restaurant last evening, my boyfriend asked me to be his steady date. I became anxious, fearful, intruded upon, violated. I felt that I was losing myself. I disconnected, became enraged and ended up lying under the table in a fetal position (Possible coding is the Rapprochement Phase).
3 I am not interested in sex. I like to spend time together sitting on the couch, being held, cuddled, being next to each other, and watching TV. I don't get enough of him. (Possible coding is the Symbiotic Phase as there is an insatiable need for emotional closeness and sensual contact).

### *Characteristic (Developmental) Position*

**Definition and description:** Position refers to one's place on a continuum regarding two developmental positions (Klein). One position (Paranoid-Schizoid Position) represents an individual who is angry, uses splitting, sees others as part-objects, relates from self as a part-self, lacks empathy for others, and has not established boundary between self and other. The second position (Depression Position) represents an individual who has developed empathy, fears losing the love object, repairs injuries caused to the person loved, uses repression rather than splitting, is beginning to see others and self as whole persons, and has established boundaries between self and other. An infant/child's subjective experiences, behaviors and relational interactions may be characterized by the Paranoid-Schizoid Position because of inadequate parenting, the experience of mental, physical and sexual abuse, emotional neglect, and trauma.

**Operational definition and coding procedure:** Determine where the client is on the bi-polar developmental continuum. Use a 5-point scale to indicate at which end on the continuum the client is at with 1 = Paranoid Schizoid Position and 5 = Depressive Position. If the client clearly meets the criteria for the Paranoid Schizoid Position, assign a score between 1 and 3. If the client clearly meets the criteria for the Depressive Position assign a score between 4 and 5. If the client manifests characteristics of both the Paranoid Schizoid Position and the Depressive Position or fluctuates between the two positions, assign a value of 3.

*Examples:*

1 I truly regret the way that I treated the women that I dated in the past. They were good women; I was not ready for a committed relationship. I regret how I hurt them and I wish that I could say that to them (Possible coding is 4 because the individual expresses compassion for those he hurt and would like to repair the relationship).
2 When my partner asks me to put away my empty coffee mug and plate or to pick up after myself, I feel treated like a kid and I become so enraged. Does she not know that I have bigger things to do than to pick up dishes? She is like a sergeant major (Possible coding is 2 because he is easily triggered to rage, he has not integrated the good and bad representations, and is not able to comply to her wishes – he is short on empathy).

### *Level of Personality Organization*

**Definition and description:** SIRP views emotional problems in terms of personality organization and its underlying dynamics. It has modified Kernberg's (1976) approach by replacing the concept instinct by the core needs.

The level of personality organization is determined by the manner in which the core needs have been integrated, the quality of the superego (reasonable, severe, harsh), the nature of defenses used to deal with conflicts and anxieties, and by the quality of relationships that have been formed (Kernberg, 1976). Based on these criteria, three levels of personality organization have been identified. Briefly these are: (1) Higher-Level: core needs are integrated with genital primacy, superego is well integrated but severe, defenses are organized around repression, internalized objects are stable, and concept of other and self is well integrated. This level is manifested in neurotics; (2) Intermediate-Level: pre-genital fixations points are present, superego is less developed, defenses are organized around repression but some primitive defenses are present, internal objects are conflicted, ego identity is established and there is a stable concept of other and self. This level is manifested in passive-aggressive, sado-masochistic, narcissistic personalities; and (3) Lower-Level: there is a pathological condensation of genital and pre-genital strivings, predominance of pre-genital aggression, unintegrated and sadistic superego, primitive defenses that are organization around splitting, internalized part-objects, identity fusion and lack of object constancy. This level is manifested in borderline, schizoid, pre-psychotic, and antisocial personality disorders.

**Operational definition and coding procedure:** Using the above criteria, identify the appropriate level of personality organization and place a check mark in the space in front of it.

## Psychometric Characteristics of SIRP-AF

The psychometric characteristics of the SIRP-AF have been studied for the level of "inter-rater agreement" which represents "the extent to which the different judges tend to make exactly the same judgments about the same rated subject" (Tinsley & Weiss, 1975, p. 359). The authors suggest that when the researcher is interested in the absolute value of rating, or the meaning of the ratings as defined by the points on the scale, it is also important to report the inter-rater agreement on the ratings.

The method used to compute the extent of inter-rater agreement was the Lawlis-Lu chi-square (Lawlis & Lu, 1972). Tinsley and Weiss (1975) recommend that a significant chi-square be followed by a T-index to indicate whether the inter-rater agreement is high, moderate, or low. The T-index is expressed as a value ranging from −1 to +1. Positive values indicate the observed agreement is greater than chance agreement while negative values indicate that the observed value is less than chance agreement. A high T-index, as .85 or higher, indicates high inter-rater agreement whereas a low T-index, as .20 or lower, indicates low inter-rater agreement (Tinsley & Weiss, 1975, pp. 367–368).

Four studies were conducted to assess the level of inter-rater agreement the results of which were computed using the Lawlis-Lu chi-square and the T-index. For each study there were four post graduate therapists. They took the course in Self-in-Relationship Psychotherapy and therefore were well acquainted with its constructs. They were trained to use the SIRP-AF to code three protocols. For each of the protocols, they independently coded them, and then met for two hours to review their codes and arrived a consensus. Following the training, they were given a protocol which they independently coded.

The results from the studies were as follows (the degree of freedom for the chi-square was 1 for all four studies).

Study 1: chi-square = 108.91; $p < .001$; T-index = .90.
Study 2: chi-square = 98.46; $p < .001$; T-index = .86.
Study 3: chi-square = 129.00; $p < .001$; T-index = .93.
Study 4: chi-square = 98.46; $p < .001$; T-index = .86.

The results show that all chi-squares were significant beyond the .001 level and that the T-index values ranged from .86 to .93 indicating high and positive agreement among raters. The results, in brief, demonstrate that well trained coders can reliably use the SIRP-AF to code clinical material.

This chapter presented the Self-in-Relationship Psychotherapy Assessment Form (SIRP-AF), its Coding Guidelines and Procedures and the Operational Criteria. Research provided evidence that clinical protocols can be reliably coded using the SIRP-AF. The following chapter demonstrates how a clinical protocol can be assessed using the SIRP Assessment Form.

## References

Cashdan, S. (1988). *Object relations therapy: Using the relationship*. London, UK: W.W. Norton & Company.

Brinich, P., & Shelley, C. (2002). *The self and personality structure: Core concepts in therapy*. Buckingham, England: Open University Press.

Freud, S. (1923). The ego and the id. *Standard Edition, 19*, 12–63.

Kaplan, H. I., & Sadock, B. J. (1991). *Synopsis of psychiatry: Behavioral sciences clinical psychiatry*. Sixth Edition. London: Williams & Wilkins.

Kernberg, O. (1976). *Object relations theory and clinical psychoanalysis*. New York: Aronson.

Klein, M. (1952). Some theoretical conclusions regarding the emotional life of the infant. In Melanie Klein (Ed.) (1975), *Envy and gratitude and other works 1946–1963* (pp. 61–93). London: Delcorte Press/Seymour Lawrence.

Klein, M. (1959). Our adult world and its roots infancy. In *Envy and gratitude and other works, 1946–1963* (pp. 247–263). London, UK: Hogarth Press.

Kohut, H. (1977). *The restoration of the self*. New York: International Universities Press.

Lawlis, G. F., & Lu, E. (1972). Judgment of counseling process: Reliability, agreement and error. *Psychological Bulletin, 78*, 17–20.

Mahler, M. S., Pine, F., & Bergman, A. (1975). *Psychological birth of the human infant*. New York: Basic Books.

Masterson, J. F. (1976). *Psychotherapy of the borderline adult: A developmental approach*. New York: Brunner/Mazel Publishers.

Meier, A., & Boivin, M. (2011). *Counselling and therapy techniques: Theory and practice*. London: SAGE.

Meier, A., & Boivin, M. (2013). *The operational criteria and coding procedures for SIRP assessment form*. Unpublished manuscript. Ottawa, Ontario.

Meier, A., & Boivin, M. (2021a). *Self-in-relationship psychotherapy semi-structured assessment interview (SSAI)*. Ottawa, Ontario. Unpublished document.

Meier, A., & Boivin, M. (2021b). *Self-in-relationship psychotherapy assessment form (SIRP-AF)*. Unpublished manuscript. Ottawa, Ontario.
Sadock, B. J., Sadock, V. A., & Ruiz, P. (2014). *Kaplan and Sadock's synopsis of psychiatry. Behavioral sciences clinical psychiatry*. 11th Edition. New York: Walter Kluwer.
Tinsley, H. E. A., & Weiss, D. J. (1975). Interrater reliability and agreement of subjective judgments. *Journal of Counseling Psychology*, *22*(4), 358–376.
White, R., & Watt, N. F. (1981). *The abnormal personality*. Chichester, West Sussex, England: Whiley & Sons.
Winnicott, D. (1965). *The family and individual development*. London: Tavistock Publishers.

## Appendix 5.1: Self-in-Relationship Psychotherapy Assessment Form (SIRP-AF)

Augustine Meier, Ph.D. and Micheline Boivin, M.A, Ottawa, Ontario, 2021.

Name: ____________________ DOB: _________ Tel: _____________
Address: __________________________ Email: __________________
Education ________________ Occupation______________________
Single ___; Married ___; Widow(er) ___; Separated ___; Divorced ___; Remarried ____
(Place a check mark in appropriate space(s))
Date: ______________ Analysis by: ___________________________

The development of Self-in-Relationship Psychotherapy Assessment Form (SIRP-AF) was influenced by theoretical constructs from Self-in-Relationship Psychotherapy. Its use, therefore, assumes familiarity with these concepts. The SIRP-AF has been designed specifically for clinicians to aid them in their understanding of the individual with whom they work and to facilitate their growth and development through appropriately planned and selected interventions.

The SIRP-AF comprises four parts. In Part I, the examiner is asked to provide descriptive data regarding the core self, relational, and physical intimacy needs influencing the person's behaviors and attitudes, the individual's representations of significant others and of self, the affects linking these representations, and the quality of his childhood interactions with his/her parents. Part II comprises scaled data regarding the manner of relating to others, psychic organization, self-structure, coping strategies, the quality of the emotional bond, object constancy, characteristic emotion, projective identifications, characteristic (developmental) phase, characteristic (development) position, and level of personality organization. In Part III, the examiner is asked to conceptualize the person's current problems in light of past and current experiences and events and the constructs from Self-in-Relationship Psychotherapy. The conceptualization typically includes precipitating, predisposing, perpetuating, and protective factors. Part IV presents the issues that need to be addressed in psychotherapy and indicates the form of therapy and possible interventions.

**Part I. Descriptive Data:** For each of the dimensions presented in the following table, provide descriptive material for the persons (e.g., mother and father) entered in the top row of the table. If other figures were or are important to the client's life (e.g., grandmother, stepfather, and so on), additional columns can be created and assessed for each topic under Dimension.



| *Dimension* | *Father* | *Mother* |
|---|---|---|
| 1 The striving of self, relational, and physical intimacy needs relative to: | | |
| 2 Internal representation of: | | |
| 3 Internal representations of self relative to: (How I view myself when with:) | | |
| 4 Affect linking representation of other to self: (How I felt my father, mother, etc. felt about me) | | |
| 5 Affect linking representation of self to other: (How I felt about my father, mother, etc.) | | |
| 6 How I felt/feel about being in the presence of: | | |
| 7 Quality or degree of good enough parenting: | | |

**Part II. Scaled Data:** Rate dimensions 1, 4, 7, and 11 on a 5-point scale. For dimensions 2 and 3 indicate the strength of each component using a 5-point scale with 1 = barely and 5 = greatly. For dimension 10, indicate the characteristic phase and indicate the strength of its presence using the 5-point scale as indicated earlier. For the remainder dimensions, check off those that are relevant. See Operational Criteria for more precise instructions. If the dimension is not relevant, leave the space blank. (PO = part object; WO = whole object; PSP = paranoid/schizoid position; DP = depressive position; EB = need for emotional bonding; SC = need for sensual contact; AU = need for autonomy; SI = need for sexual intimacy.)

| | | | | | |
|---|---|---|---|---|---|
| 1 Manner of relating to: | Father: _1 (PO) | 2 | 3 | 4 | 5_ (WO) |
| | Mother: _1 | 2 | 3 | 4 | 5_ |
| 2 Psychic- oganization | Core Needs: ___ EB<br>___AU | ___ SC<br>___ SI | ___ego | ___superego | |
| 3 Self-structure | __ striving for competency | | __ striving for significance | ___ capacity to maintain significance and competency | |
| 4 True self (Living from) | _1<br>Minimally | 2 | 3 | 4 | 5_<br>Strongly |
| 5 Coping mechanisms | ___ repression<br>___ denial<br>___ dissociation | ___ splitting<br>___ introjection<br>___ projection | ___ regression<br>___ sublimation<br>___ idealization | ___ devaluation<br>___ other<br>___ other | |
| 6 Quality of emotional bond | ___ emotionally connected | ___ striving for emotional connection | ___ avoiding emotional connection | ___ emotionally disconnected | |
| 7 Object constancy | _1<br>Not Formed | 2 | 3<br>Partially Formed | 4 | 5_<br>Fully Formed |
| 8 Characteristic emotional state | ___ angry<br>___ abandoned | | ___ anxious<br>___ smothered | ___ depressed<br>___ oppressed | ___ sad<br>Other___ |
| 9 Projective identifications | ___ dependency<br>___ other | ___ power | ___ ingratiation | ___ sex | |
| 10 Characteristic phase | ___ symbiosis | ___differentiation | ___ practicing | ___rapprochement | ___consolidation |
| 11 Characteristic position | _1<br>(PSP) | 2 | 3 | 4 | 5_<br>(DP) |
| 12 Level of personality organization | ___ higher | ___ intermediate | | ___ lower | |

**Part III. Conceptualization:** Prepare a conceptualization of the person's current problems using concepts from Self-in-Relationship Psychotherapy. This means to tell the client's story using the language of theory. The conceptualization links how the current problems and symptoms are related to predisposing, precipitating, perpetuating, and protective factors. The conceptualization is by nature abstract and hypothetical and not descriptive.

______________________________________________________________________

______________________________________________________________________

______________________________________________________________________

______________________________________________________________________

______________________________________________________________________

______________________________________________________________________

**Part IV. Treatment Aspects:** Based on your assessment, indicate the issues (e.g., splitting, caretaking, separation-individuation, abandonment, etc.) that need to be addressed in therapy and indicate primary therapeutic approaches and potential interventions.

______________________________________________________________________

______________________________________________________________________

______________________________________________________________________

______________________________________________________________________

______________________________________________________________________

______________________________________________________________________

Chapter 6

# Application of the SIRP Assessment Form – The Case of Colleen

The purpose of this chapter is to demonstrate the application of the Self-in-Relationship Psychotherapy Assessment Form (SIRP-AF) and its Operational Criteria and Coding Procedures (SIRP-OCCP) to the analysis of the contents from the psychosocial history of a young woman, Colleen.

The first part of this chapter presents the psychosocial history of Colleen. The second part presents the codes for the SIRP-AF constructs as derived from the psychosocial history. This is followed by an explanation for the codes given to the constructs. The fourth part demonstrates how to use the results from the analysis to formulate a conceptualization of her presenting problems and concerns and to plan treatment.

## Psychosocial History

Colleen sought counselling to overcome her depressed mood and sadness, to feel better in being away from home and to improve her university grades. She was enrolled in an art program in U.S.A. which took her away from home for the school year. She missed her family, felt alone and did poorly at school obtaining a C+ average. During the school year she visited her family about ten times and each time she left home to return to the college, she felt depressed and sad which she experienced about once every three weeks. During the assessment sessions, Colleen took a battery of psychological tests and background information was gathered using the semi-structured interview (Meier & Boivin, 2021; Appendix 4.A, Chapter 4).

### *Results from Psychological Tests*

On the Wechsler Adult Intelligence Scale (Wechsler, 1955), Colleen scored at the high average level of intelligence with her Verbal Score (e.g., arithmetic, vocabulary) and Performance Score (e.g., picture completion, object assembly) being relatively equal. The results from the Strong-Campbell Interest Inventory (Strong & Campbell, 1974) strongly indicated that her interests were in the area of the arts including music/dramatics, art, and writing.

DOI: 10.4324/9781003272502-8

The results from Minnesota Multiphasic Personality Inventory (Hathaway & McKinley, 1949) and the Personality Research Form (Jackson, 1974) suggest that Colleen can easily become intensely angry, argumentative, combative, and impulsive. She tends to seek attention, to blame others for her problems, to experience helplessness and to repress her feelings. She is lacking in curiosity and analytic interests and is somewhat limited in terms of insight into her own problems. The results from the Rorschach projective test (Klopfer & Davidson, 1960), Thematic Apperception Test (Bellak, 1993), and the House-Tree-Person Tests (Buck & Warren, 1992) suggest that Colleen often feels a lack of psychological warmth from family, feels inadequate and depressed, harbors guilt feelings, sees her social world as being bleak, has difficulty integrating her impulses (e.g., sensual, affection) with a set of values, and is conflicted. The positive qualities are that she is outgoing, charming, engaging, attentive, and sensitive.

## Background Information

Colleen, 20 years of age, came to therapy dressed in colorful attire and non-traditional hairdos. She wore broad brim hats (red, white, blue), colored high-heel shoes (green, red, and white), and tops, skirts, dresses, jeans of varied colors and styles. She was the kind of person who would not go unnoticed.

### *Family of Origin*

Colleen, the youngest of four girls, is closest to her youngest sister. She considers her sisters to be more talented and better than her, particularly the eldest sister.

Her father, a retired project manager for a large construction firm, was often home only for the weekends because his work took him to different parts of Canada. Her father set high standards for his children and expected them to be successful. She describes her father as being selfish, sly, and childish, controlling, and did not allow Colleen to be her own person. She is angry at her father and hates him for the times he has emotionally hurt and neglected her. He had the power to emotionally crush her for which she had no defenses. She felt that he had not given her anything. She recalled that when she was young, she approached her father to be close to him and that he was so unemotional and non-affectionate that she felt pushed aside. She did not feel close to her father who picked on her and favored her sisters.

Colleen's mother, in reality, brought up the children. She enforced the rules and standards. Colleen's mother was neither a sensual nor an affectionate person and kept distant from the children. It was important to Colleen that her mother provide precise feedback on her performance as a person so as to avoid being scolded by both the mother and the father. When Colleen experienced a fear of losing a relationship, she craved to be close to her mother whom she pictured as holding and rocking her and reassuring her that all will be well.

During her year at the art school, Colleen went home about ten times. She felt guilty as she thought that once you leave home, you should make it on your own and that she had to take care of herself. She could not expect her mother to continue to do things for her. These thoughts were painful for her.

Colleen set high standards for herself but often failed to live up to these self-imposed standards. In failing to live up to her standards, Colleen became confused, discouraged, down on herself, and depressed. She was suspicious and did not trust easily. She saw herself as a person who did not plan but liked to do things on the spur of the moment. She described herself as being like her father in that she has his temper and impatience.

### *Education*

Colleen completed secondary school and one year of college. She did poorly from Grades 9 to 12 but very well in Grade 13 winning a scholarship to attend an art school in the U.S.A. She found the first year at the art school boring and frustrating since she expected it to be like it was when she was in Grade 13. She began her second year but dropped out at the beginning of the year. She applied to other art schools, was accepted, and was enrolled.

Colleen's interest in art began while in grade school. Art was the subject at which she did the best; however, she was not the best student in art. While in grade school, an artist from the community came to the school to evaluate the art of the students. The artist picked the painting of one of Colleen's friends. This challenged Colleen to excel in art which she began to do in Grade 13. This led to her winning a scholarship to continue with art.

She described herself as a perfectionist. When doing art, she could not allow herself to play with her work, to experiment with it, and to restart it. At times painting did not come naturally, but she forced herself to paint. One of the reasons that Colleen found the first year at the art school difficult was because she did not receive clear feedback from her art teachers. This caused her to feel uncertain, indecisive and down on herself. Ironically, when she did receive feedback, she seldom accepted it wanting to do it her own way as she did not like to become dependent on others.

### *Work*

Colleen has limited work experience. During the summer following her first year at the school of art and during the first year of therapy, Colleen had a job at a clothing store. She did not get along well with the supervisor and resented being told to take her lunch break in the early afternoon.

*Social*

She tends to be a loner although she has one close female friend. She likes to spend her time alone watching T.V. or listening to music which is how she takes care of herself and how she escapes from the unpleasant. During the year at the art school, she lived with a roommate and went out only with her. By choice, she had no other friends.

She had difficulty with heterosexual relationships. She longed for intimacy but was afraid that in getting close to a guy her neediness would push him away and thereby she would lose him. Colleen said that she liked to charm guys and when they paid attention to her, she wanted no more from them. That is, she began to cool things and withdraw and be less interested. For her, the charming in itself brought on the desired pleasure.

She has a boyfriend who is very jealous and possessive of her and intrusive in wanting to know the things she did when at a party which she wanted to conceal from him. Although she found certain aspects of the relationship difficult, she could not leave him. At times she feared that because she was miserable toward him, she would lose him. When they had a conflict, she could not be assertive and open with him. Instead, she typically left the scene and spoke about it to him later.

## The Codes on the SIRP Assessment Form

The SIRP Assessment Form (SIRP-AF) and the Operational Criteria and Coding Procedures (OCCP) (Meier & Boivin, 2013) were used to analyze the information provided by the report of Colleen's psychosocial history. The information was first analyzed for Descriptive Data according to the SIRP constructs using the operational criteria. Secondly the Psychosocial History was analyzed for the Scaled Data using the SIRP constructs. Descriptive Data provides information about the home in which Colleen was raised and the Scaled Data provides information about Colleen's inner world and how she internalized her experiences in terms of the psychic organization.

### *Descriptive Data Codes*

The Descriptive Data are based on the analysis of the information directly communicated to the therapist by the client or on inferences drawn from the information. The inferences, however, are grounded in the clinical material. In coding the SIRP dimensions, the coder used the definitions and coding procedures presented in the OCCP. Table 6.1 summarizes the Descriptive Data for Colleen's father and mother as perceived by her. The dimensions include unmet self, relational and physical intimacy needs, representations of father, mother, and self, feelings associated with the representations and description of the family environment in which Colleen was raised.

*Table 6.1* Descriptive data for Colleen using the SIRP-AF

| *Dimension* | *Father* | *Mother* |
|---|---|---|
| 1. The striving of relational, self, and physical intimacy needs relative to: | Emotional closeness; be seen; be affirmed for being lovable | Emotional closeness; guidance; support without demand, reassurance, be held, connection |
| 2. Internal representation of: | Selfish, controlling, domineering, unfair, cold, sly, childish, distant | Distant, withholding, inconsistent, disciplinarian, scolding; protector, supporter |
| 3. Internal representation of self relative to: (How I experience myself when with …) | Inadequate, unlovable, powerless, not worth caring about, crushed, unimportant | Unlovable, overly dependent, demanding, burdensome; worthwhile, lovable |
| 4. Affect linking representation of other to self: (How I felt my father, mother, etc. felt about me) | Angry, not accepting, impatient | Burden, hanging on to her apron strings, impatient, dependent, obliged |
| 5. Affect linking representation of self to other: (How I felt about my father, mother, etc.) | Hateful, angry, hurt, frustrated, love/hate | Emotionally empty, angry, sad, lonely, shameful |
| 6. How I felt/feel about myself when with: | Insignificant, inadequate, unsafe, guarded | Safe, secure, childlike, protected, reassured |
| 7. Quality of being parented: (Degree of good enough parenting) | Demanding, distant, rigid | Restricting, inconsistent in emotional availability, demanding |

### *Scaled Data Codes*

Similar to the Descriptive Data, the Scaled Data are grounded on the verbal communications of the client or on inferences drawn from these communications. The results from this analysis are presented in Table 6.2. The dimensions assessed include the manner in which Colleen relates to her parents, psychic organization, self-structure, true self, coping mechanisms, quality of emotional bond, object constancy, characteristic emotion, projective identification (relational patterns), characteristic (developmental) phase, characteristic (developmental) position, and level of personality organization.

## Explanations for the SIRP-AF Codes

The explanation for the SIRP-AF codes for both the Descriptive Data and the the Scaled Data are presented. It should be noted that when there is insufficient clinical material to code a specific dimension, one can still make inferences regarding that dimension based on the clinical material and on the codes for other

*Table 6.2* Scaled data using the SIRP-AF

| | | | | | |
|---|---|---|---|---|---|
| 1. Manner of relating to: | Father: 1 (PO) | 2 ___ X | 3 | 4 | 5 (WO) |
| | Mother: 1 | 2 | 3 | 4 | 5 |
| 2. Psychic organization | Core Needs: | 3.5 EB<br>___ AU | 3.5 SC<br>___ SI | 2 ego | 3.5 superego |
| 3. Self structure | 3.5 striving for competency | | 3.5 striving for significance | 2.5 capacity to maintain significance and competency | |
| 4. True Self (Living from) | 1 Minimally | 2 | 3 | 4 | 5 Strongly |
| 5. Coping mechanisms | ___ denial<br>3 projection<br>___ other | 2 splitting<br>___ regression | 1 repression<br>___ idealization | ___ introjection<br>4 devaluation | |
| 6. Quality of emotional bond | ___ emotionally connected | X striving for emotional connection | ___ avoiding emotional connection | ___ emotionally disconnected | |
| 7. Object Constancy | 1 Fully Absent | 2 | 3 Weakly Present | 4 | 5 Fully Present |
| 8. Characteristic Emotion | ___ anger<br>___ frustration | ___ anxiety | X sadness<br>___ depressed | ___ abandoned<br>Other ___ | |
| 9. Projective identification | X dependency<br>___ other | ___ power | ___ ingratiation | ___ sex | |
| 10. Characteristic phase | ___ symbiosis | 2 differentiation | ___ practicing | 1 rapprochement | ___ consolidation |
| 11. Characteristic position | 1 (PSP) | 2 | 3 | 4 | 5 (DP) |
| 12. Level of personality organization | ___ higher | | X intermediate | | ___ lower |

Rate dimensions 1, 4, 7, and 11 on a 5-point scale. For dimensions 2, 3, and10 indicate the strength of each component using a 5-point scale with 1 = barely and 5 = greatly. For the remainder dimensions check off those that are relevant. See Operational Criteria for more precise instructions. If the dimension is not relevant, leave the space blank. PO = part object; WO = whole object; PSP = paranoid/schizoid position; DP = depressive position; EB = need for emotional bonding; SC = need for sensual contact; AU = need for autonomy; SI = need for sexual intimacy dimensions. For example, if the client is using the defense mechanism of splitting, one can assume that the client rages, sees others as part-objects and either idealizes or devalues them and she might still be in the paranoid/schizoid position. This type of reasoning would be included in the explanation for coding a dimension in a specific way. The explanation for the codes given to a dimension is presented separately for the Descriptive Data and for the Scaled Data.

### Codes for Descriptive Data

The descriptive data presents, in a global fashion, the client's perception of her childhood relationship with significant others, her perception of others and of herself, and the general atmosphere of the home environment in which she was raised. It presents, in general, what it was like to have lived with others in the home of her childhood. These experiences also provide in a general way how the child might have responded to them and tried to make sense of them all of which is reflected in her inner world as depicted in the scaled data.

#### *The striving unmet relational, self, and physical intimacy needs*

This dimension identifies the unmet core relational, self, and physical intimacy needs that are pushing for satiation in relationships. The relational needs include the needs for emotional bonding and for autonomy. The self needs include the needs to be competent and to be significant. The physical intimacy needs include the need for sensual contact (e.g., touch, hugs) and the need for sexual intimacy.

Colleen's psychosocial history suggests that her two core needs are for emotional bonding and for being a significant person who people like to be with. Her history indicates that Colleen tends to seek out persons on whom she can become dependent and receive from them guidance, support, approval, recognition and advice. This is demonstrated in her relationship with her mother and art teacher. Thus, one can say that one of her significant interpersonal motives is for emotional connection or bonding, to be in relationship on which she can depend for approval, guidance, support and direction. It has also been seen that she does not accept having to figure things out for herself. Yet there is a struggle here since she wants to be autonomous as well. Another core need is for sensual contact as she pictured her mother holding and rocking her. The needs for emotional bonding, to be a significant person, and for sensual contact shape and influence her relationships to the point that the needs will not cease until satisfied.

#### *Internal representations of others*

The internal representations of the other are cognitive and affective images formed from the infant/child's experience with significant caregivers.

The representations can bear a positive, negative or a mixed positive/negative valence. Representations are not to be confused with the feelings that one has for others.

The significant figures in Colleen's life are her mother and her father. Her representations of her mother are mixed in nature. She sees her mother as someone to whom she can go for emotional support, protection, and love. This is particularly so when Colleen feels anxious and insecure in losing a relationship. She also sees her mother as not being there for her particularly when Colleen does things that her mother does not approve of such as clinging and wanting her mother's time. Thus, Colleen, as an adult, has mixed representations of her mother, the mother who can be present in times of insecurity and the mother who pushes her out when Colleen becomes too clinging. Regarding her father, Colleen sees him in a very negative light, as someone who is selfish, domineering, childish, sly, unfair, and emotionally distant. For her, he is a bad object who was not and is not there for her. She sees him as a person who has emotionally oppressed her in the past and continues to have the power to crush her in the present.

#### *Representation of self*

The internal representation of self is a cognitive and affective image of self formed from the infant/child's experience with significant caregivers. The mental representation is very much influenced by the quality and nature of the caregiver's responses to the infant/child's needs, feelings and behaviors. If the responses are positive the infant/child thinks of herself as a good person and as having caused the positive behaviors on part of the caregiver. The reverse happens when the caregiver's responses are negative. These self-representations might include seeing one as lovable, competent, wanted, and intelligent or their opposites. Self-representations are also formed from the comments and feedback from others.

Relative to her mother, Colleen sees herself in a mixed way. At one time, she sees herself as being a worthwhile and lovable person since her mother is there for her. At another time she sees herself as not being good enough, a burden, overly dependent, and not lovable because her mother does not respond to her needs and Colleen feels pushed aside. As for her representation of herself relative to her father, she sees herself as not meeting his standards, letting him down, inadequate, and not being good enough.

#### *Affect linking representation of other to self*

This refers to the feeling that the individual perceives the other (e.g., caregivers) had toward her when she was an infant/child. Regarding the mother's feelings toward her, the mother is perceived to feel that Colleen is a burden and is impatient with Colleen's dependency needs. As for her father,

Colleen perceives him to be angry at her, not accepting of her and is impatient. She is too needy for both the father and the mother and they are at a loss how to respond adequately to her feelings and needs.

### *Affect linking representation of self to other*

This construct assesses the feelings that the client, as an infant/child, had toward a significant caregiver and might still have the same feelings toward them today. As for her relationship with her mother, Colleen feels good about herself when she can turn to her mother for comfort, support, and direction. However, she feels negative toward her mother when the mother is not emotionally available. In situations such as these, it can be hypothesized that she becomes needy and feels emotionally neglected, empty, discouraged, pouts, whines, and may throw temper-tantrums. Regarding her father, she feels angry toward him and hates him for constantly asking for more from her and for favoring her sisters over her. Her feeling about self is that she is not good enough, not adequate; she feels hurt and frustrated.

### *How I felt/feel about myself when with the other*

This dimension assesses how the person felt when in the presence of the significant other such as father and mother. Regarding the father, Colleen felt anxious, insecure, and unsafe around him because of his selfish, sly, childish, and controlling behaviors. She also felt helpless because she could not elicit from him emotional closeness and caring behaviors. As for her mother, Colleen feels safe, secure, protected, and reassured despite not receiving the love she needed. The reason for this might be that the mother's positive responses toward Colleen outweighed the negative responses.

### *Quality of being parented*

The quality of being parented refers to the infant/child's experience of how she was brought up by the parents. This would include parental behaviors such as being supportive, caring, consistent, validating, peace loving and protective, or their opposites. Of importance is whether the positive responses outweigh the negative responses because no family upbringing is without its conflicts, hurts, anxieties, and so on. Given the aforementioned criteria, it appears that her parents did not adequately respond to Colleen's need for emotional connection and validation for being a lovable person. It appears as well that they failed to help her to separate and individuate to become an autonomous person. The home can be characterized as having been intense, demanding, restricting, inconsistent, and rigid because of the father's anger and the mother's impatience and emotional neglect.

## *Codes for Scaled Data*

The results from the scaled data provide a picture of the person's inner world that was formed in large part through her interactions with significant others. The inner world is composed of memories, affects, motives, images, perceptions, and sensations that influence, to a great extent, how the person processes incoming information and shapes her interactions with others and with the world.

### *Manner of relating to significant others*

This dimension addresses the manner in which persons are perceived and/or related to. When an individual relates to the other as inordinately needing them (e.g., for direction, emotional support) and is very dependent on them, the other is referred to as a part-object. That is, an individual relates to the other not as a person in her own right (whole-object) with her needs, feelings, strengths, and shortcomings, but as the latter is needed.

Colleen relates to both her father and mother as she needs them rather than to who they are with their own needs, feelings, thoughts, and so on. She is not able to relate to them in a give and take manner. Colleen is given scores of 2.5 and 3 for the manner in which she relates to father and mother, respectively. This indicates that she might at one time relate to the mother as a part-object and at another time relate to the mother as a whole-object. It also indicates that she has achieved partial psychological separation and a partial sense of autonomy.

### *Psychic organization*

The construct, psychic organization, refers to the psychic structure formed from an infant/child's experiences in her interactions with significant others and the world. The psychic organization is comprised of the internalized parent (i.e., superego), the internalized inner child (i.e., core needs), and her adaptive capacities (i.e., ego). The internalized parent can be thought of as demanding/critical or as affirming/validating and displaying values and ideals to live by. The former is referred to as the conscience and the latter as ego-ideal. The inner child can be conceived as the child craving for emotional bonding, sensual contact, and for autonomy.

More specifically, the superego represents the internal parent that can be demanding, critical, and harsh and restrict, oppose, and/or oppress the needs of the child. The superego determines the unacceptable and acceptable behaviors and conduct.

The parent and child are internalized as separate but interdependent agents that can come in to conflict with each other. The demands of the superego and the needs of the child can overpower the resources of the ego and thereby create internal conflicts.

The psychosocial history suggests that Colleen has internalized a demanding and critical superego (similar to that of her parents) as she has adopted values and ideals (e.g., become autonomous) that, when she does not live up to them, she becomes discouraged and critical of herself. At the same time, she is left with an inner child that craves emotional bonding and sensual contact and autonomy. She tends to be impulsive and pouts and whines when her needs are not responded to. In such moments, the ego loses control of both the internal demands and neediness. For this reason, Colleen has been given scores of 3.5 on the strivings for emotional bonding. 3.5 on need for sensual contact, a score of 3.5 on superego and a score of 2 on ego which appears not able to reconcile the external demands with her own strivings.

### *Self-structure*

The self comprises an internal sense of being competent (able to pursue meaningful goals) and being significant and having the capacity to maintain this sense. It represents an enduring experience of being competent and significant and it does not fundamentally depend on affirmations and validations from others and is not easily destabilized. How one perceives oneself to be competent and significant might change across time, however, the fundamental feelings endure. The self is the product initially of the evaluations of others and later from the person reflecting on herself in context of her interactions with the significant others. The feeling of being competent and significant and the capacity to maintain these are referred to as self-structure which adapts itself to situations. The sense of competency and feeling significant are in harmony and support each other.

It appears that Colleen struggles with both a sense of competency and feeling significant (and lovable). She strives to feel and to be seen as being competent and significant. She requires feedback for her performance from both her mother and from the art teachers. She requires validation for her work. She also struggles with feeling significant as she easily gets down on herself, becomes depressed and discouraged. She feels unlovable which erodes her self-esteem. She lacks the capacity to maintain a positive sense of her competency and being significant. For this reason, Colleen is given values of 3.5 for both as she continues to strive and yearn to feel competent and significant. She is given a value of 2.5 for her ability to maintain a sense of competency and significant.

### *True self*

Winnicott (1960) speaks of the social manner in which a person relates to others in terms of True Self and False Self. True Self refers to an individual living according to her own values, interests, ambitions and dreams that are congruent with her sense of self and identity. False self refers to a person who lives according to the demands and expectations of others with the assumed goal of pleasing them in order to be loved and liked.

For ease in assessing the extent to which a person lives from a True Self and False Self, only True Self is coded on a 5-point scale. By knowing the value for the True Self one can arrive at a value for False Self as the combined scores must equal 5. Thus, if the code for True Self is 3 then the code for False Self is 2 since the two numbers must equal five.

Colleen functions most often from the position of the False Self. That is, she lives according to the expectations of others rather than to be guided by what comes from within, that is, be guided by her inner core. It appears that, as a child, she was more focused on securing the love and attention of her parents, particularly her mother, rather than on pursuing her own interests and needs. The result has been the development of a False Self. This is not to say that she always functions from the position of a False Self. For these reasons, Colleen is given the values of 2 for the True Self and by deduction 3 for the False Self.

### *Defense Mechanisms and Coping Strategies*

To manage the frustrations, anxieties, and conflicts and to maintain and enhance self-esteem, the infant/child develops defense mechanisms and coping strategies that can be considered to be conscious and/or unconscious in nature. Conscious coping strategies might include negotiation, compromise, problem solving, endearment and empathy. On the other hand, unconscious defense mechanisms might include repression, dissociation, denial, and splitting (for definitions see Chapter 5). The pattern of coping strategies provides information regarding the nature of an individual's emotional problems and the age of their onset. The use of splitting and dissociation compared to the use of rationalization, indicates an earlier onset of the emotional problem. When early childhood problems go unresolved, the infant/child might continue to use the unconscious mechanisms when becoming an adolescent and adult.

Colleen's psychosocial history suggests the continued use of low-level splitting of the object into good and bad, repressing her feelings as manifested in her not being able to get in touch with her feelings, projection as demonstrated in transferring her feeling of not being understood on to her art teacher, and devaluation as manifested in her image of her father. The frequently used defense mechanisms, therefore, are: repression, low-level splitting, projection, and devaluation. Colleen also manifests a regressive pull as observed in picturing her mother as holding her, rocking her, and reassuring her that all will be well.

### *Quality of emotional bond*

This construct refers to the quality of an infant/child's emotional bonding to another person on whom the infant/child would normally rely for safety, security, nurturance, stability, and comfort. The infant/child can experience being emotionally bonded, and/or pursue or avoid emotional bonding, or feel emotionally disconnected from the significant other.

Based on the psychosocial history, it can be said that Colleen pursues emotional bonding and sensual contact with her mother as she pictures her mother as holding and rocking her and reassuring her that all will be well. Colleen did not establish a secure emotional bond with her mother and her father. Today, she is still in pursuit of emotionally bonding (connecting) and sensual contact in a secure way with significant others.

### *Object constancy*

Object constancy refers to the internalization of the admired traits and functions of a significant other (e.g., mother, father) who is related to as an idealized person and to whom the individual is emotionally bonded (connected). The presence of object constancy brings about the capacities for feelings of emotional well-being which fortifies the infant/child when emotionally distraught such as when the significant other is absent. Positive object constancy provides an inner resource to which to turn to for a new perspective on an issue and for self-comfort which permits the infant/child to function separately in familiar surroundings despite moderate degrees of tension and discomfort.

Colleen found it very difficult to function on her own and to be away from home as she intensely missed her mother. The client had not formed a positive cognitive and affective representation of her mother that she could carry with her and to which she could turn to self-comfort in times of stress, conflict, and loneliness. For Colleen a constant positive object to whom she can turn to self-comfort is, at best, weakly present since for her it is very painful to be away from home. Moreover, when not in the physical presence of her mother, the internal representation of mother also vanishes.

### *Characteristic emotional state*

A characteristic emotional state is one that is familiar, was first experienced intensely in the past (e.g., childhood), is carried into the present, and manifests itself in a disproportionate response to a given situation. For example, if a person becomes irate and angry when given a mild criticism for her work and her response appears to be disproportionate to the criticism, one could say that anger is the person's characteristic emotion. A characteristic emotional state is typically brought about by a persistent dissatisfaction in not having one's core relational, self, and physical intimacy needs met in infancy/childhood. The telling sign of a characteristic emotion is that it is a familiar emotion and is disproportionate to the stimulus.

Although Colleen reports being depressed, the results from the psychological tests do not support the diagnosis of being depressed. Her characteristic emotion seems to be that of sadness because of emotional disconnection from significant others, particularly her father and mother. It is possible that her emotional sadness touches on the feeling of being depressed and emotionally neglected which is supported by her tendency to split, idealize, and devalue others. Outwardly it might appear that depression is her characteristic emotion, however, this emotion is related to sadness because of being emotionally disconnected. For Colleen sadness lies deeper than depression, anger, and frustration.

### *Projective identifications*

These are compulsive and repetitive relational patterns driven by underlying unmet core needs which have as their purpose to establish and maintain relationships and to influence the nature of these relationships. The classical forms of projective identification are the need to be taken care of, the need to be in charge, the need to use one's sexuality (arouse a sexual response in the other) to begin and maintain a relationship, and the need to ingratiate others. These projective identifications are named Dependency, Power, Sexuality, and Ingratiation, respectively (Cashdan, 1988). Be it noted that projective identifications are driven by unmet core self, relational, and/or physical intimacy needs.

Colleen's primary interpersonal pattern (projective identification) is that of Dependency on others for support, advice, encouragement, and comfort. She induces others to play the role of a caretaker by her giving the message that she is helpless, needs to be comforted, and cannot make it on her own. She also uses her charm and sexuality to attract the interests of others so as to develop a relationship. However, this serves the purpose of becoming dependent on others and to have her needs for connection and lovability satisfied. Thus, the Projective Identification of Dependency is checked since it is Colleen's dominant relational pattern.

### *Characteristic (developmental) phase*

The term, characteristic developmental phase, refers to the phase that clearly describes the individual's current subjective experiences, behaviors, and relational interactions of which one or more of the pre-oedipal phases of development, that is, the Symbiosis, Differentiation, Practicing, Rapprochement and Consolidation and Object Constancy subphases, are significant. It is possible that because of trauma, abuse, emotional neglect, for example, an infant/child continues to function from one of these phases which have significant implications for development in adolescence and adulthood (see Chapter 5 for definitions and details about being stuck at a subphase).

Colleen's subjective experiences, behaviors and relational interactions appear to be impacted by the Rapprochement subphase in a significant way. This is demonstrated by her not having established object constancy and not replaced splitting by repression and not seeing others as whole persons rather than as part persons who serve her needs. It is also demonstrated by her difficulty to establish satisfying intimate relationships and lastly by her pouting behavior when things do not go her way and by her adult temper tantrums.

Her subjective experiences, behaviors and relationships appear to be impacted by the Differentiation and Practicing subphases as she experiences a difficulty to become an individuated person. She has only partially differentiated from her mother on whom she relies for comfort and guidance and she is still striving to feel competent which is associated with the Practicing subphase. In support of the latter, it appears that anxiety impeded her from experimenting with her motor skills and exploring the non-mother world. It is also supported by her fear to venture out and socialize. However, the most characteristic subphase from which Colleen is currently functioning is the Rapprochement subphase.

### *Characteristic (developmental) position*

Position refers to one of two developmental positions on a continuum with two poles. One position (Paranoid-Schizoid Position) represents an individual who is angry, uses splitting, sees others as part-objects, relates from self as a part-self, lacks empathy for others, and has not established a firm boundary between self and other. The second position (Depressive Position) represents an individual who has developed empathy and fears losing the love object, uses repression rather than splitting, begins to see others and self as whole persons, and have established firm boundaries between self and other.

According to the position from which Colleen functions, it is somewhere between the Paranoid-Schizoid and the Depressive Positions. She has developed empathy for the significant others, with the exception of her father. However, she still uses a low-level of splitting, projects negative images on others, and/or devalues them. For the reasons given, it seems appropriate to give a value of 3 on the developmental continuum.

### *Level of personality organization*

The level of personality organization is determined by the manner in which the core relational, self, and physical needs have been integrated, the quality of the superego (reasonable, severe, harsh), the nature of defenses used to deal with conflicts and anxieties, and by the quality of relationships that have been formed. Three levels of personality organization have been identified, namely, Higher-Level, Intermediate-Level, and Lower-Level (see Chapter 5 for definitions).

Based on these criteria, Colleen's personality organization can be described to be at the Intermediate-Level since pre-genital fixations points are present, superego is less developed, defenses are organized around repression but some primitive defenses are present and internal objects are conflicted. However, ego identity is established and there is a stable concept of the other and self.

In summary, Colleen's personality is characterized by the pursuit of the unmet core needs for emotional bonding and being significant, a skewed psychic organization toward superego functions, a self-structure with low self-esteem, and coping strategies dominated by projection, devaluation, splitting, and regression. In terms of her relationships, she tends to comply with the wishes of others and takes the position of dependency. She has a stronger need for a relationship than to become autonomous and pursue a life of her own.

## Conceptualization

A conceptualization is typically an explanation of an individual's presenting problem using one or more theoretical constructs. When the individual's problems are more extensive and intensive and when they are explained by a more complex theory, the conceptualization becomes more complex, and extended as well. This is the case for Colleen which explains the length of the conceptualization.

The conceptualization of Colleen's presenting problems and concerns are based on the psychosocial history and on the results from the SIRP-AF. The Descriptive Data and the Scaled Data from the SIRP-AF provide a bird's eye view of Colleen's psychological and self-organization, the unmet core needs that are pushing for satisfaction, how the unmet core needs are compensated for in relational patterns and the coping strategies. The data provides information as to which areas need to be addressed in therapy. The conceptualization comprises a report of her symptoms and the precipitating, predisposing, and the maintaining factors.

Colleen reported feeling depressed, sad, not doing well at the university, missing her family, not motivated to socialize and make new friends and spending time alone in her room watching TV. She felt deprived of and yet craved for emotional closeness, particularly with her mother, who she pictured in times of distress as holding and rocking her. She struggled with heterosexual relationships in that, on the one hand, she wanted the emotional intimacy but feared that her neediness would push them away and on the other hand when she did attract their attention by charming them with her sexuality, she lost interest in them, cooled, and terminated the relationship.

Her current difficulties and problems were precipitated with her leaving home to attend university and by a lack of structure in her program of studies. Being in a new city, she did not have a network of friends from whom she could receive emotional support and reassurance.

Colleen appears to be predisposed to feel sad, disconnected, alone, and unhappy because of her childhood experiences in having had parents who were not emotionally available to her, a father who was critical of her and favored her sisters over her, and a mother who was inconsistent in her caregiving behaviors. The home atmosphere was tense, restrictive, cold, and demanding. Neither parent adequately responded to the needs and feelings of Colleen. She did not have adults who cherished her and who she admired and identified with and whose personal qualities and relational and emotional capacities she internalized.

Due to her relational experiences as a child and as a pre-teen, she developed the impression that she was not loved and accepted for who she was and that she was less capable than her sisters. She felt that she was a burden and not good enough (i.e., low self-esteem). This experience led her to develop a psychic organization that reflected her lived experience with significant others. That is, she developed a severe superego that reflected her demanding and critical parents (e.g., father) and a needy inner child that reflected her real needy child. Because of the demands of her superego, she maintained tight control of her feelings and needs and complied with the wishes and expectations of others so as to obtain the craved emotional connection. In virtue of her severe superego, she is hard on herself and tends toward perfectionism. As for her internal child, it craves for emotional connection and recognition that that she matters (i.e., is significant). These needs are the driving forces in pursuit of her relationships.

As a child, she did not have the cognitive resources to form an ego that could adaptively respond to the demands of the parents and needs of the child. In terms of dealing with frustrations, conflicts and anxieties, she fluctuated between repressing them and complying with the demands of the situation and acting out behaviorally by pouting, whining, throwing temper tantrums and by experiencing sadness. These mechanisms were used to attract the attention of the significant others who temporally responded to her feelings and needs. In most stressful situations, she craved to be held by her mother; she yearned for a sensual contact.

In not having adults who she could admire, treasure, and identify with, she failed to develop object constancy which provides a resource to be libidinally connected to the loved person whether they are present or absent. In not having developed object constancy, she was deprived of the capacity to remain emotionally connected to the loved person which led to her feeling of sadness in being away from her family. In not having formed object constancy, she lacked the capacity to take distance from an event to see it in a different perspective and to regulate her emotions including sadness.

Her core needs to form an emotional bond and to feel significant are reflected in her struggles to form intimate relationships. Her social interactions were driven by her unmet core needs for emotional connection and for being significant. In relationships, she presented herself as being dependent on others for their validations to nurture her core need for significance and to bolster her self-esteem and self-worth. Because of her past experiences in not having her need for connection and significance adequately and consistently responded to, she feared emotional intimacy although she craved it. When relationships become too intimate, she terminated them for fear that if they progress her neediness will become burdensome and cause the person to break up the relationship and bring to full bloom her sadness, a feeling that she has experienced for all of her life.

Her problems are perpetuated, that is maintained, by being away from home, by her (irrational) belief that in having left the home, she had no right to lean on her family for emotional support, by the fear that her neediness, if expressed, would alienate others and by her critical and demanding nature of herself. Another factor is that she was not motivated to develop new relationships thus she remained disconnected from others and alone. She made no efforts to form relationships with guys for fear that her neediness would lead to rejections.

In terms of her strengths, she has very good relational skills, is intelligent, creative and imaginative, caring and empathic toward others, and grounded in reality. Since she tends to please others, she has the capacity to form relationships although they often do not last.

In summary, Colleen is still struggling to complete the separation and individuation process, to psychologically separate and to achieve a sense of autonomy while still maintaining an emotional bond with the significant other. Colleen remains emotionally attached to her mother as it seems that she did not experience her mother's love to the full and, in some fashion, is still craving it. Because of her intense need for emotional bonding and the need to feel important, she finds it hard to move forward to build a life of her own. Her unmet childhood needs for emotional connection and for sensual contact outweigh her need for autonomy and independence and prevent her from investing energy in the development of her sense of self.

## Therapeutic Aspects

Regarding therapy, short-term goals should include the establishment of a solid, safe, secure, and accepting therapeutic relationship to help her to become aware of and articulate her feelings, thoughts, and needs regarding the current situation including her relationships so as to feel validated for her concerns. It is also important to help her to manage her symptoms of sadness and loneliness and help her to expand her social network.

Long-term goals should include working through and completing the separation-individuation process with a focus on achieving a sense of psychological separation and autonomy and thus becoming her own person. A second goal is to develop ego resources to assertively and courageously articulate her needs and feelings and to harmonize the internal demands with her affectionate needs. A third goal is to develop object constancy so as to increase the capacity to regulate affect and better tolerate the absence of significant others, that is, to have them psychologically present even though they are physically absent. A fourth goal is to develop the capacity for intimacy which entails negotiating time spent together with time spent being separate. The ultimate goal is for her to become her own person, live from her true sense of self, form meaningful relationships, feel competent and lovable, and creatively and courageously deal with the problems of daily living.

The therapist could use Experiential Focusing to help Colleen uncover her underlying unmet core needs and Task-Directed Imagery to develop Object Constancy and a sense of being worthwhile. To aid her to connect her current emotional state of being sad and emotionally deprived, to an earlier childhood state, the therapist could engage the client in Ego State Therapy to heal the early wounds of rejection and emotional neglect. Task-Directed Imagery could be used to develop the capacity for healthy intimacy that entails maintaining her individuality in the presence and absence of a loved one. The Gestalt Two Chair technique could be used to give voice to and empower the child within and bring about greater intrapersonal harmony (for descriptions and demonstrations of these techniques, see Meier & Boivin, 2011).

The purpose of this chapter was to demonstrate how to use the SIRP Assessment Form (SIRP-AF) and Operational Criteria and Coding Procedures to code the contents of a written psychosocial assessment report using constructs from Self-in-Relationship Psychotherapy. The results from the psychosocial assessment and the coding using the SIRP-AF were conceptualized and treatment issues and appropriate treatment strategies were proposed. The following chapters present the application of Self-in-Relationship Psychotherapy in working with clients.

## References

Bellak, L. (1993). *The T.A.T., C.A.T., and S.A.T. in clinical use.* Toronto, Canada: Allyn and Bacon.

Buck, J. N., & Warren, W. L. (1992). *The house-tree-person projective drawing technique. Manual and interpretive guide.* Los Angeles, CA: Western Psychological Services.

Cashdan, S. (1988). *Object relations therapy: Using the relationship*. New York: W.W. Norton.

Hathaway, S. R., & McKinley, J. C. (1949). *Minnesota multiphasic personality inventory*. New York: Psychological Corporation.

Jackson, D. (1974). *Personality research form*. New York: Research Psychologists Press.

Klopfer, B., & Davidson, H. H. (1960). *The Rorschach method of personality diagnosis*. New York: Harcourt, Brace & World.

Meier, A., & Boivin, M. (2011). *Counselling and therapy techniques: Theory and practice*. London, UK: Sage.

Meier, A., & Boivin, M. (2013). *The operational criteria and coding procedures for SIRP assessment form*. Unpublished manuscript. Ottawa, Ontario.

Meier, A., & Boivin, M. (2021). *Self-in-relationship psychotherapy semi-structured assessment interview (SSAI)*. Ottawa, Ontario. Unpublished document.

Strong, E. K., & Campbell, D. P. (1974). *Strong-Campbell interest inventory*. Montreal, QC: Institute of Psychological Research. 1977.

Wechsler, D. (1955). *Wechsler adult intelligence scale*. Washington, D.C.: The American Psychological Corporation.

Winnicott, D. (1960). Ego distortion in terms of true and false self. In D. Winnicott (Ed.), (1965), *The maturational processes and the facilitating environment* (pp. 140–152). New York: International Universities Press.

# Part III

# Psychotherapy Process

Chapter 7

# Psychotherapy Goals, Processes, and Techniques

This chapter presents the goals, processes, and techniques of Self-in-Relationship Psychotherapy (SIRP). The chapter begins by presenting principal and subsidiary psychotherapy goals of SIRP. This is followed by a summary of the essential qualities and characteristics of a SIRP-oriented psychotherapist. The qualities and characteristics of clients who are suited for SIRP are then presented. The characteristics that define the SIRP approach are briefly described. The last part of this chapter presents the main therapeutic techniques used by the SIRP approach.

## Goals of Psychotherapy

The psychotherapeutic tasks of SIRP are multiple as they are keyed to its constructs that represent various human conditions such as internal conflicts, low self-esteem, being demanding and critical of oneself, to mention a few. The principal goal is to help clients to uncover, recognize, and accept their core relational, self, and physical intimacy needs and to assert and integrate them in their relationships and in their daily living. The realization of the unmet core needs is often accompanied by obstacles which have to be addressed and negotiated prior to focusing directly on accepting and integrating the unmet childhood and/or growth needs (see Chapter 8 for a discussion of some barriers). The SIRP approach presents the psychotherapy goals according to its principal and subsidiary goals.

### *Principal Psychotherapy Goal*

The principal goal of SIRP is for the individual to uncover, reclaim, and assert his core unmet relational, self, and physical intimacy needs and to reorient his life according to these needs. In the same way that cognitions and affects play significant roles in cognitive and experiential therapies, respectively, so too, needs play a significant role in SIRP. The SIRP approach links unmet needs to many of the emotional and behavioral problems presented by clients. The core needs are often not apparent as they are

DOI: 10.4324/9781003272502-10

disguised in compensated behaviors such as excelling in the academics and sports and being a caretaker and when in reality, they seek to have their relational, self, and/or physical intimacy needs met through the compensatory behaviors.

The example of a client who had multiple conflicting unmet core needs that kept him from moving forward is the teenager, Carlos, who is the eldest of four children. With the birth of his sister, when he was eighteen months of age, he felt displaced and abandoned by the mother who paid more attention to the newborn. This experience had a profound effect on him emotionally and socially. He sought therapy because he felt anxious, found it difficult to be away from home, did not know what he wanted to do with his life, and felt that he was losing out on life. In the course of therapy, Carlos provided three clues to his emotional unrest, namely, he did not want to be tied down, he had a desire to excel in something but he could not bring himself around to commit, and he felt that he was missing out on something and that others were having more fun. The three unmet core needs were he wanting his space (i.e., autonomy), being competent, and being emotionally connected.

The three unmet core needs can be understood within the context of the separation and individuation process (Mahler et al., 1975). It can be assumed that prior to the birth of his sister, Carlos was on the way to individuation and autonomous behavior as he liked having his own space (i.e., autonomy) and began to experience mastery over things (i.e., competency). However, the birth of his sister raised the fear of losing his mother and his attention turned to securing this relationship. The threat of losing the love of his mother prompted Carlos to relinquish his autonomous strivings and revert to dependent behaviors. He was caught in the pursuit of the three conflicting unmet core needs, namely, to be emotionally connected to the caregiver, to be autonomous, and to be competent. However, the need to have the continued relationship with his mother appeared to dominate.

### *Subsidiary Psychotherapy Goals*

The subsidiary psychotherapy goals are those that present themselves at individual therapy sessions and are intimately connected to the principal goal. One can visualize the relationship between the principal goal and subsidiary goals similar to the relationship of the spokes of a wheel to its hub. All of the spokes lead to the hub. In the same way the subsidiary goals lead to the principal goal as described above. In working with subsidiary goals, one indirectly works on the principal goal.

The subsidiary goals included in this presentation are adopted from object relation psychotherapists and self psychologists who extended and modified psychoanalysis in their work with a unique population. The psychotherapists observed that the goal of their work was often determined by the nature of the problem that the client presented. Among the subsidiary goals are: (a) gain an awareness of the nature of the presenting problem, (b) unfreeze earlier emotional failures, (c) transform bad objects and their effects, (d) transform psychic organizations, (e) transform self-organization, (f) develop a genuine true and integrated self, and (g) increase the capacity for relatedness. The subsidiary goals, which overlap are often worked through by offering the client opportunities to experience self and other in a new and fresh way. Among the goals presented, there is not one that is more important than the other, their importance is dependent upon the concern presented by the client.

### *Gaining awareness of the nature of the problem*

In using the SIRP approach, it is essential that clients have an insight into the nature of the problem and its predisposing, precipitating, perpetuating, and protective factors. Predisposing factors (e.g., low self-esteem) are the internal or underlying factors that condition a person to be vulnerable to experience a particular psychological problem. Precipitating factors (e.g., events, situations) are those that trigger a psychological problem. Perpetuating factors (e.g., secondary gains; toxic environment) are the factors that keep a person in the present situation and prevent him from moving forward. Protective factors include an individual's areas of interest, talents, competencies that counteract the predisposing, precipitating and perpetuating factors and reduce the intensity of the problems.

The SIRP approach is characterized by its emphasis on the predisposing factors and how they impact current problems without negating the importance of the precipitating, perpetuating, and protective factors. Predisposing factors are internalizations of repeated negative experiences of early childhood, adolescence and adulthood that condition a person to respond in a specific way to external stressors or events. Included among these factors may be low self-esteem, harsh superego, and feeling inadequate. It is important to assess how a predisposing factor relates to a current problem. For example, an employee may feel compelled to constantly request validation from his director for the quality of his work. A goal of therapy is to examine the motives underlying the need for constant validations. It might be related to the fact that as a child he was constantly criticized and felt inferior to his siblings. Thus, it is important for the client to link his need for constant validation at the workplace to his unmet childhood need for validation. This unmet need functions as a predisposing factor that continues to push for validation.

An example that illustrates gaining an awareness of her relational problems is Yolande, single, in her thirties and from a large family. During the course of therapy, she had been in and out of five heterosexual relationships. Each began the same way with the client idealizing the male partner and eventually ending the relationship with her being angry and hateful toward him for not being emotionally available and responding to her needs. A turning point came when the client, in reviewing her relationships, observed that the same pattern emerged each time and added that there must be something about herself that influences how relationships are formed and broken. She became aware that her relational problems were related to her taking care of the other and not letting others take care of her although she craved for it. She became aware that when she was very young, she tried to get the attention of her emotionally unavailable mother by taking care of her and responding to her needs. Yolande did not experience what it was like to be taken care of. She was able to link her caretaking behaviors of men to her caretaking behaviors toward her mother to get her attention. She was able to understand that her caretaking behavior was a predisposing factor in the way she indirectly sought the love and attention in her relationships and in the manner that she formed significant relationships.

### *Unfreezing earlier emotional failures*

Frozen early emotional failures refer to developmental stages that were not worked through at the appropriate age. These may include failures to achieve emotional bonding (connection), to experiment with and practice new developing motor skills, and to psychologically separate, individuate and become one's own person (Mahler et al., 1975). A goal of therapy is to "unfreeze the early emotional failure" (Winnicott, 1959–1964, p. 128) by providing a successful experience of emotional connection, opportunities to practice skills, and to psychologically separate and individuate in a healthy way. Certain aspects of the environment that originally failed are relived with the environment but this time succeeding to facilitate the individual's inherited tendencies for growth and maturity. This is accomplished by a process of controlled regression to early dependence and to the stage of environmental failure. This regression can be accomplished by the use of Regression Therapy, Ego State Therapy and Experiential Focusing (These techniques are described later). The successful negotiation of a developmental failure serves as a building block for continued growth and development.

The case of Andrew, married, Caucasian, and in his thirties, illustrates how a frozen earlier failure kept him from forming a committed, satisfying, and emotionally intimate relationship. At his work place, he met a young woman, Ashley, who emotionally gripped and disoriented him. He could not get her out of his mind. She was his obsession. He could not understand why she gripped him so strongly. In the early phase of psychotherapy, he dismissed the idea that being smitten by Ashley was linked to early childhood experiences. Further therapy, however, brought to light that he was raised by a cold and distant mother and a critical and demanding father. Without being conscious of it, Andrew, for most of his life searched for the love, affection and validation that he did not receive from his parents. His relationships with women prior to meeting Ashley left him unfulfilled and empty. Ashley, however, embodied the love, affection, and validation that Andrew sought. In her he found the completion of himself. Therapy helped Andrew to become aware that to form meaningful, healthy, and satisfying relations with women, it is essential that he work through (i.e., unfreeze) the early emotional failure in not having formed emotional and physical bonds. Andrew's unmet childhood need for emotional and physical bonding prevented him from forming emotionally intimate adult heterosexual relationships.

### *Transforming psychic structure and ego building*

A good number of clients seek psychotherapy because they push themselves to perform and succeed, feel guilty, and are critical of themselves when they do not excel at their expected level or at the expected level of others. These experiences bring to the forefront the concept of psychic organization and how it has been skewed in the direction of duties and obligations and minimizes the place of pleasure and play.

The psyche is formed by a child from the interactions that he has with the parents. The affects, memories, thoughts, sensations, and motives of these interactions are internalized to form ego states from which emerges a psychic organization. That which is experienced out-there is internalized in-here. The internal replicates the external.

The psychic organization comprises three inner forces, namely, Child, Parent, and Adult (Berne, 1961) or Id, Superego, and Ego (Freud, 1923) to mention two systems. The Id/Child represents that which is part of one's inheritance (e.g., impulses, needs), the Parent/Superego represents that which is acquired from the social environment (e.g., duties, values), and the Adult/Ego represents reason and adaptive capacities. Depending on the nature and quality of the interactions, the child's psyche will be organized accordingly. Thus, for a child that is brought up in a very strict, oppressive, and demanding environment, his psyche might be organized having a domineering, demanding, and critical Parent/Superego. For a child who is emotionally neglected, his psyche might be organized with a needy and pleasure-seeking Child/Id. The task of the Adult/Ego is to reconcile the conflict between these two forces and bring it about that the needs of the Child/Id and demands of the Parent/Superego are achieved. When the ego fails to achieve this, the individual's psychic organization is skewed either in the direction of the Parent/Superego (e.g., being demanding, critical), Child/Id (e.g., feeling needy, neglected) or the Adult/Ego (e.g., being rational).

The following example illustrates how an individual's psychic is skewed in the direction of a demanding, critical and duty-bound Parent/Superego and the impact that it had on his relationships with women. Rick, in his late twenties, single, and a graduate student in English Literature, struggled with forming a commitment in relationships to women. He constantly carried on an internal dialogue with one part making demands and being critical of himself (which he called the Wall) when it came to relationships with women and the second part rebelling (which he called the Self) against the Wall. Rick accepted to use the Gestalt Two Chair Technique to externalize and resolve his internal conflict. He came to realize that the voice of the Wall represented the critical attitude of his mother regarding relationships with women and the voice of the Self represented his craving to have a relationship with a woman. The conflict between the demands of the Wall and needs of Self kept him from making commitments. The exercise brought to light Rick's unmet childhood need for autonomy and independence. At the end of this exercise, he picked up the chair in which the Wall sat, opened the office door and sat her outside where she remains to this day. The following sessions addressed this need and its assertion in his daily life by giving greater voice to the Self which resulted in less internal struggle and greater internal peace.

### *Transforming self-structures*

Within the context of its first human relationships, the infant/child not only develops relationships with caregivers but also forms an image of them and of self that is based on the responses from the caregivers. The images of self can be positive or negative and can be carried into adolescence and adulthood. Negative images of self often present themselves as problems with self-esteem such as feeling inadequate and incompetent or feeling unlovable, insignificant, and undeserving.

In his studies of narcissistically wounded clients, Kohut (1971, p. 11) observed that the woundedness can occur on one of two dimensions or on both: wounded at the level of feeling adequate and competent and wounded at the level of feeling lovable and significant. The self, therefore, comprises two self-needs, namely, the need to feel competent and the need to feel significant (Kohut 1977, pp, 48–50). The infant/child and later adolescents and adults seek admiration for their competencies and affirmations for they being significant. The feelings about self (i.e., self-structures) can be transformed within the transference where the therapist offers a new kind of experience for the client. Through the resolution of the transference, the client acquires additional structures within the self.

An example of being wounded both at the level of the sense of competency and significance (i.e., lovability) and the struggle to repair the woundedness are illustrated by the client Kami who was in her late twenties and married with no children. At age of six, her father left the family and Kami stayed with her depressed, demanding, critical and emotionally unavailable mother. Kami felt incompetent and not loved, thought that there was something wrong with her, that she was flawed and undeserving of the mother's love because she did not comply to the mother's demands in the way that the mother wanted it. Kami carried this view of herself into adolescence and into adulthood and it influenced her relationships and her work. She feared that others would see her as a flawed, undeserving and a bad person and would abandon her. To guard against being abandoned, she gave more of herself in relationships than what was needed but not to her satisfaction. At the workplace, she constantly put pressure on herself to accomplish more than was asked of her so as to prove to her and others that she was competent.

Kami sought therapy to address her low self-esteem which was marked by both feeling insignificant and incompetent. In the early stages of therapy, Kami idealized the therapist and struggled with her fear that he would abandon her if he saw how flawed and how a bad person she was. None of the therapist's pointing out how competent she was at work and how good of a person she was made a difference. In due time she became frustrated with therapy and with the therapist since she observed that there was little progress made in helping her to feel better about herself. This experience triggered her sense of worthlessness, incompetency, being flawed and bad person and fear of being abandoned. It was new for her to directly express her feelings and needs to a significant person, the therapist. She felt guilty about her behavior. However, in working through the transference, Kami learned how to express her feelings and her unmet needs for significance and competency and felt accepted for expressing them. This therapeutic work marked the beginning of a journey for her to achieve both a sense that she was a significant, lovable, deserving and competent person. Over time, she transformed her self-structure and addressed and integrated her unmet childhood needs for significance and competency.

### *Transforming bad objects and their effects*

Fairbairn (1943, 1944) wrote about releasing bad objects (e.g., a critical father). It might be more appropriate to speak about transforming bad objects since in the majority of cases an object is not totally bad but does possess some redeeming qualities. A repressed bad object continues to impact the individual's thoughts, feelings and behaviors until it is transformed. To transform a bad object implies bringing in something new (e.g., seeing the good aspects of the object) and seeing the person as a whole person (e.g., a whole object) with strengths and weaknesses,

A therapist can facilitate the transformation of the bad object by having the individual dialogue with the bad object using the Gestalt Two-Chair Technique (Meier & Boivin, 2011). Typically, in such dialogues, the individual becomes aware of the redeeming qualities of the bad object and becomes empathic toward the bad object both of which lead to its transformation. The therapist can also facilitate the transformation of the client's internal bad object when he becomes the target of the bad object through transference. In working through the transference and seeing the therapist with his strengths and limitations and not wanting to lose the therapist's care, the client develops empathy for the therapist and relates to him as a whole person. The client can use the experience on seeing the therapist with strengths and limitations to empathically relate to the strengths and limitations of others.

The case of Dylan illustrates the transformation of a bad object and its consequent effects. The bad object for Dylan was his highly critical and demanding father who mistreated him in childhood and early adolescence. Despite his pleasing efforts, Dylan could not obtain his father's attention, admiration, love, and positive regard. Dylan grew up feeling frustrated, angry and worthless. He was easily provoked and reacted in aggressive ways. In therapy Dylan was able to link his low self-esteem, anger, and acting out behaviors to his childhood experience with his father and expressed his wish to have a dialogue with his father using the Gestalt Two-Chair Technique. In the course of the exercise, the father apologized for his behaviors and added that he knew no other way in how to be a father as he was brought up in the same way by his own father. This empathic response on part of the father, softened Dylan's attitude toward his father and he began to have a tender heart toward him. The totally negative attitude toward the father – the bad object – was transformed to include the positive attributes of the father who was seen with both his negative and positive qualities. The presence of the bad object with its accompanying negative feelings had prevented Dylan from accessing his unmet need to be accepted as a lovable and worthwhile person.

#### *Developing a genuine true and integrated self*

Clients who have experienced very difficult childhood relationships often put aside their own feelings, needs and preferences and comply with the expectations and demands of their parents in order to have a relationship with them. The children are also not given the opportunity to work through their subjective perception of reality (i.e., illusion, sense of omnipotence) and to come to terms with objective realities (Winnicott, 1960). The capacity to differentiate one's subjective perception of reality from objective reality is also referred to as mentalization (Fonagy & Bateman, 2006). Such behaviors often lead to developing a "false self" to hide and protect the true self. A genuine true self refers to the "inherited potential that constitutes the 'kernel' of the child" (Winnicott, 1960, p. 142) and integration refers to the increased organization of the individual into a unit. An infant achieves a true sense of self when it lets go of omnipotence and illusion and when, through the meeting and confirmation of its needs, it discovers the environment and the *not-me* world and the establishment of the *me*, that is, with a true self that has a *me* and a *not-me* clearly established (Winnicott, 1960).

The struggle toward developing a true and integrated self is illustrated by Matsu, a single and professional woman in her mid-thirties. As an infant and child, her caregivers affirmed and validated her feelings, needs and self-expressions. Around the age of two or three she was expected to conform to the standards of the high society of her parents who were respected professionals in their community and often entertained guests in their home. The parents began to withhold their affirmative responses when Matsu became too needy and when she expressed her negative emotions and disappointments particularly in the presences of guests. During the course of therapy Matsu experienced something very new, however it was not "new-new" since she had experienced it up until the age of two or three. In therapy she became aware that at the age of about two, she began to accommodate to the wishes of her parents and put aside her own feelings and needs. She spent her energy living the life expected by her parents and invested minimal energy on her own personal growth and development. In the process she developed a false self (Winnicott, 1948). Therapy focused on helping Matsu to separate from the emotional bonds that kept her tied to her parents and to individuate and become her own person. Through this process, her unmet childhood needs to be an autonomous and independent person were realized which led to the development of a genuine and integrated self.

### *Increasing the capacity for relatedness*

Fairbairn believes that therapeutic change comprises in an increased capacity for relatedness, the ability to relate in new ways, and to restore the capacity to make direct and full contact with others. More explicitly, Fairbairn (1946) states that therapeutic change is characterized by "a capacity on the part of a differentiated individual for co-operative relationships with differentiated objects … It is a relationship involving evenly matched giving and taking between two differentiated individuals who are mutually dependent, and between whom there is no disparity of dependence" (p. 145).

The task of psychotherapy is to help an individual increase his capacity for relatedness. This entails drawing the attention of the individual to his way of relating, to his expectations of the relationships, and to what he is ready to give or not to give to the other. It includes as well, the client becoming aware of his unmet childhood or growth needs that are impinging upon the relationship.

With regards to couples, they often present themselves for therapy because they lack skills such as empathy and the ability to negotiate, compromise, solve conflicts and repair ruptures in their relationship. They are typically blind to the needs of the other and are focused primarily on their own self and relational needs. One or both partners might try to draw the other into playing the role of a "parent" to provide the unmet childhood needs. These endeavours have been referred to as projective identifications (Cashdan, 1988) and maladaptive cyclical patterns (Strupp & Binder, 1985).

The struggle to increase their capacity for relatedness is illustrated by the couple, Pedro and Priscilla, who had a very stormy relationship which drove them emotionally apart. Pedro was physically and mentally abused as a child and Priscilla was brought up in an oppressive home where affection was not expressed. Pedro was controlled by his emotions and Priscilla was driven by her expectations. Both had very strong opinions and saw most things in opposite terms. Pedro in particular needed to demonstrate that his view was correct which Priscilla resisted. A turning point in therapy came when Pedro, out of desperation, put his viewpoint aside and tried to understand Priscilla by placing himself in her position. This led him to become more empathic toward her. With Pedro becoming more empathic, Priscilla responded in like by being less critical of him. Both expressed the desire to improve their relationship and to become aware of their own unmet childhood needs and those of their partner and to be sensitive and responsive to them. With consistent effort to focus on their mutual unmet childhood needs, the couple made gains in their capacity to relate and their relationship began to change in very significant ways.

### *Connecting with one's inner wisdom*

An important requisite for SIRP is for the client to have the capacity to connect with his subjective experiences that include his feelings, thoughts, and needs, to mention a few. The goal of SIRP is to enable to client to accept responsibility for self-growth, to become self-determining, self-oriented and self-validating (Briere, 1992; Briere & Lanktree, 2012). In the pursuit of self-growth, the client is guided by his inner wisdom which is imbedded within a bodily felt sense of the problem and takes direction from it (Gendlin, 1996).

The following example illustrates how an individual learned how to access his subjective experiences and to assert them socially and at the workplace. The client, Ricardo, married, in his early thirties, and working in the health field, sought therapy because he could not make decisions; he procrastinated and had difficulty expressing his feelings, needs and thoughts. Ricardo was not able to get to the roots of his experiences using verbal psychotherapy, thus Gendlin's (1996) Experiential Focusing Technique was suggested and accepted. This technique helps a person to come to an understanding of his problems and difficulties through a bodily felt sense of them. There is a wisdom imbedded within a bodily felt sense that is not readily available in an intellectual understanding of a problem or difficulty.

At the beginning of the focusing technique, Ricardo experienced pressure points in various parts of his body. As he paid attention to these pressure points, he became aware that he was pressured by others to get a job, by society to conform to its standards, by his wife, and by himself to meet standards. He sensed two conflicting parts within him, a child-like part and a controlling part. The child-like part wanted to say to the controlling part "get off from my back and let me alone." The controlling part, in turn, tuned out and shut the child-like part out. He recalled that as a teenager, he was expected to conform and not to protest. He was validated for compliance to parental expectations, but not for his need for autonomy and independence. The exercise shed light on his current problems and allowed him to access his unmet childhood needs for autonomy and independence and to assert them in his relationships. He was guided by his inner wisdom that was embedded within a bodily felt sense. By the end of the exercise, the two "split off parts" of himself reconciled and agree to work together.

## Therapist Qualities and Characteristics

It is assumed that the SIRP-oriented psychotherapist embodies the three Rogers (1957, 1959) core conditions of unconditional positive regard, empathy, and congruence and that he has the ability to collaborate with the client to establish the psychotherapy goals and work toward achieving them (Beck et al., 1979). In addition, it is assumed that the therapist is able to provide a safe, secure, and protective environment for the client to access and disclose very private and intimate thoughts, feelings and needs. This section addresses additional qualities and abilities that are essential for psychotherapists who adopt the SIRP approach. These include capacity for emotional intimacy, capacity to emotionally engage with the client, being present in the moment, being attuned to the client's developmental needs, and be able to work with client transference and psychotherapist countertransference (Meier, 2010a).

### *Capacity for Emotional Intimacy*

A SIRP oriented therapist tries to feel what it is like to live in the client's inner world and not to stand outside of it as an observer. To be with a client by identifying with his inner world is an emotionally intimate moment. One can conceive of the Rogerian notion of empathic responding and Kohut's concept of "empathic immersion" as representing psychotherapist's capacity for emotional intimacy. The two, however, are different. Roger's concept of empathic responding is more cognitive as it asks the psychotherapist to pay attention to the emotional content of the client's statement and to mirror it back to the client. Kohut's concept of empathic immersion entails immersing oneself into the experience of the client, moving around in that experience, living it with the client, and allowing that which is essential to emerge. The concept of emotional intimacy is closer to Kohut's notion of empathic immersion than it is to Roger's idea of empathic responding. The big challenge for the therapist is not to lose who he is, that is, his identity, his self-hood, when deeply and intimately engaged with the client's narrative of her life. At the same time, it is crucial for the psychotherapist to maintain relational boundaries.

### *Capacity to Emotionally Engage with the Client*

For the therapist adopting the SIRP approach, it is essential that he have the capacity to emotionally engage with the client. To engage with the client, it is essential that he meet the person of the client before addressing the presenting issues. The meeting of the person of the client provides the broad context within which healing is to take place. Clients who present themselves in therapy with histories of developmental injuries, emotional, physical and sexual abuse, and trauma often report feelings of emotional brokenness, being flawed, loathing self, despair, helplessness, rage, anger, and terror. To help clients heal the experiences from which these feelings derive, it is important for the therapist to emotionally engage with these experiences, to empathically understand them, and to have a bodily felt sense of what it is like to be emotionally broken and feeling worthless, for example. It is important for the therapist to know what it "feels like to be a client" (Winnicott, 1963d, p. 229) and to bring to these painful places, inner strength, hope, understanding and care. These attributes can serve as the beginning of a client's healing and empowerment.

Klein emphasized the importance for child psychoanalysts to become emotionally engaged with the children who they treat. The children were from dysfunctional homes and presented with destructive fantasies and aggressive impulses (Klein, 1952/1975). The analyst was to be prepared to be the target of the child's aggressive projections or of the comforting and caring parent. Klein's relational approach has been extended to working with adult clients struggling with personality disorders such as borderline personality disorder (Kernberg et al., 1989; Masterson, 1976), narcissistic personality disorder (Kohut, 1977; Masterson & Klein, 1995), and schizoid personality disorder (Fairbairn, 1940, 1941). In the Kleinian approach, the "psychotherapist and the client are more fundamentally enmeshed with the two struggling to organize and make meaningful the affective life of the patient into which the analyst is inevitably and usefully drawn" (Mitchell & Black, 1995, p. 107).

### *Be Present in the Moment*

The SIRP approach to psychotherapy requires focused concentration, being present in the moment, awareness and acceptance of self and the other, a sense of inner tranquility, and a sense of being effective. The therapist makes all efforts to try to understand the client's mood, feelings thoughts, behaviors and needs from the client's frame of reference. The psychotherapist observes the interaction between himself and client and makes use of this information to provide a broader context within which to understand the client's presenting concerns and difficulties. The therapist tries to obtain a bodily felt sense, in addition to an intellectual understanding, of the client's inner world and real-life struggles.

In order to develop the ability to be present in the moment, it might be helpful for the therapist to set aside some time prior to seeing a client to prepare himself to receive the client. This is particularly true for clients who have developmental injuries and histories of abuse and trauma and who perceive them to be flawed, being a bad person and feel shamed by these experiences and react out in an angry way. This procedure is illustrated by the therapist in seeing Gabrielle who was emotionally neglected as a child and harshly disciplined. During the course of therapy, Gabrielle often vented her rage and anger toward the people in her life but resisted to explore their source. To provide the kind of therapy that she needed and to receive her in whatever mood she was, the therapist spent some time before seeing her to understand where she was stuck developmentally, to determine her unmet childhood need, and to brace himself to receive her negative emotions. This reflection, before seeing the client, helped the therapist to be present in the moment, not to take the client's acting out personally and to be creative in therapeutic work with the client. With the therapist responding in an understanding and caring way rather than to be defensive, the client was disarmed as she did not know how to respond to this new way of relating. This facilitated a sense of safety and protection which allowed the client to become vulnerable and be open to disclose intimate thoughts, feelings and needs.

### *Be Attuned to the Client's Developmental Needs*

For clients who present with feelings of anxiety, anger, and depression that are of longstanding or are chronic, it is important to determine whether the feelings are related to situational stressors or whether they are linked to the client's failure to achieve appropriate childhood developmental tasks such as emotional bonding and becoming a separate and autonomous person but yet be relationally connected. In such cases, a SIRP oriented psychotherapist pays particular attention to the developmental needs of the client, identifies the missed stages of development, and provides the necessary conditions for the client to move forward at his pace (Mahler & Furer, 1968, p. 184).

To help the client reverse the developmental failures, the therapist offers the client opportunities to re-experience the missed early stage of development with the therapist serving as an auxiliary ego and performing the necessary healing functions. The therapist acts as a "catalyst" for the client's growth and development, and balances "nurturing" and "nudging" within the therapeutic relationship. This enables the client to go deeper and to reach higher levels of relationships (Mahler & Furer, 1968, p. 167).

The importance of being attuned to the developmental needs of the client can be illustrated by the specific needs of two different clients, one struggling with borderline personality disorder (BPD) and the other struggling with narcissistic personality disorder (NPD). A significant struggle of the client with BPD is feeling abandoned and a significant struggle of the client with NPD is feeling inadequate and worthless. The developmental need of the former is to be securely connected in a relationship and that of the latter is to be competent and worthwhile. The injury of the former is primarily a relational issue and injury of the latter is primarily an injury to the self. In terms of treatment for the BPD, it is necessary to foster (nurture) therapeutic bonding before challenging and nudging the client toward individuation, separateness and interdependency. The client needs to bond before she can leave the "nest." As for the treatment for the NPD, it is necessary to validate and affirm the client and to build self-esteem before challenging his behaviors such as entitlement. Therefore, the developmental needs of the client determine the therapeutic goals of psychotherapy and guide its process. For a lively discussion of this topic, see Masterson et al. (1991).

### *Work with Client Transference*

It is inevitable that clients who are struggling with unmet childhood needs will pressure the therapist to fulfill these needs. The therapist must have the fortitude to work with the client's transference. Freud (1940) described a transference as an individual directing his emotional feelings and wishes toward the therapist as though he was the original object which caused the feelings. He considered transferences to be ambivalent as they comprise positive (affectionate) as well as negative (hostile) attitudes toward the analyst, who as a rule is put in the place of one or other of the patient's parents, his father or mother (Freud, 1938). Included in the notion of transference are "the client's attempts to draw the therapist into assuming different roles such as being a rescuer, caretaker, and sexual partner" (Meier, 2010b, p. 52). Such client behaviors have been referred to as projective identifications (Cashdan, 1988).

There are no specific criteria to clearly and unambiguously differentiate transference from an expected emotional reaction that transpires in therapy (Meier, 2010b). However, one can assume that there is transference when the client's emotional response is disproportionate to what the therapist said or did, tries to draw the therapist into unwanted behaviors, and/or idealizes or devalues the therapist. Regardless of the nature of the client's responses, it is important to address them according to the client's capacity to deal with them and at the same time provide a new perspective.

There are authors (Smith, 2003) who claim that transferences are artifacts of psychoanalytic treatment, that is, they are unconscious creations of the analyst. Freud (1925) disagrees with them and says that a transference is not created by analysis, rather, transference is "merely uncovered and isolated by analysis" (p. 42) and that "psychoanalytic treatment does not create transferences, it merely brings them to light" (Freud, 1905, p. 117).

It can be argued that both the therapist and client contribute to the creation of transference. Barranger and Barranger (1996) claim that "everything that happens in the analytic situation is a product of three factors: the psychoanalytic setting, the internal world of the patient, and the internal world of the analyst, thus creating a 'bi-personal field' in which the analyst shapes the patient's experience at least as much as the patient shapes the analyst's" (cited by Smith, 2003, p. 120). It is important for the psychotherapist to be able to work with transferences and to enable the client to work through the original conflict (Freud, 1938).

### *Manage Countertransference*

When confronted with a client's transference, a therapist is bound to have an emotional reaction. This emotional reaction is referred to as countertransference. In recent years the discussion on countertransference has been about its content and source, its usefulness in therapy, and the need to expand its definition (Meier, 2010b).

There is extensive agreement among authors about the usefulness of a therapist's countertransference in psychotherapy. Freud (1913) argued that all persons have an unconscious capacity to understand the unconscious concerns of the other and that everyone "possesses in his own unconscious an instrument with which he can interpret the utterances of the unconscious in other people" (p. 320). This statement implies a positive aspect of emotional knowing, or in short, a capacity for countertransference. Other authors suggest that countertransference is an adaptive process (Hartmann, 1939), is an "instrument of research into the patient's unconscious" (Heimann, 1950, p. 81), is an invaluable tool to understand the patient (Basch, 1988, p. 149), can deepen a therapist's awareness of relational dynamics (Hayes et al., 1998), and is a natural response to the client's projective identification (Cashdan, 1988, p. 97).

There is disagreement as how to define countertransference and various modifications have been offered. The impetus to revise and extend the concept of countertransference came from the application of psychoanalysis to emotionally disturbed children and to adults suffering from emotional problems more severe than neurosis and to respond to the pre-Oedipal emotional needs of patients and to address their impoverished ego organization. Four definitions of countertransference have been offered, namely, the classical, totalistic, integrative and moderate concepts. (Meier, 2010b).

Freud (1910), the originator of the concept, defined countertransference as resulting from "the patient's influence on his [psychoanalyst) unconscious feelings ... [which need] ... to be overcome" (pp. 144–145). This definition maintains that countertransference is unconscious, is located in the psychoanalyst, and is triggered by the patient. This is referred to as the *Classical Definition* of countertransference.

The *Totalistic Definition* views countertransference as being evoked by the patient and includes all of the therapist's emotional reactions to the client, whether conscious or unconscious, conflict-based, or reality based (Gabbard, 2001; Hayes, 2004; Wolitzky, 1995). The *Integrative Concept* describes countertransference as a therapist's conscious or unconscious reactions to clients that are based on the therapist's unresolved conflicts. This approach locates the source of the therapist's reactions within the therapist (Hayes, 2004, p. 7). The *Moderate Concept* views countertransference as "therapist's idiosyncratic reactions ... to clients that are based primarily in the therapist's own personal conflicts, biases, or difficulties ... These reactions can be conscious or unconscious and triggered by transference" (Fauth, 2006, p. 17).

### Two-dimensional model of countertransference

The attempts made thus far to define countertransference have not been successful and can lead to confusion among therapists. It might be useful to view countertransference along two dimensions, namely, the therapist's degree of awareness of his countertransference feelings and wishes (i.e., unmet needs) and the therapist's degree of awareness of the origin of the countertransference. Using these two dimensions, one can think of four different types of countertransference (Types 1–4) (Meier 2010b). A brief description of each of the four types follows.

**Type 1.** *No awareness of countertransferential experiences*: This type refers to a therapist not having any awareness of his emotional reactions to the client's responses. The therapist considers his response to be typical of that of any therapist in the same situation. This type overlaps with the classic definition of countertransference. Type 1 countertransference can be destructive and is not an acceptable part of the therapist client-relationship.

**Type 2.** *Aware of emotional reaction but not of its origin:* In this type of countertransference, the therapist is aware of his emotional reactions and realizes that something is amiss but he does not have any awareness of the origin of the emotional feelings and needs or control over them.

**Type 3.** *Aware of emotional reaction and of its origin*: The therapist is aware of his emotional reactions and unmet needs and is also aware of their origin and attempts to keep the countertransference in check. This type of countertransference can be of great help to the therapist to understand the deeper issues of the client and to guide the therapy process.

**Type 4.** *Integrated experience*: The therapist is aware of the potential for a countertransferential response but because it has been worked through earlier, the therapist is able to maintain his composure while at the same time encouraging the client to describe his transference and work it through.

The advantage of using the 4-Type Model is that one avoids trying to come up with a definition of countertransference that covers all situations. The 4-Type Model provides a good instrument for any therapist to assess the quality of his countertransference and to decide what action, if any, needs to take place.

## Client Qualities and Characteristics

Not all clients are suited for SIRP with its focus on the treatment of developmental injuries and long-term aftereffects of abuse and trauma. Not suited for the SIRP approach includes clients who are in the acute state of psychosis and are suicidal, homicidal, abusive and violent. However, when these symptoms are managed, the client can benefit from the SIRP approach as it helps them to link their behaviors to problematic childhood experiences. The qualities and abilities of clients suited for the SIRP approach include the capacity for reflection and self-awareness, tolerance for psychologically painful experiences, commitment to growth of self, and the ability to use the therapist as an alter-ego (Meier, 2010b).

### *Capacity for Self-Reflection and Self-Awareness*

SIRP promotes behavioral, attitudinal, and relational changes through the transformation of internal organizations such as psychic structure and self-organizations. In order to achieve these transformations, it is essential that the client have the capacity to reflect on his subjective experiences (e.g., thoughts, feelings, motives) and become aware how these subjective experiences might act as predisposing factors that influence his current problems. It is also essential that the client become aware that these subjective experiences were formed, at least in part, by the childhood interactions with significant persons in his life and that the subjective experiences have been shaped to form the internal organizations such as the psychic and self-organizations. These organizations serve as a mindset, lens or template through which information is processed and they act as a motivator that influences behaviors and relationships. For a client with developmental injuries and is a survivor of abuse and trauma, it is important for the client to have the capacity to assess and understand how these have affected him and bring about the necessary changes in order to address the presenting concerns and problems.

The case of Andrew illustrates the role that awareness plays in understanding a relational problem. At his place of work, Andrew met a young woman, Ashley, who emotionally gripped him and he did not understand what happened nor could he get her out of his mind. She became his obsession. In the course of therapy, he mentioned that he was brought up by an emotionally cold and distant mother and a critical and demanding father. Yet for all of his life he searched for the love, affection, and validation that he did not receive from his parents. Ashley embodied the love, affection, and validation that he has sought for all of his life; he needed her affection to feel complete as a person. Andrew became aware that therapy must focus on the unmet needs from childhood in order to have a fulfilling and satisfying adult relationship. But he had no idea as how to go about achieving this.

### *Tolerance for Psychologically Painful Experiences*

Clients who present with developmental injuries and experiences of abuse and trauma often report feeling anxious, flawed, worthless, broken, disorganized and insignificant and painfully fear being abandoned. The client's natural tendency is to avoid these very painful experiences and not to bring them up in therapy. They fear that they might be judged, not be understood, be a burden to the therapist, and/or that the therapist will not be able to go with them into the depth of their painful experiences. To address these psychologically painful feelings, the client must possess the capacity to tolerate them. It is important for the therapist not to encourage the client to open up these painful experiences or use techniques to open them up unless both the client and therapist are ready and able to go to these places. To be with the client in the depth of his painful experiences and help him to tolerate them, the therapist must be able to be present in hope, understanding, inner strength and care and provide safety, security and protection.

The case of Kami illustrates a client's ambivalence in talking to the therapist about her painful experiences trying to comply to the wishes and demands of her critical and demanding mother. In not being able to satisfy her mother's wishes, Kami felt that there was something wrong with her, that she was flawed and a bad person. She wanted to talk about the experience to the therapist and yet hesitated not knowing whether the therapist would think of her as being "flawed" and a "bad person" in not being able to comply to her mother's wishes. She feared that the therapist would judge her and reject her as did her mother. Feeling safe, secure, understood and cared for, Kami shared her experience and in doing so gradually developed a tolerance to endure the pain of disclosing the experiences. It was important for the client to experience that therapist was able to engage in the client's deep lying pain.

### *Commitment to Therapy and their Self-Growth*

SIRP presents a unique challenge to clients to remain committed to therapy and to their self-growth because of its focus on internal transformation (e.g., softening the internalized critical parent) rather than only on behavior change. When clients experience and observe that their therapy is helping them to bring about their desired personal and/or interpersonal changes, they remain committed to the process and to their personal growth despite how painful and difficult it might be. However, for clients whose efforts seem to have failed to bring about the desired changes and when they come to realize that to bring them about, they need to make changes within themselves (e.g., softening the internalized critical parent), they can become discouraged, impatient, question the value of therapy, and lose motivation. It is easier for clients to remain committed to therapy and self-development when they are able to observe and experience the changes, but it is more difficult for a client who must make internal transformations to remain committed because these transformations are not tangible and immediate changes are difficult to perceive.

Ingrid, in her early twenties and single, illustrates commitment to psychotherapy. As a teenager, Ingrid was promiscuous, used street drugs, and attempted suicide several times. In her late teens, she became aware how she had messed up her life and she was determined to turn her life around. In the course of therapy, she addressed her use of street drugs and her sexual behaviors. She also explored her painful childhood experiences and how the use of drugs and sexuality was her way to deal with them. Despite how painful it was to address these issues, Ingrid's experiences of internal transformations held her committed to psychotherapy and to her personal growth and development.

### *Ability to Use the Therapist as an Alter-Ego*

Mahler and Furer (1968), when discussing the origin of infantile psychoses, make the point that some children are not able to internalize their mother and use what she offers for their growth and development. The point is that in order for a child to grow and develop he must have the capacity to utilize what is given to him.

Analogously, the same can be said for an adult client seeking therapy. The client must have the capacity to utilize what is being offered in therapy and use the therapist as an alter ego to develop the necessary skills, understandings, and attitudes to address his issues and move forward in life. The client experiences that the therapist offers a different reality from what the client has experienced in the past. In interacting with the therapist, the client might feel understood, accepted, significant, and cared for and might learn skills of assertiveness, open communication, and solving conflicts and problems. These therapist's qualities might serve as a strong impetus for the client to rethink and modify his own perceptions of self and other, style of communication, and relational patterns. The client uses the therapist as a model for change and transformations. Therapists often report that clients, when they find themselves in difficult situation, will ask themselves, "What would my therapist say?" This is an example of how clients use their therapists as an alter ego.

## The Therapeutic Change Process

Three of the characteristics that define the SIRP' change process, include fostering a self-discovery and action-oriented approach, focusing on psychotherapeutic themes, and viewing treatment in terms of phases that unfold across space and time. These three characteristics are briefly described.

### *Self-Discovery and Action-Oriented Approach to Psychotherapy*

SIRP subscribes to a self-discovery and action-oriented therapeutic approach. It postulates that personal growth and development are a function of one's capacity to gain awareness of the life-giving forces within oneself and then to take action and orient one's life around these forces (Maslow, 1954; Rogers, 1961). In the SIRP approach the "life-giving forces" are the core relational, self and physical intimacy needs.

The self-discovery aspect of the SIRP approach facilitates the personal discovery of a set of feelings, motives, cognitions, values and meanings that enhance personal growth and the discovery of a similar set that inhibit personal growth and development. It also includes the discovery of abilities, competencies, and style of interpersonal behaviors (Meier & Boivin, 1987). The action-oriented aspect of the SIRP approach includes experiential, behavioral and/or cognitive exercises and techniques to help clients to translate their personal discoveries (i.e., insight, awareness) into meaningful behaviors, actions, and relationships.

The SIRP approach assumes that insight and awareness are therapeutically meaningful if they lead to new and more effective actions and behaviors. Equally, the SIRP approach assumes that new actions and behaviors need to be informed by insights and awareness for them to endure. Resourceful clients are often able to translate, on their own, the new insights and awareness into new actions and behaviors.

### *Thematic Approach to Psychotherapy*

SIRP approaches the treatment of emotional and behavioral disorders in terms of themes. It does not directly treat a diagnostic category such as major depressive disorder, but rather it treats its constituents or themes.

Themes "comprise the personal or interpersonal difficulties, concerns, and/or problems and troubling thoughts, disturbing emotions, and experiences of loss *explicitly* or *implicitly* raised and/or worked on by the client within the course of psychotherapy" (Meier & Boivin, 2000, p. 59).

Themes are conceptualized as "being bi-polar with one end of the continuum representing the problematic pole and the other end representing the [latent positive] pole towards which to strive" (Meier & Boivin, 2000, p. 59). The positive pole is opposite to the explicit or implicit stated problem. For example, in the client statement, "I feel constrained by my partner," the implicit message might be the desire to be freed from constraint and exercise autonomy and independence. Thus, the above theme, in its bi-polar form, would read "feeling constrained versus feeling freed." Both poles comprise the theme (p. 59).

The treatment of obsessive-compulsive disorder and major depressive disorder illustrate the thematic approach to psychotherapy. In the case of obsessive-compulsive disorder (American Psychiatric Association, 2013), one might treat avoidance behavior, proneness to guilt, checking behavior, anxiety and unrealistic expectations (Meier & Boivin, 1998a). The deeper lying core theme for the client struggling with obsessive-compulsive disorder might be to protect oneself from being found at fault, reprimanded and judged.

As for a client struggling with major depressive disorder, one might treat lack of self-care, feeling obligated, sense of helplessness, and need to please (Meier et al., 2006). The core theme for the client struggling with major depressive disorder might be the fear to be true to herself.

### *Phases of the Therapeutic Change Process*

SIRP views psychotherapy as a process characterized by significant client moments that are referred to as phases of the change process. The change process is thought to comprise seven phases that have been operationalized to form The Seven-Phase Model of the Change Process (SPMCP) (Meier & Boivin, 1992, 1993, 1998b, 2000; Meier et al., 2006). The combined seven phases represent a progressive forward movement in working through psychotherapeutic themes. A client does not progress linearly through the seven phases, but cyclically.

The SPMCP can be thought of from two different perspectives. First it can be thought of as describing a client's step by step process in resolving an issue. From this perspective, the SPMCP is descriptive. Second SPMCP can be thought of the steps through which a psychotherapist guides a client, particularly, when the problem dealt with is of long duration. From this perspective, the first three phases, Problem definition, Exploration, and Awareness/Insight, trace the client's presenting concerns, such as depression, back to their origins which may include factors and stressors in the person's life and/or to unresolved childhood experiences. In the fourth and fifth phases of therapy (Commitment/Decision, Experimentation/Action) the therapist helps a client, while being in the regressed and vulnerable state, to become empowered to deal with the factors and stressors underlying the problem and then use this skill and competency to deal with current problems.

Qualitative research using single samples has demonstrated that the seven phases are significant aspects of the change process for clients struggling with becoming their own person (Meier & Boivin, 2000), overcoming depression (Meier et al., 2006), resolving obsessive and compulsive behaviors (Meier & Boivin, 1998c), and working out transference (Meier, Boivin, & Meier, 2010). The seven-phase model provides a road map of the therapy process. It accounts for ninety-seven percent of the client responses and statements (Meier & Boivin, 1998b). A brief description of the seven phases follows.

### *Problem definition phase*

The client presents and discloses personal and/or interpersonal difficulties, concerns, feelings and behaviors. The therapist helps the client to identify and articulate the parameters of the problem in terms of its nature, intensity, duration, and extent. Psychotherapy goals are then established.

### *Exploration phase*

At this phase, the psychotherapist and client, together, begin to address the personal and/or interpersonal concerns and difficulties and troubling feelings particularly within the context of the client's relationships including childhood relationships and current relationships. They attempt to uncover the underlying dynamics in terms of their predisposing, precipitating, perpetuating and protective factors with reference to affective, cognitive, motivational and behavioral constituents. Particular attention is given to uncovering unmet childhood and/or growth needs that underlie the presenting concerns. This phase can extend over a long period of time as new themes emerge that need to be explored. This phase can be described as a "taking apart" or an "undoing" phase because of the analysis of the factors related to the presenting concerns. The undoing can lead to clients feeling temporarily worse when compared to how they felt when they began therapy.

### *Awareness/insight phase*

As the client explores his concerns, problems, and troubling feelings, he begins to make links between them and to the current stressors (i.e., precipitating factors) in his life and to his past experiences (i.e., predisposing factors). These linkages gradually lead to greater awareness and insight into the origin, maintenance, and meaning of his concerns, problems, and troubling feelings. The client also gains a better understanding how inappropriate cognitions, unfulfilled needs, lost meanings and unexpressed feelings relate to his current concerns and problems. This new awareness, insight and perspective on his concerns and problems provides a handle for assuming responsibility to bring about the desired changes and at the same time provides a direction for change.

### *Commitment/decision phase*

The client's new awareness, insight and perspective on his presenting concerns, problems and troubled feelings, often lead to an explicit or implicit statement and/or determination to change things in his life. He assumes responsibility for the direction that change will take in his life. Often this phase is not apparent and is subsumed either in the Awareness/Insight Phase or the Experimentation/Action phases. This phase, however, brief, is indicated by the client's motivation to change things in his life.

### *Experimentation/action phase*

The new perspective on his concerns and problems and his motivation to make the necessary changes in his life, leads the client to think, respond, and act in new and different ways. For many clients, to relate in new ways is an unchartered territory and often fraught with anxiety. Often, the clients need help to develop new skills such as assertiveness skills which can be rehearsed and practiced in the therapy sessions. The client tries to implement the new awareness by trying out and experimenting with new ways of relating, behaving and acting. Resourceful clients are able, on their own, to implement their new perspective regarding their concerns and problems.

### *Integration/consolidation*

Whereas in the Exploration Phase, the client took things apart through analysis, in the Integration/Consolidation Phase, the client reconfigures his new actions, behaviors, perceptions and feelings in a way that is consistent with his growing sense of self. This phase represents a bringing together and a solidifying of the new experiences that emerge from the Experimentation/Action phase. This phase brings about a transformation of the person's perceptions, thoughts, feelings, motives, attitudes and behaviors.

### *Termination phase*

Having achieved the goals of psychotherapy, the client begins to prepare himself to live without the support of the therapy sessions. The client's feelings and concerns regarding the termination of therapy are addressed and worked through. In the termination phase of therapy, sessions are typically scheduled further and further apart until termination. The client is informed that he is always welcome to contact the therapist for follow up sessions.

## Psychotherapy Techniques

SIRP incorporates techniques from various theoretical orientations including psychodynamic, relational, experiential, cognitive, behavioral, and social learning therapies. SIRP makes use of the basic interviewing skills (Ivey et al., 2006). Among the basic interviewing skills, empathic responding holds a significant place. However, empathic responding has been broadened to include all of a client's subjective experiences including feelings, perceptions, thoughts, meanings, values, needs, determinations, and commitments.

SIRP also incorporates advanced techniques such as Experiential Focusing, Gestalt Two-Chair Technique, Ego State Therapy, Task-Directed Imagery and Regression Therapy (Meier & Boivin, 2011). In addition to these techniques, the authors have developed exercises and/or techniques that emerged from applying the SIRP approach in their clinical practice. These include the following: Wholesomeness exercise, Progressive forward exercise and the Track record technique. It should be noted that the techniques are always used to accomplish a counselling goal which is theoretically based.

### *Experiential Focusing Technique*

Experiential focusing (Gendlin, 1996) is designed to uncover the deeper layers of presenting problems by paying attention to a bodily felt sense of them. The client begins the technique by being asked to clear a psychological space by putting aside the worries of the day. As the client creates this space, he enters into a semi-hypnotic state and arrives at a bodily felt sense of the problem. The crucial point in this technique is the fifth step where the client is asked what is needed to make the bodily felt sense of the problem better. The articulation of the need marks the beginning of accepting the unmet childhood or growth need and integrating it into his daily life. As an example, Simone in the focusing technique, became aware of her unmet childhood need to be loved, nurtured and cared for, that she needed to feel significant (Meier & Boivin, 2011).

### *Ego State Therapy*

Ego state therapy (Lawrence, 1999; Watkins & Watkins, 1997) attempts to link chronic emotional states (e.g., anxiety) to underlying problematic ego states (e.g., feeling inadequate and incompetent) that were formed in early childhood and/or through abuse and trauma at a later age. The client is asked, through imagery, to re-experience and to describe the life situation in which the problematic ego state was formed. This is followed by the client being asked to make the problematic ego state better by doing what is needed. The result is the formation of a healthy ego state whereby the person perceives himself differently (e.g., feeling adequate and competent). The change in perception leads to the realization of a fundamental need which is to be competent, autonomous and independent. The observed behavior change of the client is due to uncovering and transforming a problematic ego state. To illustrate, Sonja was able to transform a problematic ego state that she was inadequate into a healthy ego state of feeling competent and adequate. For most of her life she tried to prove to herself and to others that she was a competent and adequate person. She was able to apply the transformed problematic ego state into her current life (Meier & Boivin, 2011).

### *Gestalt Two-Chair Technique*

The Gestalt Two-Chair technique (Perls, 1969) was designed to resolve intrapsychic (i.e., internal) conflicts by engaging the two parts (e.g., Topdog and Underdog) in a meaningful and focused dialogue. The goal is to encourage the Underdog (e.g., Child) to express its needs and for the Topdog (e.g., demanding parent) to hear and respect them. In presenting and respecting their mutual needs and making compromises, the Topdog and Underdog come to a resolution of their conflict. The resolution of the internal conflict brings with it a transformation of the psychic organization resulting in greater harmony among its parts (e.g., Id, Ego, and Superego), which can be a specific and concrete goal of SIRP. A significant moment in the resolution comprises the Topdog empathically understanding the position of the Underdog and stating it as such. An example of the transformation of psychic organization is Rick (Meier & Boivin, 2011) whose Underdog (i.e., Self) expressed his need to have a voice in his life, to be autonomous, and with Topdog (i.e., Wall) empathically hearing and respecting this unmet relational need.

### *Task-Directed Imagery*

Task-Directed Imagery (Meier & Boivin, 2011) is a flexible technique that can be used for countless goals and purposes. It has been found to be effective to help clients to self-soothe, let go of excessive control in relationships, and to build trust in intimate relationships (Meier & Boivin, 2010a, 2010b, 2010c). Task-Directed Imagery can also be used to help clients to develop new behaviors such as setting limits in their social interactions. The procedures to apply Task-Directed Imagery are given in Attachment 7.1, below.

### *Regression Therapy*

It is important that therapy be attuned to the developmental needs of the client, be it a child or an adult (Mahler & Furer, 1968, p. 167, n.3). Therapy enables a client to re-experience the early missed stages of development and progress through them with the help of the therapist. To re-experience missed stages of development implies regression to these earlier stages.

Therapy is perceived as a process of controlled regression to early dependence and to the stage of environmental (i.e., parental) failure (Winnicott, 1959–1964). The therapist fosters the client's regression so that he can revisit and relive the aspects of the environment that originally failed with the environment this time succeeding to facilitate the inherited tendencies for growth and maturity.

Regression is facilitated by the client having confidence in the therapist to provide the right environment and the necessary provisions in a reliable and patient way. This includes providing a safe and protective therapeutic relationship and validating the client's relational, self, and physical intimacy needs. In regression, the client gives up the false self; the true self emerges. This is a "time of great dependence and true risk, and the patient is naturally in a deeply regressed state" (Winnicott, 1955–1956, p. 275). The goal of therapy, according to Winnicott (1959–1964), is to unfreeze the early emotional failure by providing a successful experience of empowerment (i.e., omnipotence). Regression to an earlier stage of development can be induced by techniques such as Task-Directed Imagery or it can come on gradually and spontaneously as the client feels safe, secure and protected in therapy.

An example that illustrates regression occurring gradually and spontaneously in therapy is that of Adala who was single and in her mid-thirties. She was the middle child of a large family. Her father was an alcoholic and was mean when inebriated and caring when sober. As for her mother, Adala felt unwanted, not trusted, unfairly treated, and not validated for her achievements. During the course of therapy, there was a sign of impending regression as she reported that she sees herself in a fetal position, sucking her thumb, and under the skin of the therapist. As therapy progressed, she gradually became emotionally dependent upon the therapist and regressed first to the "rapprochement phase" and then back to the "differentiation phase" (Mahler et al., 1975). Feeling safe, secure, protected and cared for, Adala began efforts to shape the therapeutic relationship according to the dynamics of her earlier unresolved rapprochement phase. She engaged in a power struggle with the therapist. She resented the time limits and location (i.e., office) of therapy and reacted strongly to them by expressing feelings of hatred and love toward the therapist, wanting to terminate and yet hold on to therapy, and by having fits of rage (i.e., an adult temper tantrum) wherein she physically abused herself. Unable to resolve the rapprochement crisis, she regressed further to the differentiation phase and was hospitalized on two different occasions. Following her last hospitalization, Adala continued with therapy and worked through the missed stages of development and her unmet childhood needs for emotional bonding, feeling lovable, and having a voice. She went on to become a significant figure in the reorganization of the health institution in which she was employed.

### *Wholesomeness Exercise*

Some clients present themselves for therapy thinking that they are flawed and bad persons and have low self-esteem and negative images of themselves. Their negative perceptions come from negative messages received in their early childhood transactions with significant others. These negative perceptions are perpetuated through internalizations to form their psychic organization where their critical and demanding part (e.g., Superego) criticizes their legitimate feelings, needs, preferences (e.g., Id) in the same way that they were criticized by real people. No amount of trying rationally to help them to change their perception of self is productive. The task, then, is to provide an experiential exercise wherein they are asked to experience themselves as a wholesome, lovable, worthwhile, and competent person. This exercise is called the Wholesomeness Exercise. The goal of this exercise is for the clients to become aware of their sense of goodness and wholesomeness and to challenge and/or replace the negative perceptions which often mask their sense of wholesomeness.

In the Wholesomeness Exercise the client is asked to take a comfortable position in the chair, relax, and let go of the daily worries. He is then asked to name the qualities and traits about himself that he likes. When he has mentioned a good number of them, the therapist asks the client to restate them. The client is then asked to embrace the qualities and traits that he likes about himself, and to have a bodily felt sense of these qualities and to experience them as being part of him. When the exercise has been completed, the client is asked for his comments.

The case of Dylan illustrates the use of the Wholesomeness exercise. Dylan, in his early 40s, was brought up in a very abusive home. His father constantly put him down, ridiculed him, and mistreated him. His mother was not able to help Dylan develop skills to effectively deal with his father's negatives as she herself felt intimidated by her own husband. Dylan came to think of himself as being inadequate, unlovable, and incompetent and being a bad and worthless person. In using the Wholesomeness exercise, Dylan at first found it difficult to say anything that he liked about himself. With prompting from the therapist based on material from the past sessions, Dylan began to describe what he liked about himself. He said, "I am a good person," "I am a generous person," "I am a competent person" and so on.

Dylan was asked to repeat these statements slowly and to embrace them experientially and bodily. It is important for the client not just to say them, but to experience and own them. Following the exercise, Dylan experienced inner peace, calmness, and greater self-confidence, was easy going, and had warm feelings for himself and for his wife, and was not bothered by things as in the past. He became more proactive and less reactive.

### *Progressive Forward Exercise*

Progressive forward exercise refers to helping a client to determine the extent to which a new feeling, thought, need, and/or experience that emerged in therapy has been part of his life across all ages without he knowing it. The client might on his own state that it is not a new experience, thought, feeling or need or the therapist might ask if he has felt something like this in the past. The client is asked when he first had such an experience. This is followed by asking the client to proceed forward from the age at which he had this experience and determine when he experienced it again. He might have experienced this at different ages such as at the age of 11, 18, and 25. He is asked to describe his experience at each age when he had the experience.

The case of Matsu, single, in her mid-thirties illustrates the use a Progressive forward exercise. During a therapy session, Matsu became aware of a new experience. However, she added that it was not new-new as she experienced this earlier in her life. She described this experience as feeling strong, accepted, capable and carefree. She reported that the last time she had this experience was when she was two years of age. It is at this age that she began to comply with the wishes of her professional parents and put aside her own feelings, needs and preferences. The therapist asked her to get in touch with the experience that she had at the age of two and move forward in time to childhood, adolescence, and adulthood and see if she experienced it anytime during the later years. As she moved forward from age two, she stopped at the following years: 4, 10, 18, 25, and 33, her current age. At each of these ages, she momentarily felt that she was herself, was able to do what she wanted to do, had the freedom to be herself, and was accepted for being herself. She was asked to go through these ages two more times and each time to hold on to her sense of strength, freedom and acceptance and to have a bodily felt sense of them. The purpose was to consolidate the impression that the experience she had at the age of two was always present. Matsu was surprised that the experiences remained with her through all the years from childhood to adulthood without her knowing it. Rather than living completely according to the expectations of others, Matsu realized that, in a limited way, she continually exercised her need for autonomy and independence. In uncovering this unmet need, she was able to assert it and take greater charge of her life.

### *Track Record Technique*

The inspiration for this technique came from the idea that if a person wants to know how well a horse will do on a race, one need only look at its track record, that is, on its past performances. This technique can be helpful for persons who struggle with feelings such as abandonment.

Richard, in his thirties, struggled to begin and maintain meaningful relationships for fear that the women he dated would leave him. Thus, he did not allow himself to become emotionally close and yet he craved such closeness. In due course, Richard met a woman with whom he was smitten and he could not disengage himself from the relationship. Both were professionals with busy schedules. They lived in separate apartments. They began to date. Richard did not get enough of their closeness when together. When he did not hear from her in due course, he felt that she lost interest in him; he felt abandoned. In due time, she connected with him to explain her reason for not responding sooner. Incidents such as these happened repeatedly and after each lapse of time the woman returned the call and provided legitimate reasons for the delayed response. Such responses challenged Richard's thought that her delays in responding meant that she was abandoning him. By remembering the outcome of each of the occasions where he felt that she was abandoning him (the track record), Richard was able to work through his feelings of abandonment and come to realize that to the same degree that he wanted her in his life, she also wanted him in her life. In working out his fears of being abandoned by the woman in his current relationship, he also addressed the origin of his abandonment feelings and worked toward healing them.

This chapter presented the goals of therapy and the essential qualities and characteristics of psychotherapists and clients. It also presented the theoretical approach to therapy and therapeutic techniques. The next chapter addresses the strategies in working with core self, relational, and physical intimacy needs and the barriers that the client may confront in this process.

## References

American Psychiatric Association (2013). *Diagnostic and statistical manual of mental disorders* (DSM-5). Fifth edition. Washington, D.C.: American Psychiatric Association.

Barranger, M., & Barranger, W. (1996). Insight in the analytic situation. In R. Litman (Ed.), *Psychoanalysis in the Americas*. New York: International Universities Press.

Basch, M. F. (1988). *Understanding psychotherapy: The science behind the art*. New York: Basic Books.

Beck, A. T., Rush, A. J., Shaw, B. F., & Emery, G. (1979). *Cognitive therapy of depression*. New York: Guilford Press.

Berne, E. (1961). *Transactional analysis in psychotherapy*. New York: Grove Press.

Briere, J. N. (1992). *Child abuse trauma: Theory and treatment of lasting effects.* New York: Sage Publications.

Briere, J. N., & Lanktree, C. B. (2012). *Treating complex trauma in adolescents and young adults.* New York: Sage Publications.

Cashdan, S. (1988). *Object relations therapy: Using the relationship.* New York: Norton.

Edward, J., Ruskin, N., & Turrini, P. (1981). *Separation-individuation: Theory and application.* New York, NY: Gardner Press.

Fairbairn, W. R. D. (1940). Schizoid factors in the personality. In *Psychoanalytic studies of personality* (pp. 3–27). New York: Basic Books.

Fairbairn, W. R. D. (1941). A revised psychopathology of the psychoses and psychoneuroses. In *Psychoanalytic studies of personality* (pp. 28–58). New York, NY: Basic Books.

Fairbairn, W. R. D. (1943). The repression and the return of bad objects. *British Journal of Medical Psychology, 19.*

Fairbairn, W. R. D. (1944). Endopsychic structure considered in terms of object relationships. In *An object-relations theory of the personality* (pp. 82–136). New York: Basic Books.

Fairbairn, W. R. D. (1946). Object relations and dynamic structure. In W. R. D. Fairbairn (Ed.), *Psychoanalytic studies of the* personality (pp. 137–151). New York: Routledge.

Fauth, J. (2006). Toward more (and) better countertransference research. *Psychotherapy: Theory, Research, Practice, Training, 43*(1), 16–31.

Fonagy, P., & Bateman, A. (2006). Mechanism of change in mentalization based treatment of borderline personality disorder. *Journal of clinical Psychology, 62*, 411–430.

Freud, S. (1905). Fragment of an analysis of a case of hysteria. *Standard Edition, 7*, 7–111.

Freud, S. (1910). Future prospects of psychoanalytic psychotherapy. *Standard Edition, 2*, 139–151.

Freud, S. (1913). The disposition to obsessional neurosis: A contribution to the problem of choice of neurosis. *Standard Edition, 12*, 317–326.

Freud, S. (1914). On the history of the psychoanalytic movement. *Standard Edition, 14*, 7–66.

Freud, S. (1923). The Ego and the Id. *Standard Edition, 19*, 12–63.

Freud, S. (1925). An autobiographical study. *Standard Edition, 20*, 7–70.

Freud, S. (1940). An outline of psychoanalysis. *Standard Edition, 23* (1953) 144–207.

Gabbard, G. O. (2001). A contemporary psychoanalytic model of countertransference. *Psychotherapy in Practice, 57*(8), 983–991.

Gendlin, E. T. (1996). *Focusing-oriented psychotherapy: A manual of the experiential method.* New York: Guilford Press.

Hartmann, H. (1939). *Ego psychology and the problem of adaptation.* New York: International Universities Press.

Hayes, J. (2004). Therapist know thyself: Recent research on countertransference. *Psychotherapy Bulletin, 39*(4), 6–12.

Hayes, J. A., McCracken, J. E., McClanahan, M. K., Hill, C. E., Harp, J. S., & Carozzini, P. (1998). Therapists' perspectives on countertransference: Qualitative data in search of a theory. *Journal of Counseling Psychology, 45*, 468–482.

Heimann, P. (1950). Countertransference. *British Journal of Medical Psychology, 33*, 9–15.

Ivey, A. E., Gluckstern, N. B., & Ivey, M. B. (2006). *Basic attending skills*. Third edition. North Amherst, Massachusetts: Microtraining Associates.

Kernberg, O. F., Selzer, M. A., Koenigsberg, H. W., Carr, A. C., & Appelbaum, A. H. (1989). *Psychodynamic psychotherapy of borderline patients*. Basic Books.

Klein, M. (1952/1975). The origins of transference. In M. Klein (Ed.), *Envy and gratitude and other works 1946–1963*. 48–56. London: Hogarth Press (Volume 3).

Kohut, H. (1971). *The analysis of self*. New York: International Universities Press.

Kohut, H. (1977). *The restoration of the self*. New York: International Universities Press.

Lawrence, M. A. (1999). *The use of imagery and ego state therapy in holistic healing*. Paper presented at the annual meeting of the American Association for the Study of Mental Imagery, Orlando, Florida, April.

Mahler, M., & Furer, M. (1968). *On human symbiosis and the vicissitudes of individuation*. New York: International Universities Press.

Mahler, M., Pine, F., & Bergman, A. (1975). *The psychological birth of the human infant*. New York: Basic Books.

Maslow, A. (1954). *Motivation and personality*. New York: Harper & Row.

Masterson, J. F. (1976). *Psychotherapy of the borderline adult: A developmental approach*. New York, NY: Brunner/Mazel.

Masterson, J. F., & Klein, R. (1995). *Disorders of the self: New therapeutic horizons – The Masterson approach*. New York: Brunner/Mazel.

Masterson, J. F., Tolpin, M., & Sifneos, P. E. (1991). *Comparing psychoanalytic psychotherapies*. New York: Brunner/Mazel.

Meier, A. (2001). Adult survivors of incest and the capacity to forgive: An object relations perspective. In A. Meier & P. VanKatwyk (Eds.), *The challenge of forgiveness* (pp. 87–123). Saint Paul University, Ottawa, Ontario: Novalis.

Meier, A., Boivin, M., & Meier, M. (2010). Working through the transference of an unresolved separation/individuation pattern: A case study using theme-analysis. In A. Meier & M. Rovers, (Eds.) *The helping relationship: Healing and change in community context* (pp. 109–129). Ottawa, Ontario: University of Ottawa Press.

Meier, A. (2010a). The therapeutic relationship and techniques: How the clients bring about the desired change. In A. Meier & M. Rovers, (Eds.), *The helping relationship: Healing and change in community context* (pp. 1–31). Ottawa, Ontario: University of Ottawa Press.

Meier, A. (2010b). Transference and countertransference revisited. In A. Meier & M. Rovers, (Eds.), *The helping relationship: Healing and change in community context* (pp. 47–78). Ottawa, Ontario: University of Ottawa Press.

Meier, A., & Boivin, M. (1987). Self-discovery approach to counselling. *Pastoral Sciences, 6*, 145–168.

Meier, A., & Boivin, M. (1992). *A seven-phase model of the change process and its clinical applications*. Paper presented at the 8th Annual Conference of the Society for the Exploration of Psychotherapy Integration, San Diego, California, April 3.

Meier, A., & Boivin, M. (1993). *The interplay of affect, cognitions, and needs in a model of psychotherapeutic change*. Paper presented at the 9th Annual Conference of the Society for the Exploration of Psychotherapy Integration. New York: NY. April 23.

Meier, A., & Boivin, M. (1998a). *Treatment changes to compulsive behaviors in obsessive compulsive disorders: A case study using theme-analysis*. Paper presented at the 29th annual meeting of the Society for Psychotherapy Research. Snowbird, Utah, June 24–28.

Meier, A., & Boivin, M. (1998b). *The seven-phase model of the change process: Theoretical foundation, definitions, coding guidelines, training procedures, and research* data. 5th Edition. Unpublished manuscript. Ottawa, Ontario: Saint Paul University.

Meier, A., & Boivin, M. (2000). The achievement of greater selfhood: The application of theme-analysis to a case study. *Psychotherapy Research*, *10*(1), 57–77.

Meier, A., & Boivin, M. (2006). Intrapsychic conflicts: Their formation, underlying dynamics and resolution: An object relations perspective. In A. Meier & M. Rovers (Eds.), *Through conflict to reconciliation* (pp. 295–328). Ottawa, Ontario: Novalis.

Meier, A., & Boivin, M. (2010a). *The effectiveness of task-directed imagery, dialectical behavior therapy and empathic responding to develop the capacity to self-soothe*. Unpublished manuscript.

Meier, A., & Boivin M. (2010b). *The effectiveness of task-directed imagery and behavior rehearsal to develop competency to let-go of controlling behavior in intimate relationships*. Unpublished manuscript.

Meier, A., & Boivin M. (2010c). *Task-directed imagery: Its effectiveness to develop trust in intimate relationships*. Unpublished manuscript.

Meier, A., & Boivin, M. (2011). *Counselling and therapy techniques: Theory and Practice*. London, England: Sage Publishers.

Meier, A., Boivin, M., & Meier, A. (2006). The treatment of depression: A case study using theme-analysis. *Counselling and Psychotherapy Research*, *6*(2), 115–125,

Mitchell, S. A., & Black, M. L. (1995). *Freud and beyond: A history of modern psychoanalytic thought* (pp. 124–134). New York: Basic Books.

Perls, F. S. (1969). *Gestalt therapy verbatim*. Toronto: Bantam Books.

Rogers, C. (1957) The necessary and sufficient conditions of therapeutic personality change. *Journal of Consulting Psychology*, *21*(2): 95–103.

Rogers, C. (1959). A Theory of Therapy, Personality and Interpersonal Relationships as Developed in the Client-centered Framework. In S. Koch (Ed.), *Psychology: A Study of a Science. Vol. 3: Formulations of the Person and the Social Context*. New York: McGraw Hill.

Rogers, C. R. (1961). *On becoming a person: A therapist's view of psychotherapy*. Boston: Houghton Mifflin.

Smith, D. L. (2003). *Psychoanalysis in focus*. London: Sage Publications.

Strupp, H. H., & Binder, J. L. (1985). *Psychotherapy in a new key: A guide to time-limited dynamic psychotherapy*. New York: Basic Books.

Watkins, J. G., & Watkins, H. H. (1997). *Ego states: Theory and therapy*. New York: Norton.

Winnicott, D. (1948). Paediatrics and psychiatry. In D. Winnicott (Ed.), (1975), *Through paediatrics to psychoanalysis* (pp. 157–173). New York: Basic Books.

Winnicott, D. (1955–1956). Clinical varieties of transference. In D. Winnicott (Ed.), (1975), *Through paediatrics to psychoanalysis* (pp. 295–299). New York: Basic Books.

Winnicott, D. (1959-1964). Classification: Is there a psycho-analytic contribution to psychiatric classification. In D. Winnicott (Ed.), (1965), *The maturational processes and the facilitating environment* (pp. 124–139). New York: International Universities Press.
Winnicott, D. (1960). Ego distortion in terms of true and false self. In D. Winnicott (Ed.), (1965), *The maturational processes and the facilitating environment* (pp. 140–152). New York: International Universities Press.
Winnicott, D. (1962). Ego integration in child development. In D. Winnicott (Ed.), (1965), *The maturational processes and the facilitating environment* (pp. 56–63). New York: International Universities Press.
Winnicott, D. (1963). The mentally ill in your caseload. In D. Winnicott (Ed.), (1965), *The maturational processes and the facilitating environment* (pp. 217–229). New York: International Universities Press.
Wolitzky, D. L. (1995). The theory and practice of traditional psychoanalytic psychotherapy. In A. S. Gurman & S. B. Messer (Eds.), *Essential psychotherapies: Theory and practice* (pp. 12–15). New York: Guilford Press.

## Appendix 7.1: Task-Directed Imagery: Procedures

The distinguishing characteristic of Task-Directed Imagery is that the client is empowered prior to being asked to carry out a difficult task. The focus of Task-Directed Imagery is for the client to become aware of unmet needs and to express them. Task-Directed Imagery consists of the following four steps:

Step 1: Finding a place wherein one feels oneself and empowered: In this step, the client is asked to imagine being in some concrete setting or situation where she feels comfortable in being herself and empowered. The client is asked to describe the setting in terms of what is seen, heard, and smelled. To help the client with this step, the therapist might offer the following instructions:

1 I would like you to make yourself comfortable in your chair, close your eyes if you wish, and allow yourself to become relaxed.
2 In your mind, imagine being some place where you are able to be comfortable being yourself. It can be a place you have already been at. It could also be at a place that you have never been at before. Let me know when you have formed such an image.
3 (When the client indicates that she has formed an image, add) I would like you to describe the image for me. What do you see? Feel? Smell? Hear? Are you alone? Who are you with?

Step 2: Describing the feeling in being in the imagined setting: When the client has presented a sensorial description of the setting, ask how it is for her to be in this imagined setting. The client is asked to describe her state of mind, thoughts, and feelings being in that place where she can be herself. This state of mind represents a helpful ego state. Pay attention to words such as feeling strong, relieved, free, at peace, and so on as these words complete the description of the helpful ego state and will be used to design the task for the following step. The goal in having the client describe in detail her thoughts and feelings is for the client to come from a position of strength to deal with a difficult task.

Step 3: Carrying feelings and attitudes from imagined setting to the difficult task: In the third step, the client is asked to stay connected with the good feelings and attitudes experienced at the imagined setting and to carry them to a real, but often difficult, setting such as to assert herself with her partner. This task is usually difficult to execute and the client is encouraged to proceed slowly and take the time needed. If the client meets an obstacle, she is asked to circumvent or surmount the obstacle. Even if the client says that she cannot surmount it, encourage the client to continue a little while longer. To help the client negotiate this task, the therapist might provide the following instructions:

4 I would like you to hold onto all of these experiences of feeling empowered and feeling good inside and imagine being with the difficult situation that you described earlier (name the incident). As you are with the difficult situation, do not lose the good feeling about yourself and the feeling of being empowered. Take your time! If you feel that you are losing your good feelings, stop, go back, and pick them up again. Proceed gradually and go back and forth between the two if you have to. Let me know when you have been able to imagine being with the difficult task and at the same time feel good with yourself in how you succeeded to manage it.

5 (When the client has indicated that she has completed the difficult task, continue as follows). What image do you have in mind? Where do you find yourself? Describe the setting for me.

Step 4: Client's description of the experience: When the client has completed the third step, she is invited to describe how she achieved the task and how she feels in having been able to achieve it. The therapist is interested in two aspects of the experience, namely, how the client managed to bring it around so as to achieve the task and how the client feels having achieved the task. This is explored in great depth to assess the process and dynamics in using TDI to bring about change. To guide this process, the therapist might ask the following questions: (if the client's eyes are closed, invite the client to open them and be present.)

6 How did you manage to bring it about so that you were able to hold on to the good feelings and thoughts and address the difficult situation? (Listen carefully as to how the client proceeded to achieve the task. Do not rehash the exercise but focus on the process and dynamics of the imagery exercise. Listen for what is new in this

experience.) Is there anything else that you would like to say about this experience? (If the client says no, then bring the session to an end.)

7 What was this experience like for you? (Listen to what the client has to say, summarize it, and ask for clarification if needed. Then, bring the session to a close.)

Chapter 8

# Working with Unmet Core Needs in Psychotherapy

A primary goal of Self-in-Relationship Psychotherapy (SIRP) is for the therapist to help individuals to uncover and reclaim their unmet core relational, self, and physical intimacy needs, reorient their lives according to these needs, become agents of their own lives, and establish meaningful and wholesome relationships. In the same way that cognitions and affects play significant roles in cognitive and experiential therapies, respectively, core needs play a significant role in SIRP.

SIRP assumes that unmet childhood core needs and unmet growth needs are at the root of emotional, relational, self, and behavioral problems and that these needs are to be addressed to alleviate symptoms and bring about lasting change. The needs are often not apparent but are disguised in compensated behaviors such as being a caretaker, excelling in academics and sports and in disorders such as eating disorders and addictions which serve to temporarily meet their relational, self, and/or physical intimacy needs.

SIRP classifies core needs according to three groups, namely, relational, self, and physical intimacy needs (see Chapter 3). The relational needs comprise the need to emotionally bond with a significant other (e.g., caregiver) and the need to be autonomous. Self needs comprise the core need to experience being competent and to master of one's life and environment and the need to feel significant, lovable, and worthwhile. Physical intimacy needs include the need for sensual contact and for physical touch and closeness, such as embracing, hugging, and holding hands, and the need for sexual intimacy refers to the need to express oneself fully as a sexual being. These needs, in one way or another, remain with a person throughout her life.

SIRP pays particular attention to working with unmet core needs, but it does not in any fashion minimize the importance of working with cognitions and affects. On the contrary, SIRP assumes that the triad of cognitions, affects, and needs impact all aspects of human life and that they form three interdependent systems that interact in the acquisition and modification of behaviors, actions, and attitudes.

Within the triad of needs, cognitions, and affects, needs are conceived to be directional and the prime motivators of behavior, cognitive processes

DOI: 10.4324/9781003272502-11

pertain to the unique way to understand reality, solve problems, manage reality, and evaluate experiences and bring meaning to them, and feelings are thought to be responses to the satisfaction or the frustration of needs. Like a thermometer that indicates when it is too hot or too cold, so feelings act as a thermometer and indicate when things are or are not going well, that is, when needs are met or go unmet (Meier & Boivin, 1983, 2001).

In beginning of a therapy session, a SIRP-oriented psychotherapist carefully listens to the individual's concerns and problems since within these narratives reside the client's cognitive attempts to make sense of the problems, the emotional reactions to the situation, and the core relational, self, and physical intimacy needs that are unmet or threatened. Using this as a frame of reference, working with unmet needs can be understood to entail four steps.

The first step is for the therapist to listen to the individual's narrative or story which can be about an incident (e.g., poor work performance evaluation), event (e.g., an extramarital affair), action (e.g., domestic assault), relationship (e.g., feeling abandoned), or experience (e.g., failed licensing exam). The therapist invites the individual to provide appropriate information so that the therapist has a context within which to understand the presenting concerns and to assess the interaction of affect, cognitions, and needs.

In the second step, the therapist focuses on how the individual is trying to make sense of his concerns (e.g., of compulsive handwashing), that is, the therapist focuses on how an individual is cognitively processing the concerns. Often the client does not speak about how she is trying to make sense of the experience, but the therapist infers it from the manner in which the clinical material is presented.

In the third step, the psychotherapist pays attention to the individual's emotional response to the event or situation. The emotional response is an outcome of the meaning that the individual gives to the event. As a rule, pleasant experiences generate pleasant emotions and unpleasant experiences generate unpleasant emotions. An exception to this rule is when a client during the course of therapy gains awareness of a painful experience, which is construed as being pleasant because it led the client to uncovering a personal truth about her problem.

The fourth step pays attention to the needs that the individual perceives to be unmet, threatened, challenged, and/or fears to be lost. In the case of extramarital affair, for example, the individual might fear that her need to be loved and emotionally connected to a significant other will go unmet and that she will live a life of loneliness.

Relational, self, and physical intimacy needs form part of a more complex taxonomy of human needs (Maslow, 1968, 1970), but the focus in SIRP is on the relational, self, and physical intimacy needs. The manner in which these needs are integrated into one's life may be guided by higher-order needs such as one's values (e.g., generosity, compassion, equality), which serve as a broader and more significant context. The expression and integration of the needs is also guided by what Rogers called the "organismic valuing process" (Raskin & Rogers, 1989, p. 170) that assesses the personal and social appropriateness of a need. Needs typically go unexpressed because they are not validated and/or not responded to by others and/or are repressed by one's inner forces that inhibit their expression. These inner forces have been given the names of child, adult, and parent (Berne, 1961), id, ego, and superego (Freud, 1923), or libidinal, central, and antilibidinal ego states (Fairbairn, 1944). It is typically the internalized demanding parent that does not accept and inhibits the expression of the child's needs. These unmet needs, nevertheless, continue to push to be heard as the child moves into adolescence and adulthood.

This chapter focuses on the fourth step and begins by describing how unmet needs persistently push for expression and realization. This is followed by differentiating unmet childhood needs from unmet growth needs, uncovering, naming and accepting unmet needs, barriers to accepting of one's needs, weaning the unrealistic pursuit of needs, mourning and healing unmet childhood needs, and asserting and integrating needs into one's daily life. The cases used for the purpose of illustration do not refer to any particular persons and the names given to them are pseudonyms.

It should be noted that the majority of the cases are presented within the context of parents not being emotionally present to the child as needed. There is no attempt made to explain why the parents were not present as needed, nor is there any attempt made to indicate that the parents actually might have been present as needed but the child could not make use of what the parents offered her. Hypothetically, the parents might not have been present as needed due to factors such as illness, loss of job, death in the family, to mention a few. There is no intention to blame parents for the child's problems. Nevertheless, it is important to be mindful that a person's first significant relationships are with her parents and it is within these relationships that a person forms a sense of self and other and develops relational skills.

## Unmet Needs Relentlessly Push for Expression

Unmet needs, be they unmet childhood needs or unmet growth needs, persist and push for response because they represent the energy and forces that bring life to the individual, give direction to life, and lead an individual to living life to its fullness. Even though the unmet needs are repressed or suppressed, they continue to push to be heard and responded to. Unmet childhood needs persist and demand satisfaction from childhood into adolescence and adulthood. The unmet needs may lie dormant for many years and then suddenly are activated by visual, auditory, or olfactory stimuli or through a particular form of relational interaction. The unmet childhood and growth needs reside in the part of self that is referred to as the inner child (Berne, 1961), the id (Freud, 1923), or the oral libidinal ego state (Fairbairn, 1944).

The case of Louis illustrates how unmet childhood needs push until they are heard and responded to. Louis, single, 36 years of age, struggled for all of his life with issues of abandonment (Meier, 2014). When he was two years of age, his mother gave birth to his sister and he felt displaced by her. Prior to that Louis and his mother had a special relationship. In addition to the experience of being abandoned, Louis was sexually abused by a female relative when he was very young and by a girl four years older than himself when he was seven years of age. He also witnessed abuse and violence to animals that, to him, were like real people. He was traumatized, particularly, by the abuse to animals that he was fond of. His fear of abandonment and sexual abuse caused him to be cautious and avoidant in relationships. Yet the need to feel wanted and to be intimately connected drove his relationships. He met a number of women his age during his 20s, but he was not able to get close to them. When he tried to share his experiences, they did not want to hear about them and recommended that he see a psychotherapist. This is not what he wanted; he wanted to have a relationship with a woman friend. He felt pushed aside. His need to feel wanted and be in a relationship at times led him into wrong relationships. But for him, a bad relationship was better than no relationship.

Then one day he met a woman, Sonia, in her late 20s and they immediately connected emotionally. He sensed that she had something that he needed in life – that she could respond to his unmet childhood need for connection and to feel wanted and thereby heal his experience of abandonment. In due course, all of his sexual abuses and traumas emerged and he could talk to her about them without feeling pushed aside, judged, and abandoned. He felt that in the same way that he wanted to have her in his life, she also wanted to have him in her life. This relationship provided a healing presence. She often appeared in his dreams when he was having horrifying nightmares and provided a healing presence to him. In one of his dreams, he was sitting on a curb by the side of the road waiting for a dog to be killed; for him a dog was like a real person. He agonized over this and dreaded what was to take place; he could see the sadness in the eyes of the dog. As he sat there, Sonia quietly appeared in his dream. She sat on the curb about ten feet from him but remained silent. She was simply present to him. He felt a connection with her that he has not felt in the past. This was for him a healing presence. In the course of the following years, he was able to process his abuses, traumas, and feeling of abandonment and eventually was freed from them. The childhood needs to feel wanted and connected turned into a growth need to be wanted and connected in a mature way.

This example illustrates how Louis's unmet childhood need to feel wanted and connected pressed for a response and did not relent until the need was satisfied. Unmet needs not only press to be heard, but they also provide the direction as to how they are to be heard and satisfied in the healing process.

## Differentiating between Unmet Childhood Needs and Growth Needs

A fundamental goal of the SIRP approach is to help individuals become aware how their individual and relational problems are related to their unmet core relational, self, and physical intimacy needs. In working with unmet needs, it is important to differentiate between unmet childhood needs and unmet growth needs because the way they are addressed differs. Unmet childhood needs refer to the legitimate child needs such as the need for connection, competency, lovability, and autonomy for which the child was not validated and these needs continue to push for validation. Growth needs refer to the needs that were met in childhood but continue to be essential for continued growth and development in adolescent and adult relationships.

One criterion to differentiate the two sets of needs is to consider whether the unmet need has an insatiable quality to it and is disproportionate to what is expected from others. Unmet childhood needs tend to be insatiable in that they might be satisfied for the moment, but it does not last. They also do not get enough of an emotional connection when with another person. Unmet growth needs are satiable and require only small attention for their satisfaction.

A second criterion to differentiate unmet childhood needs from growth needs is to determine whether the need has a long history. Unmet childhood needs tend to have been part of the individual from as early as she can remember whereas growth needs may have their beginning in adolescence or adulthood. For example, if an individual constantly seeks validation for being competent and the validation quickly evaporates and she needs more of the same, this is referred to as an unmet childhood need. On the other hand, if an individual, from time to time, seeks validation for her competency but does not need constant validation as she can self-validate, this suggests a growth need.

A third criterion is to determine whether the unmet needs are reasonable or unreasonable. Unmet childhood needs tend to be unreasonable in the sense that no one can satisfy them regardless how much they might give of themselves whereas growth needs are reasonable and easily responded to.

A fourth criterion is to determine whether the need is phantasy based or reality based. Unmet childhood needs tend to be colored by phantasy and are idealistic whereas growth needs tend to be practical and reality based.

To illustrate the difference between unmet childhood needs and unmet growth needs, two examples will be given. The first example is that of a couple, Mario and Anita, who struggled with unmet growth needs and the second example is that of a couple, Bill and Colleen, who experienced continuous marital conflicts because of mutual unmet childhood needs.

Mario and Anita were married for ten years and had three young children. Anita took leave from work to bring up her young children. Mario was a salesperson and spent many evenings away from home seeing customers. Both were brought up in families that were loving, caring, and supportive. They sought couple therapy to address their concerns. Anita complained about Mario's absences and that she felt alone and not important to her husband. She felt mildly depressed. Mario complained about feeling pressured to spend more time with Anita with the consequence that he would not generate enough revenue to support the family and would not be promoted if he did not put in extra time at work. He also needed time and space away from the family to emotionally recharge. In the course of couple therapy, both expressed their concerns and their growth needs which for Anita was to spend more time together (i.e., for emotional connection) and for Mario to have time for himself (i.e., for autonomy). They worked toward a compromise which addressed their growth needs, improved their relationship, and restored their marital satisfactions. Their growth needs were not colored by unmet childhood needs.

Both Bill and Colleen were in their second marriage and had adult children from their first marriages and a young child from their current marriage. Colleen was a public servant and held a very responsible position. Bill was a very successful entrepreneur and was very involved, more accurately, over involved, in community affairs and in fund raising. They spent their evenings separately with Colleen watching her favorite TV programs and Bill working on the computer attending to his business. Both came from dysfunctional homes. Bill was the youngest of four brothers and always felt inferior to them. Colleen was the eldest of three girls and felt that she was taken for granted and not appreciated. Colleen complained that she and Bill did not spend enough time together which Bill did not understand as they spent two long vacations together each year. Colleen often spoke of the need for emotional connection which was incomprehensible to Bill. For Bill, spending time together, like traveling, was emotional connection. Bill complained that Colleen ignored and made light of his success at business. They had huge arguments and both threatened, at one time or another, to leave the marriage. To try to resolve their marital discord, they sought couple therapy.

In the course of therapy, it became apparent that both Bill and Colleen were driven by unmet childhood needs. Neither Bill nor Colleen was able or willing to provide what the other needed. Colleen described Bill as being like a young boy and she did not need another child in her life. Bill complained that Colleen was like his cold mother and not responsive to his sexual needs. As therapy progressed, it became clear that Bill was driven by the need to prove himself as he felt inferior to his siblings. He worked long hours at his business and community activities. The motive behind these unrelenting efforts was to feel that he is a competent and capable person which he received from the community organizers for the funds that he generated. He resented Colleen for not validating his successes which he interpreted to mean that he is an incompetent person and not good enough. Colleen, on her part, felt that the only time she mattered to Bill was when he invited her to join him for important business functions. He often did not express his appreciation for the "small" things that Colleen did such as prepare special meals and attend to Bill when he was ill. In summary, Bill's unmet childhood need was to be competent and Colleen's unmet childhood need was to matter and be significant to him. These unmet needs pushed to be satisfied and impacted the couple's relationship. When the couple became aware of their unmet childhood needs, therapy took on a new direction that focused particularly on the barriers standing in the way of responding to each other's unmet childhood needs and how to integrate them in their evolving relationship.

## Uncovering, Naming, and Accepting Unmet Needs

The first task in working with unmet needs is to help the individual to uncover an unmet need. This is often accomplished indirectly rather than directly since unmet needs are often disguised and lie outside of one's level of awareness. The uncovering of needs entails helping the person to differentiate between feelings, needs, and thoughts that individuals seldom do, particularly between feelings and needs. It is important for the individual to become aware that how one thinks about something is very different from how one feels about something and both are very different from what one needs. The use of terms such as "hot cognitions" (Safran & Greenberg, 1982, p. 83) and "emotional needs" (Gottman & Silver, 1999) are not very helpful to conceptually understand an individual's concerns because they do not clearly differentiate between the roles of the three interdependent systems, namely, cognitive, affective, and motivational systems and how they influence relational interactions.

The process of uncovering unmet needs begins by listening to the individual's narrative of her concerns, problems, difficulties and symptoms. Interwoven with the concerns and problems are to be found the individual's efforts to make sense of them, her emotional reactions to them, and implicit statements about that which she feels is threatened, challenged, absent or fears to be lost.

How, then, to get to the unmet needs? Where to look for the unmet needs? Entrance to the unmet needs can be made through many different avenues such as through analyzing feeling states, the manner of communicating, relational patterns, transferences, and body language. The psychotherapist's countertransference is yet another way to access a client's unmet needs. This section will limit itself to demonstrating how analyzing feeling states, the manner of communicating, relational patterns, emotional reaction, and making sense of one's concerns, can serve as avenues to help an individual to uncover, name, and accept unmet needs.

### *Uncovering Unmet Needs through Feelings*

An effective way to access unmet needs is through an individual's affective system, that is, through her feelings. Feelings can lead an individual to her unmet needs and to connect with them. Feelings are about something, but they are not the something that underlies an individual's concerns and difficulties. Thus, one needs to dig deeper than feelings as feelings are perceived to be responses to either the satisfaction or the frustration of needs, that is, they indicate whether one's needs are met or unmet.

Often clients begin therapy by reporting something that has deeply bothered them. One carefully listens to the incident, situation, event, and/or the behaviors of others with an eye keyed to the unmet need that has generated the feeling about the situation. In listening to an event or experience reported by an individual, the therapist listens for the feelings, the meaning given to the event, and to the needs that are unmet, threatened or lost, but the focus is on the unmet or threatened need. The following example illustrates this point.

Let's imagine that Siegfried lost his best friend in a car accident. The event is the accident. The meaning given to this accident might be that Siegfried has not only lost a friend, but he also lost what the two shared with each other, he lost the experience and the good feelings about himself that he had in being with his friend. With the loss of his friend, Siegfried experiences an inner void and emptiness and the loss of an important connection to a loved person. Siegfried's need is to be connected meaningfully to a significant other and to be loved by that person. To focus only on the feelings changes little. To try to change the meaning given to the event by saying that eventually all people have to face their mortality or that Siegfried can find others to befriend, is not helpful. It is only by focusing on the loss, mourning the loss and learning how to fill the emptiness created by the loss that will make a difference. The loss represents an unmet need for a meaningful connection. It is in addressing the unmet need and finding a response to it that will make a difference.

As the individual expresses his feelings regarding a situation, the therapist tries to get a sense of the unmet need that activated the feeling. To achieve this, the therapist listens to the individual's implicit message and tone of voice and pays attention to body gestures and posture. In addition to the client's articulation of his feelings, the therapist might also ask the individual to pay attention to her body, to get a bodily felt sense of what lies deeper

(Gendlin, 1996). The therapist might also use his own experiences (e.g., countertransference) and bodily felt feeling to get a sense of what is missing in the individual's life, that is, the unmet need (Satir, 2013).

The following example illustrates how a loss in early childhood turns into an unmet childhood need that relentlessly pushes for expression and influences life beyond childhood. Carlos, a teenager, sought therapy to deal with panic attacks, depression, physical complaints, and lack of motivation for school work. He left his home to attend a university in another city. He had ambivalent feelings about being away from home. He was the eldest of five children with 16 months between himself and the second born. He was brought up by parents who were high functioning professionals. As a child and young teenager, he had the freedom to pursue his interests which included solitary winter sports such as alpine skiing. When as a child and young teenager he was emotionally troubled, he would not express his feelings but would distract himself by engaging in activities and in his solitary sports. He found it painful to be close to his family and he dealt with it by taking distance. He also found it difficult to be away from home such as being at summer camps.

In the course of therapy, he provided three cues related to his emotional unrest, namely, he feared that he was missing out on something and that others were having more fun, he had a desire to excel in something but he could not bring himself around to commit, and he did not want to be tied down. The therapist made sense of these three cues within the context of the separation and individuation process (Mahler et al., 1975). At the time of the birth of the second born, Carlos felt displaced, rejected, and abandoned. He had not yet worked through the developmental process of separation and individuation and consequently felt pushed out and became predisposed to feeling abandoned when excluded by significant others. In being pushed out, he felt distraught and thought that the second born was having more fun than he was. The fact that he did not want to be tied down and wanted to excel, suggests that prior to the birth of the second born, Carlos was moving in the direction of individuation and autonomy which he relished as a child. However, with the birth of the second-born child and feeling that his relationship with the significant caregiver (e.g., mother) was threatened, Carlos relinquished his autonomous strivings and reverted to dependent behaviors. He was caught in the pursuit of the two conflicted primary needs, to be emotionally connected to the caregiver, and yet to be autonomous and to excel. Thus, both his need to be emotionally connected and to be autonomous and excel were left unfulfilled. He became aware that these two unmet childhood needs were at the heart of his anxieties, panic attacks, depression, lack of motivation for studies, and inability to commit himself. This painful realization, however, was a positive for him as he was able to discuss his feelings more openly with his parents and siblings rather than to repress them, and it began his long journey in working out issues around emotional bonding and autonomy.

### *Entry to Unmet Needs by Analyzing the Manner of Communicating*

The manner of communication includes the extent to which the persons are collaborative, try to understand each other, are able to articulate their feelings, thoughts and needs and are able to tolerate and respect differences. It also includes the words that are used in the communication and the tone that is given to the words (Luthman, 1974; Roberto-Forman, 2008; Satir, 1972; Satir et al., 1991). When the communication becomes conflictual and when partners are not ready to listen to each other and judgmental words are exchanged, one can anticipate that their mutual needs, be they unmet childhood needs or unmet growth needs, are not being heard, validated, and responded to. Often the words that are exchanged between the two individuals provide a clue to the unmet needs. Using her countertransference and intuitive skills, the psychotherapist in the middle of a heated discussion, might share her perception of the dynamics of the relational discord in terms of unmet needs. It is important for the psychotherapist to listen to what is being spoken about and listen for their individuals' reactions to the topic and their ability to focus on it rather than to speak in parallel about two different topics in order to make their point.

The way to use a couple's manner of communicating as an entrance to their unmet needs is illustrated by the case of Sophia and Raoul who have been married for 19 years and had three teenage children. Raoul was the youngest of four brothers all of whom excelled but he did not. Sophia was the oldest girl in the family and assumed many responsibilities without being appreciated and validated. Sophia worked for a large private company and Raoul was an entrepreneur. In recent years Sophia became very anxious about their financial situation since Raoul's business enterprises were often risky and he made decisions without discussing them with her. In his slow business periods, he made improvements to the house such as building a walk to the front door. In one of their heated discussions, Sophia complained about not being included in the decisions that Raoul was making about the house and Raoul responded saying that whatever he does is not good enough. He referred to her not complimenting him on having built a beautiful walk, but instead pointed out minor defects. In the heat of this discussion, the therapist, sensing that he had a grasp of the underlying dynamics, asked them to stop arguing and he shared with them his impressions. Turning to Raoul, the psychotherapist said that he feels that whatever Raoul does is not good enough and then turning to Sophia he shared his impression that she feels that what she has to say does not matter. These comments led to a deeper discussion with Raoul expressing that since childhood he felt that he was not good enough and Sophia stating that since childhood she felt that her feelings, needs, and aspirations did not matter. Both Sophia and Raoul were reaching out to their partner to have their unmet childhood needs responded to. For the Raoul the unmet childhood needs were for autonomy and competency and for Sophia the unmet childhood needs were for feeling significant and worthwhile. The recognition of their mutual unmet childhood needs changed the course of their interactions and that of therapy. They became aware that their marital discord is related not only to their unmet growth needs but also to their unmet childhood needs.

### *Discerning Unmet Needs by Analyzing Relational Patterns*

There is an overlap in the underlying dynamics of communication styles and relational patterns. However, in relational patterns the focus is more on behavior and body clues and messages regarding the desired and expected behaviors from others (Luthman, 1974). In understanding relational patterns, the interest is about the type of relationship that an individual expects from another person, the way that an individual relates toward another, and the way an individual tries to draw the other into relating in a specific way. Thus, there are two elements in the relational pattern, namely, the manner in which an individual relates to others in word and behavior and the manner in which an individual expects the same from others. Relational patterns vary greatly and have been given different names such as placater, blamer, computer, and distracter (Satir, 1972); fusion and distancing (Roberto-Forman, 2008); dependency, power, and ingratiation (Cashdan, 1988); maladaptive cyclical patterns (Strupp & Binder, 1985); and pursuer and avoidant.

Underlying problematic relational patterns are unmet growth and/or unmet childhood needs. The relational patterns have as their goal to have these needs responded to and satisfied in a particular way. Often relationships begin with both parties anticipating that the other will provide that which is missing in their life (Hendrix, 1990, 2007). When what is missing is unmet childhood needs and the partner becomes aware that he cannot respond to them, the partners soon become frustrated with each other. The consequence is that both discontinue making efforts to respond to the needs of the other because their own needs are not being satisfied. This leads to marital dissatisfaction and outright conflict. It is very important, therefore, to differentiate relational patterns that are driven by unmet growth needs from those that are driven by unmet childhood needs as the work with them differs.

Relational patterns that are driven by unmet childhood needs can best be understood as the externalization and projection onto another of an individual's own internal struggle between his inner child needs and parental demands (Berne, 1961). These internal struggles indicate that the individual has not accepted his own child's needs, and similar to his actual parent, the child's internal parent is critical and unaccepting of his childhood needs. Thus, for example, one partner, whose unmet childhood need is to be loved and to feel worthwhile, will expect to be validated for these needs by his/her partner. The same holds true if a partner's unmet childhood need is to be competent and autonomous. Often such relationships are patterned after a parent-child relationship with one playing the role of the critical and demanding parent and the other playing the role of the needy and hurting child.

The psychotherapist can use the relationship to uncover unmet childhood and/or growth needs. In this process, the therapist pays attention to the voice of the partners and asks himself whether the voice is that of an adult, parent, or child. The therapist also pays attention to the expectations that the partners have of each other and how they are trying to draw the other into relating or behaving in a specific way. For example, a partner may do all that she can to prevent the other from leaving the house to participate in a work-related activity because the meaning given to his leaving for this activity is that she is not wanted, is not important and significant. The unmet childhood need is to be loved, to be wanted, and to be important.

To illustrate how the relational pattern can be used to uncover unmet needs, reference will be made to Stan and Cathy who have been married for 15 years and have three children. Cathy is the eldest of six children. She took great interest in her younger siblings and assumed responsibility for their care when called upon. She learned to give of herself to others but did not expect much in return from her younger siblings. She learned to be emotionally available to others without expecting them to be emotionally available to her. Stan was the youngest of four children and was brought up in a dysfunctional home. Neither of his parents was emotionally available to him as needed. His father was very critical of Stan particularly when Stan, as a child, was needy and whining. When criticized by his father for such behaviors, Stan thought of himself as being a "bad person" and unwanted and unloved. At the beginning of their relationship, Cathy validated and supported Stan in his entrepreneurial projects. As time passed, Stan needed more and more validation not just for being good at his work, but for being a good person. Cathy initially made great efforts to respond to his ever-increasing need for validation. But it was not enough. Stan would often point out to Cathy how she was to relate to him, speak to him (e.g., what words to use), and how to respond to his needs. Cathy felt that what she did was not good enough. Initially she felt that there was something wrong with her, she doubted herself and apologized for her behaviors. She began to feel oppressed, violated, and defeated. However, she came to realize that she was not the problem. She could no longer comply with his wishes.

In the course of therapy, it became clear that Stan's need for validation was not an unmet growth need, but an unmet childhood need. It also became apparent that Stan was torn and conflicted within. He had internalized his critical father which became for him his internal parent which was critical of his inner child's needs. He externalized his internal conflict in his relationship with Cathy. In the relationship Stan was the critical parent and Cathy was a happy, content, reasonable, practical, and easy-going person who did not respond to Stan's every need. She did not allow herself to be drawn into his demands to relate and behave in the expected way which escalated the conflict. At a very young age, Stan associated the failure of his father to respond to his needs and feelings to him being an unlovable, worthless, and bad person. Stan tried to repeat this relational pattern in his relationship with Cathy. Underlying their marital conflicts was Stan's unmet childhood need for lovability, being worthwhile and a good person. This became clear in the way in which he wanted Cathy to follow his instructions, talk to him using his words, and deal with conflicts.

Stan's unmet childhood needs to feel significant and to be seen as being a good person was disguised and hidden in what seemed like "controlling and manipulative behaviors." Stan learned from childhood that he could not count on his parents for his personal wellbeing thus he took charge of his life at a young age. In his relationship with Cathy, he determined how she was to speak to him and respond to his needs and demands. These requests or demands were motivated by his unmet childhood need to feel significant and worthwhile and a good person.

In order to resolve the relational issues, it is important for Stan to resolve his internal conflicts between the harsh and demanding parent and the legitimate needs of the child and to give voice to these needs. The appropriate form of therapy for Stan needs to address the interpersonal and the intrapersonal that is, the individual and the system, and bring about congruency between the two (Luthman, 1974; Napier & Whitaker, 1988; Satir, 1972).

### *Identifying Unmet Needs through Making Sense of Events and Concerns*

One can access unmet childhood and unmet growth needs by asking the individual to provide her meaning of a troubling experience (e.g., event, situation, experience) that she presented at the beginning of a therapy session. The individual is not asked to interpret the experiences but indicate how she makes subjective sense of the experience (Mahoney, 1991). This implies that the individual makes sense of the experience by applying sensations, memories, perceptions, feelings, and motives from previous experiences to a current experience. It is assumed that the memories, perceptions, and motives from previous experience have become organized as schemas (Beck et al., 2014), ego states (Watkins & Watkins, 1997) and/or internal representations (Klein, 1952). Thus, when an individual is asked how she makes sense of a current experience, she will associate it with a previous experience and apply the internal representations from the previous experience to the current experience. The meaning that an individual gives to an experience, therefore, is based in part on objective reality and in part on subjective reality such as an internal representation.

Within the meaning given to an experience, there are latent unmet childhood or unmet growth needs. The experience that the individual reported has become problematic because it either threatens one or more of her relational, self, and physical intimacy needs or it activates an unmet childhood need. In listening to the meaning given to an experience, the therapist listens for the unmet childhood and/or unmet growth need and how it was activated by a recent experience. The following example illustrates this dynamic.

Gertrude, single and in her mid-30s, is a counselor who has been providing individual and couple counseling for almost a decade. She requested psychotherapy for herself because she was stressed out by one of her clients who made critical comments about the way she arranged her office. He would also miss appointments without informing Gertrude about it. She tried to let the client's comments about the arrangement of the office slide by. One day, however, he questioned her counseling approach and professional credentials. She was very upset by his comments and began to doubt her competency as a counselor even though she knew cognitively that she was very well qualified. She began to question her competencies as a therapist as the client's comments were not the first such criticisms. The therapist asked her what meaning she brought to this experience. Her response was that she is incompetent and that her feelings did not matter. She linked this experience to her own childhood during which she often heard the message that she was slow in learning and unlike her younger brother who was quick to learn new things. She also felt that her feelings and needs were not respected but those of her brother were. Coming out of her childhood experiences, Gertrude was left with the unrelenting needs to be competent and that she mattered. Her client, by his comments and missing appointments without informing Gertrude in advance, activated the unmet childhood needs. Thus, with the psychotherapist asking Gertrude the meaning of her experience, she was able to discern her unmet childhood needs and to address them.

## Barriers to Accepting One's Needs

When one views the models of personality, psychopathology, and psychotherapy that influence research and practice, one readily sees that these models are organized around feelings, cognitive processes, and behaviors with little, if any, attention given to motives (Meier & Boivin, 2001). In our Western culture talking about one's feelings and thoughts is quite acceptable, but it is less acceptable to talk about one's needs as it is assumed adults have outgrown their childhood needs. This attitude might be based on the failure to differentiate between childhood needs and growth needs with the latter being part of one's life from womb to tomb. It has been demonstrated above how growth needs are an integral aspect of every person's life and represent the positive life force which gives direction for wholesome living. For this reason, it is important to identify the barriers that prevent a person from accepting and expressing his growth needs and orienting her life accordingly.

The barriers that stand in the way of a person accepting and expressing her needs and living from them can be thought of in terms of external factors and internal factors. External factors might include negative attitude toward needs and not having learned how to assert one's needs. Internal factors might include feeling guilty and selfish in asserting one's needs, not deserving to have one's needs met, and that needs are too painful to accept. The internal factors are often due to internal struggles or conflicts with the internal critical parent part of a person dominating the child part of the person. The following examples illustrate several barriers to accepting and asserting one's needs.

### *Negative Attitude toward Needs*

In our culture, the acceptable attitude about relationships – also about the workplace, educational institutions, and businesses – is that of independence, performance, accomplishment, and success and not about emotional bonding, friendships, and community. When the word *need* arises, the thought is about unmet childhood needs and rarely about growth needs. Since adults are expected to have outgrown their childhood needs, they are no longer expected to have relational, self, and physical intimacy needs which, in reality, are lifelong growth needs. Needs are either, not responded to or accepted, or they are minimized and dismissed. This negative attitude toward needs is a barrier for a person to have her needs accepted by others and for the individual to assert her needs for fear that they might be minimized or dismissed.

This negative attitude toward the needs of others is illustrated by the case of Ming-tun, a graduate student in a counseling program in a Canadian university. Ming-tun, from Hong Kong, took his undergraduate degree in experimental psychology and philosophy. His orientation in counseling was cognitive which conflicted with the humanistic orientation of the graduate program in counseling in which he was registered. Ming-tun was given the message by his supervisor, that, he would have to consider leaving the program as he experienced difficulty formulating empathic responses. Ming-tun was distraught by this suggestion as he felt that with more time, he could master empathic responses. He wanted his supervisor to hear and validate his feelings, desires, and needs; he wanted his need (aspiration to be a counselor) to matter to the supervisor. Ming-tun was assigned another supervisor who gave Ming-tun ample time to hone his skills which he eventually accomplished. This case illustrates the importance of respecting the needs and aspirations of others and helping them achieve their goals.

### *Not Knowing How to Assert One's Needs*

There could be three significant reasons why an individual, as a child, did not learn how to assert her needs. First, the individual was brought up in an overprotective home where decisions were made for the child. Thus, the child was not given the opportunity to learn how to ask for things or to assert her needs, feelings, and preferences. Second, the individual was brought up in a home where the atmosphere was negative, tense, and hostile and one's feelings and needs were either dismissed or criticized. Third, the individual was brought up in a loving, caring, and joyful home that was easy going where the members of the family anticipated and accepted each other's feelings and needs and felt free to assert them. How might either one of the three scenarios affect an individual's ability to assert her needs, feelings, and opinions?

The case of Ingrid, 22, a graduate student in economics, intelligent, knowledgeable, and brought up in an easy-going family, illustrates her difficulty to assert herself in a classroom which was more gregarious than the home in which she was brought up. She wanted to participate in the classroom discussions and feel as intelligent as her colleagues but she was afraid to ask questions or to make a comment on an issue for fear that it might come out wrong or seem off topic. In her mind, she would rehearse the question she wanted to ask or the comment that she wanted to make, but by the time she was ready to ask a question, the question was asked or the comment was made by another student. She felt frustrated with herself and began to think that others are cleverer than she because they were able to ask relevant questions and make meaningful comments. This case illustrates that it is not enough to know one's needs but it is also important to learn the skills how to assert them and in this case to feel as competent as her colleagues.

### *Feeling Guilty and Selfish in Asserting One's Needs*

Another barrier to the acceptance and assertion of one's needs is feeling guilty and selfish in putting one's own needs ahead of those of others. This is particularly characteristic of individuals who have an internalized parent that is prohibitive and idealistic and is not adequately moderated by the internalized adult. The internalized parent informs the person about the behaviors, actions, and attitudes that are not acceptable, and the behaviors, actions, and attitudes that one should strive toward. A fundamental (unrealistic) ideal is to place the needs, interests, and feelings of others ahead of those of one's own. A consequence of breaching this ideal is to feel guilty and selfish, which stand in the way of being true to oneself and living authentically and congruently.

This negative attitude toward the acceptance of another's need is illustrated in the case of Anselm. He was brought up in a middle-class home. His father was a college professor and laid-back and emotionally absent from the home. His mother was anxious, insecure, and demanding and rewarded him with her affection for compliance with her wishes. When Anselm expressed his need for autonomy and independence, she withdrew her affection and became critical of him. Whenever Anselm asserted his need for autonomy and independence to the displeasure of his mother, he would feel guilty, selfish, worthless, and angry and he feared that he would be punished. Anselm learned that to receive the affection of others, he had put the needs of others ahead of his own. His wish not to feel guilty and not to appear selfish kept him for asserting his own needs. In suppressing his own needs, he developed inauthentic relationships with his parents, coworkers, members of the community, and his wife.

### *Feeling Not Deserving*

Children who are emotionally neglected, maltreated, traumatized and/or sexually abused, often develop the sense that they are bad, flawed and not deserving in having their affectional needs met and good things given to them. These children internalize these external messages to form part of their own internal organization with their inner critical and uncaring parent sending the message to the inner child that she is bad and flawed and not deserving of love and affection. When such individuals, either as children, adolescents, or adults, are complimented or given awards, their natural tendency is to think that a mistake was made and that if people would understand them, they would have done differently. They are also very afraid that people will find out that they are not the person that they are thought to be. For this reason, they do not risk to ask favors and affection from others.

This feeling of not deserving good things in life is illustrated by the case of Elvira, nineteen, who was brought up by her alcoholic and emotionally disturbed and neglectful mother. In her childhood and pre-teen years, Elvira would arrive home from school to find her mother lying drunk on the couch. Elvira became the caregiver of her mother and saw to it that she had prepared meals. When lucid, the mother would be critical of Elvira and demean and shame her. Elvira began to think that she was the cause of her mother's drinking and emotional problems and began to feel that she is a bad person and that there is something terribly wrong with her. She tried to cope with her situation by turning to drugs and alcohol and when this failed to numb her feelings, she attempted suicide on three different occasions. Although she planned the last suicide very carefully, it failed. This failure was the beginning of Elvira turning her life around. She struggled most with believing that she was a good and deserving person. When she was shown kindness and given favors, she had to return them ten-fold. She would not and could not assert her needs for affection and friendship. When others showed interest in being her friend, she could not understand why they wanted it and she avoided such gestures. When she received good marks in her course, she interpreted this to have been a mistake on part of the professor. Her inability to accept herself as an intelligent, loving, good and caring person stood in the way of her asserting her needs for affection and friendship. She thought of herself as being flawed and undeserving.

### *Unmet needs are too painful to accept*

There are situations where it is too painful to address unmet childhood needs. This is particularly true for an adult, who as a child, did not feel as admired as her siblings and felt left on the sidelines. As a child, she might have gone out of her way to please her parents but without an appropriate response from them. The child was left with a broken heart and in order to deal with the pain, she disconnected from her feelings.

The avoidance of looking at painful unmet needs is illustrated by the case of Tania who was married to Andrew for eight years. Tania was brought up with three older brothers who received praise and admiration for their intellectual and athletic accomplishments. She was neither intellectual nor athletic. Her parents were accomplished professionals. Andrew was brought up by his emotionally unstable and needy mother with whom he experienced no emotional connection and yet craved for it. At his work place, Andrew met a woman who swept him off from his feet as he saw in her the love and affection that he wanted and unconsciously craved. Tania noticed that Andrew's level of intimacy with her began to change. She became suspicious of him, checked his e-mails, and to her shock, saw affectional exchanges between Andrew and his new woman friend. In the course of couple therapy, Andrew mentioned that he does not know whether he still loves or ever loved Tania. Andrew's statement cut into her heart. She could not and did not want to believe that Andrew did not love her and that he could not get the love back that they had when they were married. For Tania the thought of not being loved by Andrew activated her childhood experiences in feeling not being loved and admired by her parents, particularly, by her mother. Rather than addressing the possibility that Andrew does not love her, Tania tried to convince Andrew that he actually did love her when they were newly married and that he can get his love for her back again. This example illustrates how a childhood pain in not being loved and admired by her parents keeps Tania from realistically evaluating her relationship with Andrew.

## Weaning From the Unrealistic Pursuit of Needs

An important step in weaning from the unrealistic pursuit of needs is to determine when an individual's needs are unrealistic. An individual's needs are deemed to be unrealistic when they are insatiable, cannot be reasonably satisfied by anyone, when the person feels empty when not with a significant other, or when the person feels incompetent when not constantly validated. Associated with unrealistic needs is the assumption that when they are not responded to, the individual is no longer loved and admired, and is forgotten and abandoned.

One example of having an unrealistic need is that of Julia who had her own musical band. She was particularly close to one of the band members, Hugo. She always looked forward to their practices so as to be with Hugo. After their weekly practice, she and Hugo spent another two or more hours together. When he was about to leave, she felt that she did not have enough of him and was not ready to see him go. After he left, she felt empty and alone and she lost all sense of having been with him. Julia's unrealistic need has its origin in her childhood relationship with her inattentive and occupied mother who Julia followed around the house for love and affection.

How to wean the unrealistic pursuit of needs? First, it is important for the individual to recognize that her need is unrealistic and insatiable and to accept this as a reality. Second, the individual has to become aware of the assumption on which the unrealistic need rests and to challenge this assumption. Third, it is important for the individual to resist the impulse to pursue the unrealistic need; not to give into it and to talk herself out of it. Fourth, it is helpful for the individual to observe the consequence in resisting the impulse to pursue the unrealistic need. This helps to form a new perspective on the unrealistic pursuit of needs.

The struggle against the unrealistic pursuit of needs is illustrated by the case of Rafael who mentored Gabriela in advanced statistics. Both were graduates students. Rafael was specializing in mathematics and statistics and Gabriela was specializing in counseling psychology but struggled with statistics. Gabriela arranged to meet regularly with Rafael for help in statistics. Shortly after they begin to work together, Rafael began to develop strong feelings of affection for Gabriela. As these feelings of affection for Gabriela grew, Rafael became more troubled by his own feelings for her and by her leaving after each meeting. He had not experienced such intense feelings for someone in the past. After she left, he felt an enormous ache in his heart, he missed her intensely, he felt abandoned, and could not wait to be together with her again. At the same time, he wondered whether she liked and wanted him as much as he liked and wanted her. As the weeks went by, he noticed no change in her mood and in her manner of being with him. Her feelings about him and her relationship with him were constant. Each time she left him, he fought against his urge to call her and he looked for clues that contradicted his assumption that she is abandoning him and not liking him and wanting to be with him. With his continued struggle against the unrealistic pursuit of his need for emotional contact with Gabriela and with his challenging the assumption that being apart from each other meant she did not think of him and abandoned him, he gained a new perspective on their relationship. He came to the realization that she wanted him in his life as much as he wanted her in his life. His unrealistic needs for her subsided. Rafael's struggle with abandonment had its origin in childhood with the birth of his sister when he was eighteen months of age. He felt that his mother's attention to the new baby meant that she loved him less and was abandoning him.

## Mourning Unmet Childhood and Loss of Growth Needs

It is part of every individual's experience not to have had all of her childhood needs met. However, the extent to which one's childhood needs go unmet varies largely and ranges from not having all of the toys and sweats that one wanted, for example, to having one's need for affection and being competent dismissed. The majority of the children are able to manage their unmet needs. However, children whose relational, self, and physical intimacy needs were unmet for a prolonged period of time will enter adolescence and adulthood struggling to recapture what was lost in childhood. They will eventually come to understand what was not given to them in childhood cannot be regained. They will mourn that for which they had a right to, as a child, to receive from significant others and that which could have been theirs but will never be. For example, a child who, at the age of one year, lost her mother will forever yearn for that physical and emotional bonding that she momentarily tasted before it was taken from her.

Circumstances also arise when one is faced with mourning growth needs. Growth needs are an extension of the childhood relational, self, and physical intimacy needs. Every person needs to be significant to someone, and to feel loved and competent in order to grow as a person individually, relationally, intellectually and spiritually. Individuals grow in a relationship where they feel at home with each other, are accepted, respected, validated, and challenged. When a relationship is broken for whatever reason, the individual left behind experiences the loss of that which enriched her life and her sense of being fully alive. Lost growth needs differ from unmet childhood needs in that the former do not have the insatiable quality of the latter and are addressed satisfactorily in due time.

The situation is different for a person who is struggling with unmet child needs and at the same time is experiencing the loss of growth needs. An example is that of Thomas who was divorced ten years ago but is not able to move on and form new relationships. Thomas experienced abandonment as a child but he did not mourn the unmet need for connection because in being with his wife, she comforted and soothed him each time he experienced abandonment. He did not face his fear of abandonment. When he and his wife broke up, Thomas was left with mourning his unmet childhood needs. Not having done so, kept him from mourning the loss of his relationship with his wife and from moving forward in developing new relationships. To move forward, it was necessary for Thomas to mourn both the loss of his relationship with his wife and his unmet childhood needs.

The following example illustrates in more detail the mourning of unmet childhood needs and the loss of growth needs. Mathias, twenty-two, single, worked for his father's landscape company. He learned at a very young age to handle equipment and drive vehicles. His father was proud of his son's skills. As a child, toddler and pre-teenager, Mathias craved for more emotional closeness with his distant father. Mathias had troubled teenage years which drove an emotional wedge between him and his father. However, toward the end of his teens, Mathias settled down and enrolled in a college degree in landscaping in which he did very well. His father was proud of him and spoke highly of him to his friends. Mathias was beginning to have an emotionally closer relationship with his father and enjoyed working with him. Mathias was also proud of his successes and, in his heart, he wanted to give the joy of his academic success to his father. In a symbolic way, he wanted to give the joy of his college diploma to his father to repair the relationship of the past, rebuild the relationship of the present and build a relationship for the future. The father became suddenly ill and passed away before Mathias obtained his diploma. Mathias was in a state of shock, then angry at his father for having died before he obtained his diploma and thereby deprived him of giving the joy of his success to his father. By his father's untimely death, Mathias was left to mourn the unmet childhood need for love and affection that he craved for from his father. Mathias was also left to mourn the loss of the close and meaningful friendship-like relationship that was developing with his father. Thus, Mathias was left to mourn both his unmet childhood needs, the loss of growth needs and the opportunity to repair their childhood conflicts by symbolically "offering" his diploma to his father.

## Unmet Needs in Physical Ailments and Emotional and Behavioral Problems

As was mentioned earlier, needs push relentlessly to be responded to and when this does not occur in ordinary living, the individual, unconsciously, finds myriad ineffective behaviors to deal with them. These behaviors may range from feigning illness and somatization to opposition behaviors and emotional disorders. The following examples illustrate how unmet needs play a role in the development of physical ailments and in behavioral and emotional problems.

### *Feigning illness*

Josée, sixteen, was referred for counseling because during the past year she had been depressed, attempted suicide twice by overdosing, found school boring, had few friends, and was dissatisfied with home life. She described her parents as being strict and moralistic in their attitude and inconsistent in disciplining their children. She described her mother as being sweet, soft, and passive and at the same time controlling, nagging and laying on guilt trips. She tried to protect her mother from the father's angry outbursts. Her relationship with her father was troubled and inconsistent. At one moment he would be bossy and treat her like a two-year old and at another moment he would be thoughtful and compassionate toward her. She often stayed away from home overnight as she could not tolerate the angry and hostile home atmosphere. At different times, she tried to bring joy to the family but was criticized for this and put down. Her relationship with her siblings was non-existent. She considered herself as the scapegoat of the family.

She constantly sought the affection from her mother and when it was not given to her, Josée often followed her mother around the house, a behavior referred to as shadowing by Mahler and associates (1975). Josée also feigned illness to get the love she needed from her parents. She began at a very young age to pretend to be ill so that she did not have to go to school but could stay home with her mother. At another time she pretended that she was deaf. She was taken to the hospital to have tubes placed in her ears and provided with a hearing aid. During the course of therapy, Josée became aware that she feigned illness to be loved and accepted and for physical closeness, affection, and to be taken care of as a child; in short to feel that she mattered to her parents. As she began to be more assertive of her relational, self, and physical intimacy needs with her mother, father, siblings and boyfriend, feigning sickness to get the love that she needed, subsided.

### *Somatization*

Physical ailments such as migraine headaches, hypertension, and irritable bowel syndrome are thought to be due to a set of complex factors including stress, anxiety, and anger together with a genetic, immunological, neurological and/or physiological factors and/or predispositions (Bakal, 1992; Devi, 2013). Treatments for these disorders often involve, in addition to medication, psychological interventions such as relaxation and mindfulness meditation. Unmet needs might also contribute to some of the physical ailments as illustrated by the following example.

Donald, in his mid-forties, mechanical engineer, married with three children, was referred by his family doctor for psychological treatment because medication was not improving the client's irritable bowel syndrome. Psychological treatment began with the established hypothesis that stress and anxiety contributed to this disorder. The exploration of the client's stressors and sources of anxiety and the practice of relaxation exercises did not improve his condition. One day, in the course of therapy, he expressed his anger at his favorite daughter, Darlene, for not pursuing a traditional career, like himself. She was in a relationship with a young man who had no set goals in life and who did not encourage Darlene to pursue a career similar to that of her father. Donald felt pushed aside by his daughter and that he no longer mattered to her. He felt that his need to be mattered by his daughter was being threatened. The focus of therapy shifted from focusing on his anxiety to focusing on his anger and to addressing his unmet need to be significant and to matter not only to his daughter but to others as well. Within a couple of months, his irritable bowel syndrome subsided.

### *Oppositional and defiant behavior*

Nathan, 15, was referred for therapy because of his oppositional defiant behavior. He was the youngest of three children. He was brought up in a home where there was constant fighting and tension which eventually led to the parents' divorce. He and his two siblings were brought up by their mother who was constantly depressed and angry, emotionally demanding and critical of the children, and violated sexual boundaries. The father was emotionally absent and ineffective in enabling the children to deal with the family conflicts. Nathan's parents were inconsistent in their relationship with him and he could not rely on them to attend to his relational and self needs. He felt that his feelings and needs did not matter to his parents. In his younger years he complied with their wishes and expectations. However, when he became a teenager and was living with his father and his second wife, Nathan no longer took instructions from them. By now he had learned to fend for himself and to take charge of his life as he could not count on his father and step-mother to be there for him when needed. In his teens, when asked to carry out a chore or to behave in a particular way, his immediate reaction was to oppose their requests which led to huge arguments. He took charge of his own life and did not entrust it to his parents. Therapy focused on his need to matter, heal the early injuries to self, and learn how to assert his needs. The therapist also worked with Nathan's father and step-mother to help them to understand how Nathan was affected by his early childhood experiences. With his parents' understanding and acceptance of his needs and of him as a person, his oppositional behaviors decreased.

### *Emotional problems*

Emotional problems represent complex predisposing internal factors and precipitating external factors. Among the internal factors are cognitive processes, affective reactions and motives (e.g., unmet childhood and/or growth needs). External factors range widely to include relational, cultural and societal factors and events and situations. Unmet needs play a role in the development of emotional problems as illustrated in the following example (Meier et al., 2006).

Anselm, in his mid-forties, married for fifteen years, experienced his fourth episode with major depression during the past fifteen years. He was brought up in a middle-class home. His father, a college professor, was laid-back and emotionally absent from the home. His mother, anxious, insecure, and demanding, rewarded him with her affection, for compliance with her wishes, but withdrew her affection and became critical of him when he tried to assert his autonomy and independence. Anselm felt guilty, worthless, angry, and punished when he asserted his autonomy and felt intruded upon and violated when he complied. Anselm learned that to receive the affection of others, he had to put their needs ahead of his. As a consequence, he suppressed his need for autonomy and independence and became inauthentic in his relationships with his parents, co-workers, members of the community, and his wife. In due time, Anselm became aware that his inability to assert his autonomy and to be authentic in his relationships lay at the basis of his depression. In becoming assertive of his needs and more autonomous and independent, his depression lifted and he continued to remain free of depressive episodes for three years following psychotherapy.

## Asserting and Integrating Core Needs into One's Daily Life

After having uncovered and named the unmet childhood needs and growth needs, the task for the individual is to integrate and to assert these needs in her daily living. Before an individual is able to assert the unmet needs, it might be necessary for the individual to wean herself from unrealistic needs and to mourn the unmet childhood needs. In order to assert her needs, the person may have to work through the barriers that are keeping her from asserting her needs. The achievement of these tasks is a prerequisite to asserting and integrating one's relational, self, and physical intimacy needs in an authentic way. For most individuals, the needs are naturally, and without much concerted effort, integrated to become part of one's life. For others, who have not acquired the skills to assert their needs, they may require professional help.

An example of a person who had to acquire the skills to assert his needs, feelings, preferences, thoughts, and so on, is Anselm, cited above. He was brought up in a family where the mother, in particular, was anxious, insecure, and demanding and did not validate his movement toward autonomy and independence but affirmed his dependency on her and his compliance to her wishes. When he pursued his needs, rather than those of his mother, he felt guilty and selfish. His sense of guilt and selfishness kept him from acquiring the skills to assert his needs. Before he could begin to assert and integrate his unmet needs, Anselm had to deal with his feeling of guilt and sense of selfishness which were barriers to asserting his needs. By coming to terms with the idea that there is no justifiable reason to feel guilty and selfish in asserting his legitimate needs, he was able to accept that he could be his own person and be autonomous and independent despite the pull from his mother to remain dependent on her. In due course he was able to assert and integrate his need for autonomy and independence which brought him a great sense of freedom and inner peace.

This chapter outlined the key role that needs play in an individual's life and how to uncover them. It also indicated the barriers that can keep a person from asserting his needs, the importance of weaning the unrealistic pursuit of needs and the importance to mourn unmet childhood needs. The next chapter will address some of the therapeutic procedures involved in uncovering needs, weaning the unrealistic pursuit of needs, mourning unmet needs, and in asserting needs.

## References


Bakal, D. A. (1992). *Psychology and health.* New York: Springer Publishing Co.

Beck, A. T., Davis, D. D., & Freeman, A. (Eds.) (2014). *Cognitive therapy of personality disorders, 3rd. Edition.* New York: Guilford Press.

Berne, E. (1961). *Transactional analysis in psychotherapy.* New York: Grove Press.

Cashdan, S. (1988). *Object relations therapy: Using the relationship.* New York: Norton.

Devi, G. (2013). *A Calm Brain: How to Relax into a Stress-Free High-Powered Life.* New York: Plume Book,

Fairbairn, W. R. D. (1944). Endopsychic structure considered in terms of object relationships. In W. R. D. Fairbairn (Ed.), *An object-relations theory of the personality* (pp. 82–136). New York: Basic Books.

Freud, S. (1923). The Ego and the Id. *Standard Edition, 19*, 12–63.

Gendlin, E. T. (1996). *Focusing-oriented psychotherapy: A manual of the experiential method.* New York: Guilford Press.

Gottman, J. M., & Silver, N. (1999). *The seven principles for making marriages work.* New York: Random House.

Hendrix, H. (1990). *Getting the love you want: A guide for couples.* New York: Harper.

Hendrix, H. (2007). *Getting the love you want, 20th anniversary edition: A guide for couples.* New York: St. Martins Press.

Klein, M. (1952). Some theoretical conclusions regarding the emotional life of the infant. In M. Klein (Ed.), *Envy and gratitude and other works 1946–1963, Vol. 4* (pp. 61–93). New York: Delacorte.

Luthman, S. (1974). *The dynamic family.* Palo Alto, California: Science and Behavior Books.

Mahler, M., Pine, F., & Bergman, A. (1975). *The psychological birth of the human infant.* New York: Basic Books.

Mahoney, M. J. (1991). *Human change processes: The scientific foundations of psychotherapy*. New York: Basic Books.
Maslow, A. H. (1968). *Toward a psychology of being (2nd Edition)*. London: D. Van Nostrand.
Maslow, A. H. (1970). *Religions, values and peak-experiences*. New York: Viking Press.
Meier, A. (2014). *The healing power of relationships*. Presidential Address delivered at the annual conference of the Ottawa Institute for Object Relations Therapy, Ottawa, Ontario, June 21.
Meier, A., & Boivin, M. (1983). Towards a Synthetic Model of Psychotherapy. *Pastoral Sciences, II*, 137–176.
Meier, A., & Boivin M. (2001). Conflict resolution: The interplay of affects, cognitions, and needs in the resolution of intrapsychic conflicts. *Pastoral Sciences, 20*(1), 93–119.
Meier, A., Boivin, M., & Meier, M. (2006). The treatment of depression: A case study using theme-analysis. *Counselling & Psychotherapy Research, 6*(2), 115–125.
Meier, A., & Boivin, M. (2011b). Experiential focusing technique. In A. Meier & M. Boivin (Eds.), *Counselling and therapy techniques: Theory and Practice* (pp. 32–45). London, England: Sage Publishers.
Napier, A. Y., & Whitaker, C. A. (1988). *The family crucible*. New York: Harper & Row.
Raskin, N. J., & Rogers, C. R. (1989). Person-centered therapy. In R. J. Corsini & D. Wedding (Eds.), *Current Psychotherapies*, 4th Edition (pp. 155–194). Itasca, Illinois: F.E. Peacock Publishers.
Roberto-Forman, L. (2008). Transgenerational couple therapy. In A. S. Gurman (Ed.), *Clinical handbook of couple therapy* (pp. 196–226). New York: Guilford Press.
Rogers, C. R. (1961). *On becoming a person: A therapist's view of psychotherapy*. Boston: Houghton Mifflin.
Safran, J., & Greenberg, L. S. (1982). Eliciting "hot cognitions" in cognitive behaviour therapy: Rationale and procedural guidelines. *Canadian Psychology, 23*(2), 83–87.
Satir, V. (1972). *People making*. Palo Alto, California: Science and Behavior Books.
Satir, V. (2013). The therapist's story. In M. Baldwin (Ed.), *The use of self in therapy*, 3rd *Edition* (pp. 19–27). New York: Haworth Press.
Satir, V., Banmen, J., Gerber, J., & Gomori, M. (1991). *The Satir model: Family therapy and beyond*. Palo Alto, California: Science and Behavior Books.
Strupp, H. H., & Binder, J. L. (1985). *Psychotherapy in a new key: A guide to time-limited dynamic psychotherapy*. New York: Basic Books.
Watkins, J. G., & Watkins, H. H. (1997). *Ego states: Theory and therapy*. New York: Norton.

Chapter 9

# Relationship and Self Issues and Their Underlying Unmet Needs

This chapter presents self and relationship issues that Self-in-Relationship Psychotherapy (SIRP) typically addresses. All of the issues presented are related to one or more constructs from SIRP. It is assumed that often unmet core childhood needs underlie many of an individual's personal and relationship problems and difficulties. The unmet needs are not easily detected but are often embedded in the behavioral, emotional, and relationship difficulties that the individual presents in therapy. The unmet needs in this chapter are framed according to core relational needs (e.g., need for emotional bonding; need for autonomy), self needs (e.g., need for competency; need for significance), and physical intimacy needs (e.g., need for sensual contact; need for sexual intimacy) as presented in Chapter 3.

Needs are viewed as forming one of the three interdependent systems, namely, the cognitive, emotional, and motivational systems (Meier & Boivin, 1983, 1993). None of the systems are complete without the other, they depend on each other. The need (motivational) system, however, is deemed to be primary and underlies the emotional and cognitive systems. The three systems interact in any given behavior.

The distinction between self and relationship issues is more a question of focus rather than an actual distinction since there is no self without a relationship and no relationship without a self. Self issues refer to those that pertain to the subjective experience of self that include self-esteem, internal conflicts, being out of touch with one's body, and perceptions of self and other. Relationship issues refer to the difficulties and problems that an individual experiences within the context of relationships, particularly, close and intimate relationships. These problems may range from feeling abandoned, and not having developed a childhood emotional bond with a significant other to lacking empathy for others and using projective identifications.

It should be noted that a particular issue is not worked through in isolation from other issues. The self and relational issues are related to each other and form a unique unit for any given individual. Working on one

DOI: 10.4324/9781003272502-12

issue often indirectly addresses other issues. The self and relationship issues are not particular to any psychiatric diagnostic category; rather they are shared in different ways by a number of psychiatric categories. For example, the fear of being abandoned is an aspect of both borderline personality disorder and narcissistic personality disorder. Lastly, one does not treat a psychiatric disorder as such; rather one treats the constituents of a disorder. As an example, in helping a person overcome depression, one addresses his sense of helplessness, need to comply with expectations of others, non-assertive behavior, feeling obligated, and sense of not being authentic to self and others (Meier et al., 2006).

This chapter briefly presents examples of self and relationship issues that embody unmet core needs as understood within a SIRP perspective. More complete presentations of self and relationship issues and their embodied unmet needs are presented in the following chapter. The examples of self and relationship issues presented here are taken from the authors' clinical records, however all identifying information have been altered. For each of the self and relationship issues, there is a brief description of the issue, a statement regarding the therapeutic task and goal in working with the issue, and a presentation of possible approaches that can be used to address the issue. A case is presented that illustrates how a self and/or relationship issue has been addressed. Lastly, the underlying unmet need for each case is briefly described.

## Connecting with One's Bodily Self

### *Description*

A developmental task for the infant/child is to become an embodied psyche, that is, for the psyche to become anchored in its body so that the body and psyche become a harmonious unity (Winnicott, 1965/1981). Through coenesthetic reception, the infant develops a bodily self which comprises streams of sensations that arise within the organism – from viscera, muscles, tendons, joints, vestibular canals, and intestines (Allport, 1955/1967; Krueger, 1989; Mahler et al., 1975). The infant is first a bodily self which is the foundation for the development of a psychological self.

An infant/child can fail to embody the psyche when his desires, needs, interests, and feelings are not validated but are discounted or dismissed or when the infant/child is led to believe that his needs and feelings are bad and should be pushed aside. The disconnection between body and psyche is particularly seen in emotionally neglected and sexually abused individuals who feel ashamed of their bodies and think of their body as being bad, dirty, and evil. A disconnection between body and psyche is indicated when the person is not aware of his feelings and desires and speaks from the head and not from the head and the heart.

### *Task/Goal*

The task is to design an exercise to help an individual to pay attention to the sensations and feelings of his body, to name them and accept them. The assumption is that in accepting and owning these sensations and feelings, the individual can embody them within his sense of self.

### *Approach*

Often logical approaches are not adequate to help an individual become attuned to and aware of the sensations and feelings of his body and one must use a technique that bypasses intellectual analysis. Semi-hypnotic techniques such as experiential focusing (Gendlin, 1996) and Task-Directed Imagery (Meier & Boivin, 2011a) are effective to bring about greater bodily awareness, to connect head and heart and psyche and soma. Both of these techniques use a bodily felt feeling to uncover the underlying feelings, needs, thoughts, and personality dynamics.

### *Case: Rafal*

Rafal, in his mid-30s and married, struggled to be spontaneous in his relationships, to express affection and to make decisions. His mother died when he was five years of age and he was then placed in an orphanage for three years. He moved from school to school and had very little memory of events prior to the age of 13.

Rafal's wife came from a broken home and an alcoholic mother; she was sexually abused in childhood. She depended on her husband and she restricted his being away from home to be with his friends or to engage in sporting activities. She was sensitive to his absentees and rejections which she dealt with by going into a rage or by regressing to a fetal position. He walked on eggshells when he was around his wife.

Rafal felt pressured to fill his relational space with work rather than to let things roll along and enjoy life. He had great difficulty to get in touch with his feelings and needs and he lived mostly from the outside of his body. To help him get in touch with his bodily felt feelings, an experiential focusing exercise was designed which initially was not effective. Subsequently, an exercise which focused on becoming aware of bodily sensations was designed. For example, he was instructed to observe his feet resting on the floor, he resting against the back of the chair, his breathing and his heartbeat. This was following by the use of experiential focusing, which opened up for him a repertoire of feelings, obligations, needs, and a conflict between the inner child and the internalized parent with the latter controlling and not in tune with the needs of the former.

The use of experiential focusing eventually led to a greater awareness, acceptance, and expression of his feelings and needs and to their integration with conscious thoughts and with their assertion. For example, he began to express his need to spend time with his friends and to continue with his sporting activities. In brief, Rafal was able to bring about a greater unity between psyche and body.

### *Underlying Unmet Needs*

Rafal struggled with balancing two unmet core needs, namely, the need to remain emotionally bonded with a significant other (e.g., wife) and the need to be autonomous and pursue his interests and activities. The negative responses to his early childhood feelings and needs led Rafal to disconnect from them and to live a life which was based on complying to the demands and expectations of others.

## Connecting with the Inner Child

### *Description*

The inner child (i.e., the coherent, inherent, pristine self) may be cut off, submerged, or repressed because of social pressures to conform, or because of emotional neglect, abuse, and trauma that required the individual to invest energy to survive and therefore did not invest energy in the expansion of self and formation of healthy relationships (Fairbairn, 1944; Winnicott, 1965/1981). The inner child can be wounded, neglected, and forgotten and thereby feel abandoned, angry, and enraged. The inner child embodies the genuine self, the pristine ego and the positive energy for growth and expansion. The cut-off inner child manifests itself in behaviors, which include dependency on others for nurturance, complaints that the other is not there for him, not having life goals, searching and seeking for that which is elusive, being depressed, angry, and raging and feeling empty. The message is that there is something missing in one's life.

### *Task/Goal*

The first task is for the individual to access the cut-off part of self that has been forgotten, wounded, and neglected but which still exerts influence on the individual's behaviors, attitudes, and feelings. The second task is to help the individual to own the cut-off part of the self and to give voice to it. The factors that caused the inner child to be cut off, forgotten, wounded, neglected, and disowned have to be identified.

### *Approach*

The cut-off parts of the inner child can be accessed through the use of experiential focusing technique wherein the individual is asked to get in touch with a bodily felt feeling. The assumption is that the body remembers, that the body has an understanding of self that cannot be reached by conscious efforts (Rothschild, 2000; Van der Kolk, 2015). In other cases, the individual might bring forth material (e.g., feeling sad, abandoned) which ushers the beginning of the emergence of the cut-off parts of the inner child. In such cases one works with the material that the individual offers.

### *Case: Nita*

Nita, of East Indian origin, was brought up in a predominant Hungarian community. Her father was hospitalized with tuberculosis for the first 11 years of her life. Her mother ran a women's clothing store and therefore was not readily available to her and to her siblings. During grade school, Nita was teased to the point of humiliation for being pigeon-toed and for the color of her skin. She had no one to turn to since she did not have relatives in the community. She felt rejected, hurt, and angry, feelings that she suppressed and repressed. She was in her second marriage and experienced relationship problems. Her current partner, Bill, had an affair in the past and Nita was very suspicious of him and constantly kept track of his whereabouts and looked in his wallet for telephone numbers. When she found a suspicious telephone number, she went through all efforts with the hope of finding the person's name and address. Her inordinate need for reassurance from Bill and with he not providing it satisfactorily, led to many quarrels and squabbles to the point of violence. She sensed that she was hurting not only on the outside but also on the inside. The exploration of the inside hurt, by using experiential focusing, allowed her to enter into her subjective world and access her abandoned, angry, and hurt inner child. With deep sadness, uncontrollable weeping, and mixed emotions, Nita connected with her inner child, and promised to take care of her and to protect her from further hurts and pains. She reclaimed the cut-off part of her inner child and she began to reorient her life around the needs and wisdom of her inner child.

### *Underlying Unmet Need*

Her unmet need was to be seen as a significant person and to be loved and to be connected to her partner in a meaningful way. Her mistrust that she developed because of past relationships stood in the way of allowing her to freely have a relationship with her husband and thereby to have her needs to be found lovable and to be connected validated.

## Giving Voice to the Inner Child

### *Description*

After connecting with an inner child, it is often necessary for the client to develop a voice, to become enabled, to express his needs, feelings, and thoughts. The inner child is that part of self that has been repressed and cut off because of social pressures and/or experiences of emotional neglect, abuse, and trauma. These experiences did not permit the inner child of the individual to have a voice and did not allow him to invest energies in the growth of self and development of healthy relationships. The individual, often angry and frustrated, may know what he wants to say and do, but he fears to assert his needs and to express his thoughts and feelings because of possible rejections and criticisms. The individual expresses his readiness to have a voice when he clearly differentiates between what is expected of him and his disagreement with it and his implicit motivation to voice his concerns. That is, the individual is ready to have a voice if he engages in an internal dialogue between the demanding self and the needy self.

### *Task/Goal*

The first task is to assess the individual's implicit awareness of a bodily felt feeling that there is something within him that is pushing for release and wishes to be expressed. This is followed by providing the individual with an opportunity to become enabled and to give voice to his feelings, thoughts, and needs. As much as possible it is helpful to determine the target of the pent-up feelings as expressed by the person.

### *Approach*

To help the individual develop a voice and become empowered, one can use the Gestalt Empty Chair technique (Meier & Boivin, 2011b). This technique consists of a monologue in which the individual speaks to the targeted person who listens. The therapist can help the individual to stay focused on the task and to facilitate the monologue by restating and/or by responding empathically to the client's implicit feelings, thoughts and needs. But it is very important to help the individual to speak from his voice and express his relational needs. To add to the meaningfulness of the monologue, the therapist might ask the individual to repeat statements more intensely and empathically.

### *Case: Henri*

Henri, single, in his late 20s, expressed the wish to look at his relationship with women because he wanted to understand his difficulty with emotional intimacy. Although he recently broke off with a relationship, he had the repeated fantasy and urge of wanting to be with her romantically even though in his mind the relationship was terminated. However, when he was with her for a short time, he wanted to take distance from her because he felt invaded by her. This pattern of pushing her away and then approaching her to reconnect is a repeated pattern. He did not know whether he cared for her or whether there was some hidden motive that was driving it.

In the process of being engaged in the Gestalt empty chair technique, he felt a strong feeling that took him back to his mom who he felt had something to do about his relationships with women. The cut-off part within him, the inner child began to give voice to his feelings which were directed toward his mother. He said "I'm getting very tired of trying to please you, to make you happy, of you running everyone around you and to do the right thing for you." Henri continued with

> I feel as if you have been standing on my shoulders all of my life, you make life difficult. Get off my back and leave. If you don't want to be happy that's your responsibility. I want to be happy and I'm not going to let you mess it up. Don't bug me. I'll call you when I want to be with you.

He then added that "she doesn't want to leave." Henri then picked up the chair in which his mother imaginatively sat and placed it outside of the office to where it rests to this day.

When Henri picked up the chair, he felt a sense of empowerment, that is, a sense of autonomy. He did not know that he had the power to be in charge of his life and to have an input in relationships. He stated that he was experimenting with his power and determining its limits. His last comment was that there was something missing in the exercise which is that he would liked to have heard what his mother had to say. This statement implies that he was ready to enter into an open and real dialogue with his mother, more precisely to enter into a dialogue with the internalized mother and the internalized child which was achieved in a later session using the Gestalt two-chair technique.

### *Underlying Unmet Needs*

The underlying unmet need for Henri was to be autonomous when in the presence of his mother and yet at the same time to remain connected to her. He was ready to psychologically separate from his mother and to individuate in the sense of having the freedom to express himself and yet still remain connected to her.

## Establishing Whole-Object Representations

### *Description*

Whole-object representation refers to relating to a person as a separate, differentiated, and individuated person who has his own feelings, needs, and thoughts (Klein, 1946/1975). It refers to not idealizing nor devaluing the other and not relating to the other primarily in terms of how the person might satisfy an individual's needs. When an infant/child has negative experiences with a significant caregiver, the child might either discount the negative experiences and embellish the positive experiences (e.g., idealize the other) or the infant/child might become angry and only see the other's negative qualities (e.g., devaluate the other). Both situations are referred to relating to the other in terms of part of the person (e.g., part-object). The infant might carry these part-object representations into adolescence and adulthood and project them on future relationships and relate to them as they are needed rather than to relate to them as persons in their own right.

### *Task/Goal*

The task for an individual who relates to others as a part-object is for him to see both the strengths and the shortcomings of the other. Developing empathy for the other often facilitates the transformation of part-objects into whole-objects. Empathy tempers one's criticisms of the other. It is possible that for an individual who was abused, that he is not able, nor is expected, to see the perpetrator as a whole-object because of the injuries and hateful feelings toward him. In such cases, it is important for the survivor to see himself as a whole person, a person with specific needs, thoughts, feelings, life goals and aspirations, and values.

### *Approach*

Task-Directed Imagery is one approach that is helpful to develop whole-object representations. The individual is asked to get in touch with the goodness of the other and in being able to do this, the other is perceived as separate from self and a person in his own right. The acquisition of a more positive object representation entails the development of empathy that tempers one's criticism of the other.

### *Case: Devin*

Devin, mid-30s, married, was brought up in a home where the father was abusive toward his children and maltreated them. He was left with feelings of anger toward his father who he perceived to be a mean and hostile man. Devin, himself, was left with feelings of worthlessness, low self-esteem and feeling flawed. His wife was brought up in an oppressive, loveless, and critical home. She and Devin often had huge fights with threats of self-harm and/or leaving the relationship. Yet both wanted the relationship to endure.

In the course of therapy, Task-Directed Imagery was used to help Devin to perceive and experience himself as a wholesome person. The next step was for him to perceive and experience his wife as a wholesome person. To help Devin perceive his wife as a wholesome person, a Task-Directed Imagery was used wherein Devin was asked to get in touch with the wholesomeness of his wife. He was touched by the fact that she too was maltreated by her parents and was struggling with the childhood hurts, low self-esteem, and anger that she at times vented toward him. He became more empathic toward her and saw her through her feelings of sadness and low self-esteem and wanting to be respected and loved. He saw her as separate from himself.

Weeks later he reported that his thinking of himself as a good person and of his wife as a good person brought about warm feelings for himself and for his wife. He also reported experiencing inner calm, peace, self-confidence, was easier going, and did not have to prove himself to anyone. Things that used to bother him in the past, no longer bothered him that much; the emotional edge was taken off from these situations.

### *Underlying Unmet Needs*

Devin sought a relationship to whom he felt emotionally connected, that is, safe, secure, loved, valued, and protected. However, his tendency to project his anger and distrust on the other prevented him from having such a relationship. In being able to perceive his wife in more positive terms and as a person in her own right who wanted to be with him, he became more empathic toward her and more emotionally connected.

## Developing Object Constancy

### *Description*

Object constancy refers to an internalized representation of a person with whom one is libidinally (i.e., with love and pleasure) connected and to whom one can consistently and reliably turn (inwardly) for safety, nurturance, protection, direction, and self-comforting (Mahler et al., 1975). Object constancy implies that the perceived bad and the good qualities of a person (e.g., father) have been integrated to form a whole representation of the person. To have object constancy is similar to carrying a "friend" within our psyche and in terms of a song by Faith Hill one can say, "and everywhere

I am, there you'll be." Object constancy provides the capacity to see things in a new light, to self-comfort and self-soothe in difficult times and have the capacity to uplift oneself in troubled times.

The development of object constancy begins with the infant/child and primary caregiver relationship. In this relationship, the infant/child learns that he can confidently expect that the parent will reliably and consistently respond to his needs and emotions. Signs of having acquired object constancy are the experiences of "safe anchorage" and "confident expectation" (Mahler & Furer, 1968, p. 17), that is, the experience of being emotionally bonded and confident that his needs and emotions will be responded to.

#### *Task/Goal*

An individual who has not developed object constancy as an infant/child might find it very difficult, as an adult, to become libidinally connected to a significant person for one of two reasons: First, the individual may not know what it means to internalize a good object since he did not experience this in infancy and childhood. Second, the individual, because of painful emotional injuries of the past, might distrust and fear others and therefore lacks the inner motivation and confidence to develop object constancy.

For the individual who seeks object constancy, the therapeutic task is to help him to use current relationships to become aware of his need to be with someone with whom he feels totally comfortable, safe, secure, protected, wanted, understood (known), and loved. The task is to work through the defensive resistance that is triggered by early childhood injuries that led to the failure to develop a trusting, safe, secure, and loving relationship with a primary caregiver which are essential for the formation of object constancy. Often these individuals fear being rejected or abandoned if they were to express their needs to the other.

#### *Approach*

Developing object constancy is a challenging task that often emerges only after many months of therapy. One way to help an individual develop object constancy is to ask him to recall the good objects (persons) who were in his life but that he might have forgotten about. This is particularly helpful for individuals who still have ambivalent feelings, but more positive than negative feelings, toward persons who have been in their life even though the former might have been emotionally hurt by them. Using this approach, the therapist asks the individual to name the persons in his life who seemed to have been there for him. He is asked to describe the behaviors of these persons, their attitude toward him, and how they took him under their wing. At the same time the individual is asked to describe his own feelings, thoughts, and needs regarding the significant persons. This recalling of good objects might lead to internalizing a composite good object that serves as the basis to build other good objects.

A second approach is to use the "track-record method," particularly for a person who is struggling to become comfortable in an intimate relationship. The term "track-record" comes from horse racing and refers to a horse's performance in past races which information is used to predict how a horse will perform in future races. When applied to the development of object constancy it refers to the consistency of the meaning that one gives to a person's past behavior in order to determine the meaning of a current and future behavior. Each consistent experience contributes to a more durable object constancy (Krueger, 1989). For example, if a person does not return a text message within an hour, does this mean that the person does not care or does it mean that a person was too busy but does care? Thus a "track-record" of past meanings of a person not responding immediately to a text message can be used to determine the meaning of a current delay in responding to a text message.

### *Case: Andreas*

Andreas, single, in his mid-30s, struggled to develop trusting and emotionally close relationships with women. As a child, he felt abandoned by his mother and was sexually abused by a female adult relative. He suffered numerous traumas beginning around the age of four and was sexually abused in grade school by a girl about four years older than himself. The aftereffects of the sexual abuses and traumas manifested themselves in flashbacks, nightmares, and in being cautious in his relationships with women.

For a good part of his life and without knowing it, he sought to repair the abandonment experience by developing emotionally close relationships with women. The desire to emotionally bond with a woman was a strong driving force, more so than to free him from the long-term after effects of the sexual abuse and trauma. In his initial attempts to get emotionally close to women, he felt that he wanted them more than they wanted him and he repeatedly re-experienced feelings of being abandoned. As a compromise, he established emotional intimacy by taking care of others and in listening to their problems but not by letting others get emotionally close to him which he felt too threatening although he craved it. When the women made what he perceived to be hurtful comments about him, he took great distance from the women.

In the middle of these struggles, he met a woman, Sabina, for whom he had very special feelings; he needed her in his life, he could not let her go despite incidents when his feelings of abandonment surged. To help him to deal with his feelings of abandonment, he used, at the suggestion of the therapist, the "track-record" method. For example, the first time that Sabina did not return his text-message within an hour, he feared that she was not interested in him and that the relationship was over only to feel differently when she returned his text-message two hours later with the explanation that she was at a meeting. In processing similar situations and in establishing a "track record," Andreas began to interpret Sabina's delay in returning messages more positively and felt that she did care for him; he came to realize that he could count on Sabina – her track-record supported his conviction.

The turning point for Andreas came when he realized that Sabina wanted to be with him too as he wanted to be with her. This led to the internalization of Sabina as a good and reliable object (i.e., person) and to the development of object constancy. Over time his child-like neediness for Sabina diminished; he sensed now that he did not need Sabina in the same way as before, but he wanted her in his life.

Andreas was able to develop object constancy by using the track record method to recognize that Sabina was there for him and wanted a relationship with him. She had a history of being there and wanting a relationship with him. However, he learned that there were times when she had other things to attend to which were not indicative of her not wanting to be with him or did not think of him.

The internalization of Sabina as a good object had enormous impact on the working through of his sexual abuse and trauma. Sabina would silently appear in his nightmares and be present to him as he (often as a boy) faced a traumatic event. Over a period of six months, Andreas was totally freed of his flashbacks, nightmares, and his fear of abandonment. Consciously or unconsciously, he was able to turn to the internalized Sabina as a source for strength, direction, self-comforting and to resolve the childhood traumas, abuses, and abandonment experiences.

### *Underlying Unmet Needs*

Andreas' underlying unmet need was to become emotionally anchored (i.e., bonded) in a relationship that he could count on and one in which he felt wanted and understood. A second need was to be found significant and to be loved for who he was rather than for what he could do or give. The realization of these needs led to the development of object constancy.

## Building Self-Esteem

### *Description*

Self-esteem implies that an individual has a positive bodily sense of self and a positive psychological image of self. One gains self-esteem from feeling loved unconditionally by the principal caregivers. One also gains self-esteem from the caregiver's validation of one's innate strivings toward self-actualization and from the validation of one's sense of competency (Kohut, 1974; Maslow, 1968; White, 1967). An child also gains self-esteem from experimenting with his skills and his newly discovered abilities and experiencing oneself as being competent. Children brought up in homes where there was abuse, emotional neglect, belittling, and harsh criticism, often struggle with issues of self-esteem. Good self-esteem acts as a buffer against losses, emotional injuries and setbacks.

### *Task/Goal*

The goal, in building self-esteem, is to provide opportunities for the individual to experience himself as a worthwhile, wholesome, and competent person. Talking about it is often not enough. The individual needs to experience himself as being a competent and a wholesome person. The task is to help the individual to develop a positive interject of himself to which he can turn when things get rough and tough.

### *Approach*

Task-Directed Imagery is one technique that can be used to help an individual gain in self-esteem. In using this technique, an individual is asked to imagine being in a setting which conjures up positive feelings about himself. Another exercise is experiential focusing wherein the individual is asked to get in touch with his sense of goodness and his sense of wholesomeness. The use of these techniques is based on the assumption that the individual had some positive experience about himself in the early days, weeks, and months of his life and is able to recapture and connect with it.

### *Case: Dylan*

Dylan, married and in his early 40s, was brought up in a very abusive home. His father constantly put him down, ridiculed him, mistreated him, and had nothing good to say about him. His mother was of very little help since she too felt intimidated by her own husband. She did not teach Dylan skills to cope effectively with the father. In the process, Dylan came to think of himself as being inadequate, incompetent, and unlovable and consequently developed low self-esteem. In his relationship with his wife, he sought her affirmations that he was a competent person but because of her own personal struggles, she resisted responding to his yearnings. When he was provoked and his sense of self was attacked, he feared to be rejected and abandoned and in defense, attacked her to protect himself. When criticized and humiliated, Dylan's self-esteem did not act as a source of strength and a buffer to feeling hurt. In response to such behaviors, he acted out.

To help Dylan develop self-esteem, the wholesomeness exercise was organized (see Chapter 7). He was asked to take a comfortable position in the chair, get in touch with his sense of competency, goodness, and wholesomeness and as he attempted this, he was asked to put aside any competing thoughts or feelings that wanted his attention. At first, he found it hard to stay with the task as competing thoughts fought for his attention. The therapist encouraged him to stay with the task, and as he was with the task, to say to himself, "I am a good person," "I am a generous person," and "I'm a competent person." (These suggested statements were based on statements made by Dylan in previous sessions.) He attempted these statements and as he did his eyes began to water. He knew that he was a good and competent person, that he was a kind, thoughtful, sensitive, and compassionate. Following this exercise, Dylan experienced inner calm, peace, greater self-confidence, was easier going, had warm feelings for himself and for his wife, and things did not bother him as much as in the past. He became more proactive and less reactive.

### *Underlying Unmet Needs*

The underlying unmet need that pushed for expression was to be esteemed by others and for him to esteem himself. In SIRP terms, the underling needs were to be competent, significant, and emotionally bonded to a significant other who would accept and affirm his competency and lovability.

## Integrating Conflicted Ego States

### *Description*

An infant/child internalizes the experiences that he had with significant caregivers to form a psychic organization that reflects the lived dyadic experience. In Freudian terms, the psychic organization can be thought to comprise the critical adult part of the experience (superego), the child part of the experience (libidinal id) and the rational part of the experience (ego). When an infant/child in its upbringing is oppressed, constrained, and/or restricted by demanding caregivers, he might develop a harsh and demanding superego that does not accept the needs and feelings of the libidinal id. Conversely, indulgent parents may not help the child to learn to self-regulate his impulses and feelings. Both situations can lead to an internal conflict between the ego states.

### *Task/Goal*

The goal is to build and to empower the ego so that it can listen to and hear the demands of the superego and the needs of the libidinal id and to reconcile them and thereby establish internal harmony and peace.

### *Approach*

One approach is to use the Gestalt Two Chair Technique (Meier & Boivin, 2011b) to engage the Topdog (i.e., the superego) and the Underdog (i.e., the id) in a dialogue with the purpose of achieving harmony by applying the voice of reason to the libidinal needs and superego demands. This involves giving voice to the Underdog (i.e., inner child), strengthening the emerging ego that listens to both parties and suggests a reasonable solution. In this process, the therapist keeps both parties focused on the task, listens for the unexpressed and unmet needs, reflects these needs, and invites the two parties to respond to the needs.

### *Case: Hugo*

Hugo, 26 years old, single and Caucasian, requested therapy to help him to understand why he was not able to make commitments in relationships. Hugo was brought up to comply with the wishes and demands of his parents who at the same time dismissed and/or negated his own self-directed behaviors.

Hugo began the session saying that he felt that there was something stopping him from being happy, committed, and being who and what he would like to be. He pictured that which was stopping him as an invisible wall. There were two voices within him, that of the wall (i.e., superego) and that of the self (i.e., the id). To help resolve the conflict and to empower the ego, a dialogue between the self and the wall was set up using the Gestalt Two Chair Technique. The self expressed that he was tired of fighting the wall and for being told what to do and to be cautious with people. In his defense, the wall said that the self was just a kid and needed to be protected. Becoming empowered, the self threatened the wall saying that the day will come when he will be hurting too much and will leave. He asked the wall to trust him and to diminish the control over him. The self expressed the desire to live a more spontaneous life. Becoming more empathic and understanding of the self's feelings and needs, the wall agreed that he was too rigid and stifling and that he would work with the self toward a compromise. With the help of the voice of reason and their willingness to compromise, the wall and the self came to a satisfactory solution. Consequently, there was now greater integration among the ego states.

### *Underlying Unmet Needs*

Hugo experienced a conflict between two basic needs. One of these was the self's need for autonomy and to have a say in his life and the other, the wall, the need was for emotional bonding through control (e.g., protection, security) for fear if he let go of the control, the self in him would leave and he would be by himself.

## Working through Abandonment Issues

### *Description*

Abandonment issues are related to the loss of a loved person. Those who experience abandonment, feel being cut-off from significant others, forgotten, forsaken, given up, and lost. Typically, the feeling of being abandoned is accompanied by feelings of depression, rage, anger, helplessness, fear, guilt, emptiness, and/or void (Anderson, 2000; Masterson, 1976). Individuals who struggle with feelings of abandonment are terrified at the possibility of a significant other leaving them behind. The feeling of abandonment can be brought about by a wide range of situations such as serious emotional neglect, trauma, and abuse during infancy or childhood, being adopted at a young age, and by the position in the birth order. Regarding birth order, an oldest child might feel abandoned by the mother when a second child is born into the family because the older child might feel displaced by the second born sibling and not loved in the same way as previously.

### *Task/Goal*

The task is to provide a safe, secure, protective, and caring environment to help the individual explore his fear of abandonment with the goal of understanding its origin, accepting it as part of his experience, and learning how to cope with it. As the individual accesses his abandonment feelings, it is important for the therapist to resonate with them, immerse himself into them, provide structure for their expression and help the individual to "cry out" his feelings while at the same time to bring an internal strength to his experience.

### *Approach*

Helping an individual to work through feelings of abandonment is a long and painful process. An infant/child's response to abandonment might take one of two forms. First the infant/child might cut off emotional connection from the significant caregiver and act out in rage. Second an infant/child might relentlessly pursue emotional connection with a significant caregiver, try to please her, and resolve to be a good person and not cause a disturbance. Prior to addressing the fear of abandonment, it will be necessary to address the accompanying feelings of rage in a structured, safe, caring, and protective environment and to build internal resources to cope with both the rage and the fear of abandonment. Getting in touch with the feelings of being abandoned takes an individual to the place of greatest vulnerability and therefore it is necessary to proceed at the pace and the ability of an individual to constructively deal with these emotions.

There are three components to working through the feeling of abandonment in therapy. First, there is the enormous need on part of the individual to bond with the love object (e.g., therapist) that has become his lifeline. Being away from the love object triggers the feelings of being abandoned. The individual also wants the love object to want to be with him. The individual looks for signs and indicators as to whether the love object wants to be with him. The experience that the other wants to be with the individual is an important aspect of repairing the broken infant/child and parent relationship. Second, the individual tends to interpret emotional and physical unavailability on part of a significant other or suggestions such as how the individual can help himself, as not being wanted and loved which trigger feelings of being abandoned. To help an individual to interpret such behaviors and comments differently, one can use the "track-record" approach (see above). This involves asking the individual to recall similar incidents of the past and become aware of their outcomes. This helps the individual to put a current situation into context of previous experiences and to become aware that not being available or making suggestions do not mean that he is not loved, wanted, and cared for. Third, it is important to help the individual who cuts off a relationship to face the reality of his fears of being abandoned. The therapist might ask the individual not to cut off but to stay in touch with what he needs and to express these to the therapist. This is usually very difficult and risky for the individual to say. The individual might say something like, "I want you to stay with me as long as I need you; I don't want you to leave me." The therapist on his part reassures the individual that he will be there as long as needed.

After an individual has taken off the edge of his fear of abandonment, one might use Task-Directed Imagery to help the individual to form an emotional bond with a significant other. For an individual who resists accessing his feelings of having been abandoned, one might gently use experiential focusing to uncover it with the condition that the individual has the resources for such a task.

### *Case: Alexei*

Alexei, in his mid-30s, married, university educated, and a professional, sought therapy because he was having serious conflicts with his partner and with his parents and siblings. Alexei was extremely angry at his parents, particularly, his mother and one of his sisters.

Alexei's partner, who had significant mood swings, allied with Alexei in being angry at his mother and his sister and was instrumental in having Alexei cut-off his ties with his parents and siblings. Although he initially complied with his partner's wish to cut off ties with his family, Alexei came to the point where he wanted to settle both his relationship with his partner and with his family as he was beginning to have physical symptoms from the stress. He no longer wanted to live in a state of heightened anxiety and conflict. Arrangements were made for individual therapy for Alexei, couple therapy for Alexei and his partner, couple therapy for his parents, and family therapy for Alexei, his partner and his parents.

In the initial couple sessions, both Alexei and his partner expressed intense anger toward his parents, particularly the mother. Using narratives of Alexei's childhood behaviors, particularly with the birth of his sibling when he was two years of age, it became apparent that Alexei felt that he was displaced by his younger sibling and that he lost the love of his mother. Basically, he felt abandoned by his mother. His expressions of anger toward his mother and younger sibling were expressions of his abandonment rage. When his sister was brought home, he said "I don't want my sister. Take her away." Within the context of family therapy, Alexei was able to work through his feelings of rage toward his mother who painfully accepted his feelings. Alexei was then instructed to express what he needed from his mother. He expressed the need to be accepted and not to be thought of as being the problem in the family. His mother accepted what he said and then offered to embrace him. Alexei and his mother expressed their need for each other and reconnected through a long and intense physical embrace and expression of their love. This experience began Alexei's journey of healing from the experience of abandonment and rage to feeling connected, accepted and treasured.

### *Underlying Unmet Needs*

Underlying Alexei's anger and rage toward his parents and his conflicted relationship with his partner, was the need for emotional connection (bonding) with his mother. When he and his mother became aware of his need for emotional bonding, they then began to repair the childhood injury and the accompanying feelings of rage and abandonment.

## Transforming Projective Identifications

### *Description*

Projective identifications are repetitive and habitual ways to draw another into a particular pattern of relating (e.g., being dependent on the other and asking them to be a caretaker), particularly in close and intimate relationships (Cashdan, 1988; Ogden, 1989). The patterns of relating to others were learned at a very young age and may persist throughout adolescence and adulthood. The pattern of relating is typically driven by unmet childhood core needs.

For example, a significant caregiver might not have validated a youngster's need for autonomy but encouraged the youngster's dependency on her. An individual might emerge from this experience in one of two ways regarding relationships – either to seek someone on whom he can be dependent and the other assumes the role of a caretaker or to seek someone over whom he can exercise his sense of autonomy and the other becomes dependent on him. In an intimate relationship, a projective identification is said to be formed when one partner expresses his dependency needs and the second partner identifies with the partner's request and takes on a caretaker role.

### *Task/Goal*

The first task is to help the individuals become aware of their style of relating and how this affects their relationship. For example, one may point out that one partner is overly dependent and the other partner assumes a caretaking role. It might be important to link their tendency to draw the other into their way of relating to their early childhood experiences as this gives them a frame of reference. A clear sign that an individual tries to draw the other into her way of forming close and intimate relationships is when his partner resists the pull which leads to conflicts. It is by analyzing this conflict that helps the partners to become more aware of their pattern of relating and how it is an attempt to maintain the relationship and satisfy unmet needs. The ultimate goal is to transform the projective identification into healthy interpersonal relationships.

### *Approach*

One can begin to work with projective identifications when the individual experiences resistance from his partner to be drawn into doing things that she no longer wants to do. This resistance manifests a conflict of needs. For example, one partner might want to be taken care of and the other resists complying because he wants to be autonomous. Analyzing the style of relating and becoming aware of this pattern is often helpful in changing it. Task-Directed Imagery could be used to help an individual experience what it is like to let go of the need to draw another into their way of forming a close or intimate relationship and to let the other person free to be. This experience might also help the person to learn a different way of relating by becoming more autonomous and sensing its freedom.

### *Case: Reinhard and Steffi*

Reinhard and Steffi, married for six years, sought therapy because Steffi feared that her demands on her husband would cause him to lose interest in her and become attracted to another woman. Reinhard, the eldest of five children, comes from a caring and stable family background where he took care of his siblings and Steffi comes from a broken home where her mother did not let her grow up and, thus, she remained dependent on her mother. As a child and adolescent, Steffi feared that if she were to assert her autonomy with her mother, she would lose the emotional connection with her. Thus, Reinhard and Steffi were initially well suited for each other as he needed someone to take care of and she needed someone who would take care of her.

When Steffi entered into a close and intimate relationship her tendency was to create a relationship where she would become dependent on the partner and the partner assumed a caretaker position. She wanted to be with that person all the time and had limited interest to spend time with friends and to engage in activities without Reinhard. This is how Steffi and Reinhard's relationship began. Although Reinhard reassured her that he was interested in none other than Steffi, she could not fully believe and trust it.

In the course of therapy, Steffi became aware that she was relating to Reinhard in the same way that she related to her mother, that is, by being dependent. She no longer wanted to be dependent on her mother nor on Reinhard, but she wanted to assert her autonomy. Although she was deathly afraid to change the relationship pattern fearing that if she became more autonomous, Reinhard would lose interest in her and leave, she was determined to form her relationship of equality. Using the Task-Directed Imagery, Steffi was asked to imagine letting go of her need to depend on Reinhard and to become more autonomous. As she engaged in the exercise, she experienced a sense of inner freedom, joy, peace, and no need to manipulate Reinhard. She could let him be. This experience was the beginning of transforming their relationship into a healthy relationship. She began to develop friendships and spend time with them and she engaged in activities without Reinhard. Both became less dependent on each other.

### *Underlying Unmet Needs*

The couple experienced conflicting underlying unmet core needs with Steffi being emotionally dependent on Reinhard who needed someone to take care of so as to feel valued. The underlying unmet childhood need for Steffi was for autonomy while maintaining emotional connection whereas for Reinhard it was for emotional connection through caretaking.

## Asserting One's Needs in Relationships

### *Description*

Most of the self and relational issues presented above are about building inner resources such as self-esteem, object constancy, and connecting with one's bodily self which are assumed to be essential for healthy functioning.

An important aspect of SIRP is to enable the person to deal not only with internal states and processes but also to enable the person to deal with external realities such as intimate relationships, friendships, work, and leisure pursuits. One form of enablement in dealing with external reality is the ability to assert one's needs in relationships. To be assertive means to express openly, honestly, clearly, and authentically one's needs, opinions, feelings, rights, and expectations without feeling guilty and fearing negative consequences in expressing them and at the same time have confidence that one can effectively manage such negative responses should they occur. Thus, assertiveness entails two aspects, namely, the expression of one's needs, feelings, and thoughts and the confidence and ability to deal with the negative responses in asserting oneself.

### Task/Goal

There are several aspects in learning to become assertive. First, one needs to clearly identify and articulate the needs, rights, feelings, and thoughts that one wants to assert. That is, one has to establish a goal. Second, it is important to understand the barriers that stand in the way of being assertive. For example, a person might fear losing a relationship if he is assertive or that he will be negatively judged and evaluated. Before a person can become assertive, he will have to overcome these fears. Third, it is necessary to figure out appropriate ways of asserting oneself in each specific situation. Once this has been determined, it is then necessary to practice being assertive.

### Approach

The majority of the techniques used for assertiveness training stem primarily from cognitive and behavioral approaches. Included among the techniques are behavior rehearsal (Lange & Jakubowski, 1979; Tucker-Ladd, 1996–2011; Wolpe, 1990), role-play (Tucker-Ladd, 1996–2013), and the Laddering technique (Davis et al., 1980). The goal of these techniques is to change the behavior without addressing the subjective experiences that might underlie the difficulty to be assertive.

SIRP differs from the cognitive/behavioral approaches in developing assertiveness in that it empowers the person prior to asking him to engage in assertive behavior. One of the techniques that SIRP uses is Task-Directed Imagery which entails four steps (Meier & Boivin, 2011a). In this technique, the person is asked to go to an imaginative place where he experiences the type of empowerment required to be assertive regarding a specific task (Step 1). He is then asked to reflect on this experience of empowerment and embrace it (Step 2). Remaining in this state of empowerment, the person is asked to perform the task in imagination (Step 3). Lastly, the person is asked to provide feedback in having been assertive (Step 4).

### *Case: Catarina and Batista*

Catarina, married, in her mid-40s, and executive assistant, sought therapy to learn how to stand up to her husband, Batista, who was domineering, at times oppressive, verbally abusive, and unable to control his anger and rage. Catarina often felt intimidated by him but never physically threatened.

To help her to learn how to become assertive with Batista and stand up to him and not to let him take away her good feelings, a Task-Directed Imagery was designed. Catarina was asked to imagine being some place where she felt good about herself, where she could be herself, and in charge of her life (Step 1). She imagined being alone in their cottage and saw and smelled the beautiful flowers, saw the animals run freely; she felt the warmth of the sun and the softness of the fresh air. She felt strong and wholesome in her being. She was then asked what it was like to have this sense of inner strength and to feel this way about herself (Step 2). She found it to be freeing, relaxing, calming, and strengthening. She was then instructed to remain in touch with all of these good feelings, qualities, and inner strength and to imagine meeting Batista (Step 3). When she first met him, she found him to be critical of her. His remarks were like scratching her and causing her to bleed. As she proceeded to be with him, she fought against letting his sarcasm get to her. As they continued to be together, he became like a little boy begging her to take him up into her arms which she refused. Then he threw a temper tantrum and she said to herself that she does not have to take on his problems. She then told him that she had someplace to go to and she wanted him to come with her. She felt now that she could be with him without he getting to her and that she could take charge of the relationship. The therapist then asked her what it was like to be in this empowered state with Batista and not to let his criticisms bring her down (Step 4). She felt free and was able to be herself, to stand up to Batista; this was a new experience for her which she carried forward in her real relationship with Batista.

### *Underlying Unmet Needs*

Catarina was in a relationship where she felt disrespected by her husband and having minimal ability to moderate his acting out and abusive behaviors. In the exercise, she was able to experience asserting her needs for autonomy and to feel significant by refusing to nurture him while he was in a needy state.

In addressing self and relationship issues, it is important to conceptualize the issue within the context of SIRP, determine the task to be achieved, and to remain focused on the task as the individual struggles to work it through. It is also important to identify which of the issues are pertinent to a given individual and to determine which issues need to be addressed first before proceeding to work on other issues.

This chapter presented a number of self and relationship issues that could present themselves in a therapy session, but there are others such as establishing a whole self, integrating a split object (self), becoming empathic, triangulated relationships, and transforming anger and rage. These issues are addressed in the same manner as those presented above.

## References

Allport, G. W. (1955/1967). *Becoming: Basic considerations for a psychology of personality*. New Haven: Yale University Press.

Anderson, S. (2000). *The journey from abandonment to healing*. New York: Berkley Brooks.

Cashdan, S. (1988). *Object relations therapy: Using the relationship*. New York: W. W. Norton.

Davis, M., Eshelman, E. R., & Mckay, M. (1980). *The relaxation and stress reduction workbook* (6th ed.). Oakland, California: New Harbinger Publication.

Fairbairn, W. R. D. (1944). Endopsychic structure considered in terms of object relationships. In *An object-relations theory of the personality* (pp. 82–136). New York: Basic Books.

Gendlin, E. T. (1996). *Focusing-oriented psychotherapy: A manual of the experiential method*. New York: Guilford Press.

Klein, M. (1946/1975). Notes on some schizoid mechanisms. In *Envy and gratitude and other works 1946–1963* (pp. 1–24). New York: Delta.

Kohut, H. (1974). *The analysis of self*. New York: International Universities Press.

Krueger, D. W. (1989). *Body self and psychological self: A developmental and clinical integration of disorders of the self*. New York: Brunner/Mazel.

Lange, A. J., & Jakubowski, P. (1979). *Responsive assertive behavior: Cognitive/behavioral procedures for trainers*. Champaign, IL: Research Press.

Mahler, M., & Furer, M. (1968). *On human symbiosis and the vicissitudes of individuation*. New York: International Universities Press.

Mahler, M., Pine, F., & Bergman, A. (1975). *The psychological birth of the human infant*. New York: Basic Books.

Maslow, A. H. (1968). *Toward a psychology of being* (2nd ed.). London: D. Van Nostrand.

Masterson, J. F. (1976). *Psychotherapy of the borderline adult: A developmental approach*. New York: Brunner/Mazel.

Meier, A., & Boivin, M. (1983). Towards a synthetic model of psychotherapy. *Pastoral Sciences, II*, 137–176.

Meier, A., & Boivin, M. (1993). *The interplay of affect, cognitions, and needs in a model of psychotherapeutic change*. Paper presented at the 9th Annual Conference of the Society for the Exploration of Psychotherapy Integration. New York: NY. April 23.

Meier, A., & Boivin, M. (2011a). Task-direct imagery. In A. Meier & M. Boivin (Eds.), *Counselling and therapy techniques: Theory and Practice* (pp. 77–90). London, England: SAGE Publications.

Meier, A., & Boivin, M. (2011b). The Gestalt empty-chair and two-chair techniques.

In A. Meier & M. Boivin (Eds.), *Counselling and therapy techniques: Theory and Practice* (pp. 46–60). London, England: SAGE Publications.

Meier, A., Boivin, M., & Meier, M. (2006). The treatment of depression: A case study using theme-analysis. *Counselling and Psychotherapy Research, 6*(2), 115–125.

Ogden, T. (1989). *The primitive edge of experience.* Northvale, NJ: Jason Aronson.

Rothschild, B. (2000). *The body remembers: The psychophysiology of trauma and trauma treatment.* New York: Norton Professional Books.

Tucker-Ladd, C. (1996–2011). Methods for developing skills. In C. Tucker-Ladd (Ed.), *Psychological self-help* (pp. 1232–1334). Retrieved September 2013 from http://www.psychologicalselfhelp.org/

Van der Kolk, B. (2015). *The body keeps the score: Brain, mind and body in the healing of trauma.* New York: Penguin.

White, R. W. (1967). *Competence and the growth of personality. Science and psychoanalysis, 11, the ego.* New York: Grune & Stratton.

Winnicott, D. (1965/1981). *The family and individual development.* London: Tavistock Publishers.

Wolpe, J. (1990). *The practice of behaviour therapy* (4th ed.). New York: Pergamon Press.

Chapter 10

# Gloria: The Pursuit of Individuality

This chapter presents the case of Gloria (pseudonym) who struggled to psychologically separate from her parents, to individuate and to become her own person. She was able to achieve this task, in great part, by reworking the developmental failure through her transferential relationship with the therapist.

The chapter begins with a brief description of the separation and individuation process. This is followed by a summary of psychosocial history of Gloria and the relational and self factors that contributed to her developmental failures. The third part presents a diagnosis and the fourth part provides an assessment using the Self-in-Relationship Psychotherapy Assessment Form (SIRP-AF), which has been specifically designed for use with Self-in-Relationship Psychotherapy (SIRP). This is followed by a conceptualization of her symptoms and the treatment that helped Gloria to achieve psychological separation and individuation.

## The Separation and Individuation Process

A primary developmental task for a child is to become "emotionally bonded" with a significant other (e.g., mother) and then in due course to psychologically separate from her and to individuate and become her own person (Mahler et al., 1975). To psychologically separate refers to recognizing that there are persons separate from oneself, that is, to differentiate between the "me" and the "not me." To individuate means to develop a sense of selfhood and identity and to assert one's own preferences, values, dreams, ambitions, and needs (Masterson, 1993). It implies the ability to function in an autonomous and self-directed manner without being controlled, impaired, or feeling unduly responsible for significant others (Bowen, 1978). Parental nurturing and nudging are necessary to help a child to individuate, achieve autonomy, and to develop a sense of self (Edward et al., 1981; Mahler et al., 1975). Parental indulgence and inadequate nudging may lead to a failure to individuate and to an ill-defined sense of self.

A significant point in the separation and individuation process is the

DOI: 10.4324/9781003272502-13

rapprochement subphase during which, if it is successful, the child acquires the skills to regulate emotions and impulses, acquires the capacity to self-comfort and self-soothe, to see self and others as persons in their own right, to integrate impulses and yearnings with a positive sense of self, object constancy, and to replace the defense of splitting with the defense of repression (Masterson, 1976, 1991). A failure to achieve this developmental task can lead to deficiencies in these capacities.

## Psychosocial History and Its Contributing Factors

Gloria, of European-Canadian origin, was brought up in an upper middle-class home by parents, professionals, who were emotionally distant from her and her siblings and who did not acknowledge the children's accomplishments nor affirm them as persons. The parents expected their children to become like themselves. Both parents were rigid in their thinking and avoided engaging in emotional issues.

Regarding her relationship with her mother, Gloria did not feel emotionally bonded to her. For her mother, being dutiful was important. Gloria's childhood message from her mother was that emotions were bad and that there was a good way and a bad way of doing things. There often was a tug of war between her mother's way and Gloria's way of doing things. Gloria experienced a constant tension as to who will win the power struggle; the mother was always right. When Gloria's way of doing things conflicted with that of her mother, Gloria was accused of deliberately bugging her mother; the mother was fine when Gloria settled down and stopped bugging her. As a little girl when things got out of control, Gloria screamed, became hyperactive, spun in circles, and went into fits of rage. At times she feared that her anger and rage toward her mother would get out of control and lead her to places she did not want to go to. Gloria grew up to believe that she was inadequate, that what she wanted in life was not worthwhile and that there was something wrong with her.

As for her relationship with her father, who was depressed for a good part of his life, he expected her to behave in a particular way and if she opposed him, he criticized her, withdrew and/or retreated to his office. Often her father would entice her with something that she wanted or he would bring an interaction to the point that Gloria was vulnerable and he would then cop out. He would take her with him when he visited his clients. She felt that she had a place in his life and was valued as long as she could be pretty, well behaved and be gracious in the presence of his clients. She felt that she was very much like him. She was angry at her father and hated him for not wanting her because she was a girl and for socially exploiting her. Despite all of this, it was her father that she really loved and to whom she belonged and not to her mother. Her feelings of guilt kept her from letting go of him, to hurt him, and to take advantage of him.

Gloria had several short-term boyfriends, but she quickly broke up with them as they did not meet her standards, they were not as emotionally available as she needed them to be and/or they were too needy. She struggled to define herself as a woman and to feel free with her sexuality.

In terms of education, she pursued graduate studies in the helping profession. To support her education, she worked at an institution for special needs children.

## Diagnosis and Assessment

To assess for the severity of Gloria's current difficulties and the recovery from them, the Diagnostic and Statistical Manual of Mental Disorders (DSM-IV-TR) (American Psychiatric Association, 1994) and the Separation/Individuation Inventory (S-IPI) (Christenson & Wilson, 1994) were administered at the beginning of therapy and again at the termination of therapy. Progress in therapy was also assessed using the results from a research which analyzed transcripts of Gloria's therapy sessions for therapeutic change across time (Meier et al., 2010).

### *DSM-IV-TR*

Based on the psychosocial history, it was hypothesized that Gloria was struggling with a low-level borderline personality disorder (BPD) (Masterson, 1991). BPDs can be thought of as a full-blown personality disorder, low-level personality disorder, or as a borderline personality style (Sperry, 1995).

A BPD is described by the DSM-IV-TR (Code 301.83) as "a pervasive pattern of instability of interpersonal relationships, self-image, and affects, and marked impulsivity beginning by early adulthood and present in a variety of contexts" (American Psychiatric Association, 1994). Associated with this disorder are acting-out behaviors, which may include frantic efforts to avoid real or imagined abandonment, unstable self-image or sense of self, impulsivity (e.g., substance abuse), suicidal threats or self-mutilating behavior, inability to regulate affect, chronic feelings of emptiness, and paranoid ideations. The underlying dynamic in borderline personality disorder consists of a primitive defense against achieving self-activation or the emergence of the real self for fear of abandonment.

The low-level borderline personality client has the same underlying dynamic as the DSM-IV-TR defined BPD but differs from the latter in that it does not manifest acting-out behaviors (Masterson, 1991). A borderline personality style (Sperry, 1995) is considered to be an adaptive interpersonal pattern. Using this as a reference point, the low-level borderline personality client can be perceived to lie somewhere between a BPD and a borderline personality style.

To assess for the presence of BPD, the DSM-IV-TR was administered at the beginning of therapy and again at the termination of therapy. Prior to therapy, Gloria met the criteria for BPD (minus the acting out behavior) on the DSM-IV-TR but did not meet the criteria following therapy. As well, the client met the criteria for borderline personality style (Sperry, 1995) at the termination of therapy.

### S-IPI

Gloria's psychosocial history suggests that she remained emotionally entangled with her father and mother and did not psychologically separate from them so as to achieve a sense of individuality and self-identity. To assess for disturbances in the separation/individuation process, the S-IPI (Christenson & Wilson, 1994) was administered before therapy and at the completion of therapy. The mean score for a sample of patients diagnosed with borderline personality disorder was 201 with a standard deviation of 65.6. A sample of "normal" university employees produced a mean score of 120.6 and a standard deviation of 40. Scores higher than 190 on the S-IPI indicate separation/individuation problems. Gloria's score on the S-IPI prior to treatment was 205 and following treatment it was 130. The difference between the two scores is considered to be significant.

To summarize, Gloria met the criteria for low-level borderline personality disorder on the DSM-IV-TR and the S-IPI prior to treatment but not following treatment. The findings on the two measures indicate that Gloria had a successful therapeutic outcome.

### Theme-Analysis

Gloria's progress in therapy was assessed in a research project which analyzed transcripts from her psychotherapy sessions using Theme-Analysis (TA) which combines both a qualitative and a quantitative method (Meier et al., 2008). This multimethod approach identifies psychotherapeutic themes and traces how they change across sessions (i.e., time) using as a measure the Seven Phase Model of the Change Process (Meier & Boivin, 1998; Meier et al., 2010). The assessment entails performing (paired) correlations between phase and session for the themes organized according to their target (e.g., mother, therapist) and taken separately or combined. A Pearson r of .66 (rsq = .44) was obtained for the combined themes across all of the sessions. A Pearson r of .75 (rsq = .56) was obtained for the combined 12 themes for the two objects (e.g., mother, therapist). When taken separately, a Pearson r of .57 (rsq = .33) was obtained for the six themes for the object, mother, and a Pearson r of .86 (rsq = .73) was obtained for the six themes for the object, therapist. The strong positive correlations together with the qualitative data support the notion that themes are worked through in a progressive forward course.

## The SIRP Assessment Form

The Self-in-Relationship Psychotherapy Assessment Form (SIRP-AF) assesses a client on SIRP's major constructs by using the material from the psychosocial history. Each of the constructs has been conceptually and operationally defined (see Chapters 3 and 5). The SIRP-AF has been found to be a reliable instrument to code the constructs. This section presents the results from the application of the SIRP-AF to Gloria's psychosocial history. The task is to assess these constructs relative to Gloria's childhood, adolescence, and current experiences. The findings on the pertinent SIRP constructs are presented in Table 10.1 and briefly discussed here.

### *Relational, Self, and Physical Intimacy Needs*

Gloria's unmet childhood needs comprised the needs for emotional connection, significance, and autonomy. More specifically, she strove for emotional connection, to be valued for who she was, and have the freedom to be autonomous and independent from both of her parents. Gloria learned at a very young age, that her need for autonomy and independence conflicted with the demands and expectations of her parents and in order to have their acceptance and love, she repressed them. The parental demands and expectations deprived her of the freedom to psychologically separate and individuate. Since these needs went unanswered in childhood, they continued to press for positive responses from her significant relationships throughout her life. Among these needs, the pursuit for significance and autonomy were prominent.

### *Representations of Other and Self*

Through the relationships with her parents, Gloria began to form representations of her parents and of herself (Klein, 1948, p. 32). Her representation of her mother was that she was controlling, demanding, critical, belittling, self-righteous, and manipulative. Gloria bumped heads constantly with her mother who thought in terms of right or wrong, and black and white.

Gloria perceived her father to be weak, helpless, passive-aggressive, demanding, and manipulative. When she accompanied him on visits to his clients, he expected her to conform to his standard of behavior that is, to behave, be pretty, and be gracious. In his interactions with Gloria, her father would entice her in a conversation and/or a promise and when she became vulnerable, he would withdraw, go to his office, and let her hang high and dry.

With regards to representation of herself, in the presence of her mother, Gloria felt that there was something wrong with her and that she was a bad person. She saw herself as having to defend and explain herself.

*Table 10.1* The SIRP assessment form: results

***Part I. Descriptive data:*** *For each of the dimensions presented below provide descriptive material for the objects entered in the top row of the table. If there are other objects that have significantly influenced the person's life, add a column, and provide a name for the object.*

| *Dimension* | *Father* | *Mother* |
|---|---|---|
| 1. Organizing unmet self, relational, and physical intimacy needs relative to: | Emotionally connected, valued, autonomy | Emotionally connected, lovable, autonomy |
| 2. Internal representation of: | Weak, helpless, passive-aggressive, manipulative, demanding | Controlling, critical, demanding, belittling, manipulative, self-righteous |
| 3. Internal representations of self relative to: (How I view myself when with) | Protected, cared, accepting | On guard, fighter, defensive, oppositional, not good enough |
| 4. Affect linking representation of other to self: (How I felt my father, mother, etc. felt about me) | Conditional love, frustrated, burden | Impatient, tolerant, angry, frustrated, critical, burden |
| 5. Affect linking representation of self to other: (How I felt toward my) | Love and hate; ambivalent | Anger, hatred, not loved |
| 6. How I felt/feel when in the presence of: | On guard, vigilant, ambivalent | Not good enough, flawed, bad person, immature |
| 7. Quality or degree of good enough parenting: | Emotional neglect, oppressive; conditional love | Emotional neglect, oppressive; conditional love |

(*Continued*)

*Table 10.1* (Continued)

***Part II. Scaled data:*** *Rate dimensions 1, 4, 7, and 11 on a five-point scale. For dimensions 2, 3, and 10 indicate the strength/presence of each component using a five-point scale with 1 = barely and 5 = greatly. For the remainder dimensions check off those that are relevant. See Operational Criteria for more precise instructions. If the dimension is not relevant, leave the space blank. PO = part-object; WO = whole-object; PSP = paranoid/schizoid position; DP = depressive position; EB = need for emotional bonding; SC = need for sensual contact; AU = need for autonomy; SI = need for sexual intimacy.*

| | | | | | |
|---|---|---|---|---|---|
| 1. Manner of relating to | Father: 1 (PO) | 2 | 3 | 4 | 5 (WO) |
| | Mother: 1 | 2 | 3 | 4 | 5 |
| 2. Psychic organization | Core needs: | 3.5 EB<br>___ SC | 3 AU<br>___ SI | 2.5 Ego | 3.5 Superego<br>___ |
| 3. Self structure | 2.5 striving for significance | 2.5 striving for competency | | 2.5 capacity to secure sense of significance and competency | |
| 4. True self (living from) | 1 ___ X<br>Minimally | 2 | 3 | 4 | 5<br>Strongly |
| 5. Coping mechanisms | X repression<br>___ denial<br>___ dissociation | | X splitting<br>X introjection<br>X projection | ___ regression<br>___ sublimation<br>___ idealization | X devaluation<br>X suppression<br>___ other |
| 6. Quality of emotional bond | ___ emotionally connected | | X striving for emotional connection | ___ avoiding emotional connection | ___ emotionally disconnected |
| 7. Object constancy | 1<br>Not Formed | 2<br>Partially Formed | 3 | 4 | 5<br>Fully Formed |
| 8. Characteristic emotional state | 1 angry<br>___ abandoned | ___ anxious<br>2 smothered | | ___ depressed<br>___ oppressed | ___ sad<br>Other ___ |
| 9. Projective identifications | ___ dependency<br>___ other | X power | | ___ ingratiation | ___ sex |
| 10. Characteristic phase | ___ Symbiosis | 2 Differentiation | ___ Practicing | 1 Rapprochement | ___ Consolidation |
| 11. Characteristic position | 1<br>(PSP) | 2 | 3 | 4 | 5<br>(DP) |
| 12. Level of personality organization | ___ higher | X intermediate | | ___ lower | |

With regards to her father, she saw herself as being conditionally cared for and accepted.

### *Psychic Organization*

Gloria's psychic organization (Freud, 1923, 1938) reflected her lived childhood relationship experiences with her mother and father. That is, she internalized the demands and expectations of her parents with the message that there was something wrong with her, she was a bad person, that it was wrong to assert her needs which, when taken together, formed her *superego* that kept the internalized child with its needs in check and under control (Fairbairn, 1944/1994). She became her own internal critical parent. Gloria's ego was impoverished because neither parent provided a corrective influence on their partner's behaviors toward Gloria and nor did they help Gloria to develop relational and coping skills to deal with their behaviors. From her childhood experiences with her parents, Gloria formed a psychic organization with the ego not able to harmonize the demands of the *superego* with her core needs. As well, she was torn within as she was not able to manage the demands of the superego and to pursue individuality.

### *Self-Structure*

Gloria's self-structure is characterized by low self-esteem (i.e., insignificance), feelings of social inadequacy (i.e., incompetency), and lacking skills to maintain a positive sense of self-esteem and competency (Kohut, 1977). Her low self-esteem is reflected in Gloria thinking of herself as being a bad person and that there was something wrong with her. Her sense of inadequacy and social incompetency is reflected in her inability to influence her parents to unconditionally love her and to respond positively to her need for lovability and to her pursuit for individuality. Her anger and rage interfere with her capacity to venture out and pursue her individuality and to form meaningful and satisfying relationships. Gloria lacked the inner resources to build and maintain a healthy sense of self and a sense of social competency.

From the perspective of a social self (Winnicott, 1960/1965), Gloria's behaviors, attitudes, and interactions were very much influenced by what she thought were her parents' expectations of her. Her decisions and choices did not emanate from her sense of self but from what her parents expected; her choices and decisions were not primarily self-directed but were other-directed. Gloria's responses and interactions did not come from her true and authentic self (Jourard, 1971); she lived from a false self (Winnicott (1960/1965).

### *Defense Mechanisms and Coping Strategies*

Gloria's unconscious coping strategies appear to comprise repression, splitting, introjection, projection, and devaluation and her conscious coping strategy appears to be suppression. She repressed her own needs and feelings to avoid childhood conflicts with her mother; she internalized (i.e., introjected) the expectations, demands and mores of her parents; she was outwardly polite, pleasant and caring but internally she was frustrated and angry and projected these onto others; and she viewed others in negative terms. She consciously suppressed her feelings, preferences, and needs to placate her parents.

### *Quality of Emotional Bond*

Gloria mentioned that she did not feel emotionally bonded to her mother. In their relationship, the mother was more duty bound and intellectual in her approach and their relationship lacked warmth and emotional attunement. Gloria, in her relationships, sought "safe anchorage" and a "confident expectation" that her needs would be respected and responded to (Mahler et al., 1975). These attributes were missing in her relationship with her mother who left her with a lifelong pursuit for emotional bonding with a significant other and at the same time in a pursuit for autonomy.

### *Object Constancy*

Object constancy is formed by internalizing the admired traits and functions of the people in our life by whom we are loved and admired/cherished. Through the experience of being loved and admired/cherished, one begins to love and admire/cherish oneself, which leads to object constancy. Object constancy helps a person to be internally grounded, and it enables a person to gain a perspective on a relational or self-issue, to regulate one's affective responses and take direction from to deal with daily challenges (Mahler et al., 1975).

Based on Gloria's description of her relationship with her parents, it is quite clear that at a very young age, she did not develop "object constancy" as she had difficulty to put her experiences into perspective and to control her emotional outbursts. Her one good relationship was with her grandparents who she saw infrequently. However, in being with them and thinking about them, helped her to feel good about herself.

### *Characteristic Emotional State*

Gloria's prevailing (i.e., familiar) emotional state was that of anger (i.e., frustration) which appears to be a function of not having her childhood needs for autonomy and being significant validated. At a very young age, Gloria was expected to conform to the expectations and wishes of her parents and at the same time to put aside her own growth-oriented needs. When she was a child, she struggled to contain her feelings of anger which she acted out in temper tantrums, screaming and shouting or by repressing them to secure validations. In adolescence and adulthood, she dealt with her anger through the defense of reaction-formation which seemingly is manifested in her dedication in working with highly challenged individuals.

### *Projective Identification*

Projective identification refers to a relational dynamic by which a person repeatedly tries to draw a significant other into their way of relating (Cashdan, 1988). Underlying a projective identification is an unmet childhood need that an individual attempts to have responded to. Gloria's relationships with her parents were often stormy with her throwing temper tantrums. They were engaged in a power struggle. Thus, at a young age, Gloria tried to draw her parents into her type of relating which meant she was having the power. This style of relating appears to stem from her parents not validating her to have a voice in matters that affected her life and that what she had to say mattered.

Gloria's efforts to dominate the relationship with her parents were often not effective and thus at times she relented and complied with their wishes. However, her struggle to have a voice in a relationship, to take charge and control a relationship, continued into her adult life. Her relationships were influenced by a conflicted psychic organization that reflected her neediness and at the same time a need to control the relationship through opposition and rebelliousness. Her struggle to draw others into her way of relating is defined as the projective identification of power (Cashdan, 1988).

From another perspective, Gloria related to meaningful others in terms of how she wanted them to respond to her and how they wanted her to respond to them, that is, in the way that they needed each other. This has been referred to as relating as part-self and part-object (Klein, 1948) and as selfobjects (Kohut, 1977). That is, she did not relate to others as persons in their own right with their own needs, feelings, and preferences. She related to others as she needed them to be there for her.

### *Characteristic (Developmental) Phase*

In terms of the separation and individuation continuum (Mahler et al., 1975), Gloria was pressured to comply with the expectations and demands of her parents and to put aside the pursuit of her own needs and the expression of her feelings. This relational experience was internalized to form her psychic organization skewed toward being a demanding and critical internal parent toward herself and denying the satisfaction of her needs. This pressure to comply interfered with the development of a strong emotional bond between Gloria and her mother and working out relationships of equality and of mutual respect and acceptance. In a sense, Gloria moved out of the maternal nest too early. She failed to establish an emotional maternal bond wherein she felt "safe anchorage" and "confident expectation"; she could not count on the caregiver to respond favorably to her needs. Gloria was put in a position where she had to fight for what she needed.

She was not helped how to deal with frustrations and anger and set limits and boundaries. Since Gloria did not have the opportunity to pursue and assert her needs and express her feelings, and to establish personal goals for herself and develop relationships of equality and mutual respect and acceptance, she did not develop the social skills (e.g., setting limits and boundaries), relational skills (e.g., compromise, negotiation), and self skills (e.g., comforting self). That is, she did not develop self-directed and autonomous behaviors. She continued to seek emotional connection. In sum, Gloria's subjective experiences and relational interactions are characterized by the rapprochement subphase as well as by the differentiation subphase as she continues to pursue her autonomy and individuation. Her developmental task is to establish "safe anchorage" and to negotiate relationships that are characterized by mutual respect and acceptance of their respective self, relational, and physical intimacy needs and by equality.

### *Characteristic (Developmental) Position*

Developmental position refers to a state of psychological growth characterized by the manner in which the infant/child deals with love-hate relationships and how she experiences and relates to both internalized and externalized objects (Klein, 1935, p. 276, note; 1952). The infant/child and significant caregiver's relationship is thought of in terms of two positions (i.e., interpersonal stances), namely, the paranoid-schizoid position and the depressive position. The former is characterized by destructive (hateful) instincts and feelings and the latter by constructive (loving) instincts or feelings. The infant/child's basic conflict revolves around the instincts of these two positions, that is, between a malicious wish to destroy those close to the child and the desire to protect them. The infant/child organizes his experiences around one of these positions. The characteristic that marks a movement away from the paranoid-schizoid position and toward the depressive stance is the infant/child becoming empathic and fearing to lose the love object. The manner in which the development positions are worked through affect an individual's adult life (Klein, 1959).

Given the above, it can be stated that Gloria fluctuates between the paranoid-schizoid and depressive positions. This is based on the observation that Gloria is torn between love and hate toward her mother. When Gloria does not have her way, she becomes angry and throws temper tantrums and when she has her way, she can be loving. It is her fear to be rejected and lose the loved person that ultimately influences Gloria to suppress her destructive feelings and respond in a caring way (e.g., being empathic) to the demands and expectations of her mother.

## Conceptualization

The conceptualization of Gloria's symptoms associated with low-level borderline personality disorder and her struggle to achieve separation and individuation, is based on constructs from SIRP. Gloria's verbal reports from the therapy sessions and the results from the analysis of her reports using the SIRP-AF provide the material for the conceptualization. The conceptualization is organized according to symptoms, precipitating factors, predisposing childhood experiences, pertinent internalizations, and re-enactments.

*Symptoms:* At the beginning of therapy, Gloria expressed the desire to work through the aftereffects in being brought up by what she perceived to be controlling and domineering parents, specifically the mother, who did not validate Gloria's needs, feelings, and choices. Gloria grew up to believe that there was something wrong with her and that she was inadequate. She experienced difficulties to manage her anger particularly when it touched on her social competency and perception of self. Gloria found it difficult to form intimate relationships with persons of the opposite gender. She felt being held back from being her own person and struggled in wondering whether there was something wrong about her.

*Precipitating factors:* Gloria's recent trip overseas which took her away from connections in her home country and experiencing liberation and inner peace in being her own person, motivated her to seek therapy to help her to address the self and relational aftereffects in being brought up in a home where she was emotionally deprived and not validated for being her own person.

*Predisposing childhood experiences:* Gloria as a child was asked to conform to the expectations and demands of her parents and to give up her efforts toward her own growth and development. When Gloria began to react negatively to these constraints and act out by throwing temper tantrums, she received the message that she was hyperactive, there was something wrong with her and that she was inadequate as a person. These conflicts deprived Gloria of the opportunities to form an intimate bond with her parents and to develop positive representations of self and others. She did not achieve "safe anchorage" and "confident expectation" that her needs would be respected and responded to. She was not validated for autonomous and independent behaviors (Mahler et al., 1975).

*Pertinent internalizations:* Gloria internalized the childhood interactions with her parents to form her psychic organization, self-structure, coping strategies, perceptions of self and other, object constancy, relational dynamics, and patterns which influenced her future relational interactions. She developed a psychic organization which was skewed toward having high expectations and demands of self and others, being hard on herself (e.g., superego), feeling that there was something wrong with her when she did not comply to the wishes of her parents (e.g., negative representation of self), negating her need to receive the favors of her parents (e.g., libidinal id), and coping with the conflicts between the two forces by either complying or by acting out in frustration and anger (e.g., ineffective coping strategies).

Gloria did not form "emotional anchorage" with her mother which resulted in her not being able to develop a good representation of this relationship which is required in forming "object constancy." That is, she did not have a place within herself to turn to for perspective taking and self-soothing.

Due to the stressful relationships with her parents, Gloria did not psychologically separate from them (e.g., her anger toward them kept her engaged) and achieve her own individuality (e.g., failed to individuate). Her feeling that she was inadequate and there was something wrong with her, and her unmet needs for emotional bonding and feeling significant, inhibited her from venturing forth to become her own person (e.g., to individuate) and to feel at peace with her choices and decisions and with herself. These unmet needs lie at the roots of her current relational and personal difficulties and conflicts, including the low-level personality disorder.

*Re-enactments:* In her intimate and close relationships, Gloria re-enacted her conflicted psychic organization, self-structure, perceptions of self and other and her relational dynamics. She hesitated to assert her need for autonomy for fear that she would be rejected and abandoned for being a bad person. Yet, she resented when she felt held back from becoming autonomous and for not being accepted for being her own person. At the same time, she tried to gain control of the relationship so as to have her need for autonomy and significance met. She wanted to be autonomous and yet her skewed psychic organization was a barrier for her need to be autonomous to lead the way. Gloria's low-level borderline personality disorder appears to be related to a failure to achieve "safe anchorage" and "confident expectation" that her needs will be met and the feeling that she is a bad person when she pursues her independence. She did not acquire the skills to deal with frustrations of her needs other than to act out.

The remainder of this chapter addresses the treatment with a focus on Gloria reworking her failed negotiation of the separation and individuation process. The treatment is presented in two sections. The first section presents the goals and orientation of treatment and the therapeutic relationship. The second section focuses on the reworking of the separation and individuation process in terms of themes.

## Treatment Aspects and Approach

### *Goals of Treatment*

Gloria's principal therapeutic goal was to complete the separation and individuation process. More specifically, the subsidiary goals were to: (a) identify her unmet childhood needs (e.g., for emotional bonding, autonomy and significance) and acquire the skill to assert them, (b) bring about a greater intrapsychic harmony by empowering the ego and by giving greater voice to the inner child, (c) increase self-esteem and self-worth, (d) develop object constancy as an agent for perspective taking and regulation of affect, (e) acquire relational skills that foster mutual respect and acceptance, and (f) develop self-directed behaviors and actions. These goals were reworked simultaneously within the context of her relationship with her mother and within the context of the transferential relationship with the therapist. It was assumed that since her relational and self-issues were the outcome of a not "good enough" parental relationship, they would have to be resolved within the context of a "good enough" therapeutic relationship.

### *Description of Therapy Process*

The psychotherapy process was guided by constructs from SIRP (Meier & Boivin, 2011), self-discovery approach to counseling (Meier & Boivin, 1987), the Seven Phase Model of the Change Process (Meier & Boivin, 1992), and by the use of techniques from various theoretical orientations (see Chapter 7). The evolution of themes that emerged across therapy was assessed in terms of the Seven Phase Model of the Change Process of which the major phases are exploration, insight/awareness, experimentation/action, and integration/consolidation.

### *Therapist Orientation*

The therapist (A.M.), male, Canadian, was a doctoral-level trained and experienced psychodynamic/humanistic and developmental oriented psychotherapist who worked full-time in a university graduate psychotherapy program and had a part-time private practice. The therapist used attending and focusing skills, empathic responses, and summaries to address the client's implicit and explicit messages (Ivey, 1983), and "linking" statements (Meier & Boivin, 2000, p. 61) to connect various facets of the client's current experiences (e.g., cognitions, affects, and motives), behaviors, and relational patterns and to link the client's current experiences to his experiences of the past. The main technique used by the therapist was Task-Directed Imagery (Meier & Boivin, 2011) to help the client experience self in a new way and to become empowered and to assert her autonomy. The use of this technique in session 15 was transformative and influenced the therapeutic work for the remaining sessions.

The therapist was actively engaged in therapeutic dialogue, worked in the "here-and-now" and constantly checked back with the client to assess what she was experiencing and processing, particularly when she demonstrated changes in behavior, tone of voice, and mood (Meier & Boivin, 2000). He provided a safe and secure environment, helped the client to contain her feelings, and tried to balance nudging and nurturing (Mahler et al., 1975). The goal of therapy was to provide Gloria with opportunities to experience self and others in a new and different way and thereby foster self-understanding, a better understanding of the nature and quality of her relationships, become skilled and empowered, and to become agent of her own person within the context of her relationships.

### *Therapeutic Relationship*

The therapeutic relationship was characterized by collaboration, responsiveness to the therapist's interventions, and the client's intense motivation to change. As therapy progressed and Gloria entered more deeply into reworking the psychological separation and individuation process, she projected her problem onto the therapist and perceived him to be a barrier to her achieving separation and individuation. The client early in therapy became critical of the therapist and of therapy because therapy was moving too slowly. The therapist validated her experience understanding it to be an essential part of the recovery process. In due course she reworked the separation and individuation process and arrived at a more realistic and acceptable understanding of a real relationship. In brief, she used the therapeutic relationship to rework the separation and individuation process that she failed to negotiate with her mother in early childhood.

## Reworking the Separation and Individuation Process

Gloria's therapy took place in two parts. In the first part she was seen sporadically for 180 one-hour therapy sessions over a five-year period which primarily focused on university and work-related issues and on her desire to address difficulties to form intimate and long-lasting heterosexual relationships. Following the 180 therapy sessions, she took a leave for eight months to travel.

Upon her return from travel, she contacted the same therapist (A.M.) to continue with therapy because in her travels abroad, she experienced the freedom and pleasure of being her own person and at the same time had the opportunity to reflect on how she wanted to live her life. She wanted to rework the mindset (i.e., feelings, thoughts, representations, unmet needs) that she acquired in her troubled relationships with her parents during her childhood.

The therapy sessions, with Gloria's written permission, were audiotaped for the purpose of research. The second part of her therapy comprised 60 one-hour therapy sessions over a one-and-a-half-year period. It was during the second part of therapy, that Gloria transferred her separation and individuation difficulties with her mother onto the therapist and used this transference to resolve the earlier failed developmental task. Of the 60 therapy sessions, 37 were transcribed and together with the therapist's case notes provide the material for this part of the chapter.

The 37 audiotaped therapy sessions were analyzed using a multimethod called Theme-Analysis (Meier et al., 2008) to identify descriptive, second-order, third-order, and core themes. The results indicated that the core theme, around which all other themes converged, was the need to individuate and become her own person. The third-order themes were traced as how they were worked through across the sessions using as a criterion the Seven Phase Model of the Change Process. The results from this research have been published elsewhere (Meier et al., 2010).

In the second part of therapy, Gloria worked on her relationship with her mother and with the therapist. Most of the work regarding her mother was done after she had reworked significant issues relative to the therapist. In her real-life adult interactions with her mother, Gloria felt suffocated, put down, and as being a bad person. The mother was always right and her way was the best. Gloria was expected to comply with her mother's expectations. Gloria's wishes, needs and preferences were given no credence. Gloria and her mother continued to struggle to draw the other into their perceptions of reality. A shift in their relationship occurred when her mother was deceived and betrayed by a family member. Gloria resonated with her mother's hurt and became empathic toward her. She also learned that her mother was a victim of abuse as a child. Gloria wanted to have a better relationship with her mother.

Because of limited space, the following section presents Gloria's efforts and struggles to achieve individuality through her interaction with the therapist onto whom she projected her troubled childhood relationship. The presentation begins with Gloria forming a congenial therapeutic relationship which soon turns into her being angry toward the therapist for nudging her to look more deeply into her problems. This escalated with Gloria fearing that the gains (e.g., autonomy and individuation) she made would be taken from her and which gains she protected by pushing in the opposite direction and fighting for them. Her achievement of autonomy and individuality was an unfamiliar territory about which she at first did not know how to relate to. She then proceeded to integrate the new experiences with old experiences. The presentation ends with Gloria expressing her appreciation for the therapy, summarizing what she perceived to be the steps in the therapy process, and expressing her concerns about termination. The following presentation includes statements made by the client but none made by the therapist. The therapist's interventions comprised largely exploratory and clarifying questions and the use of Task-Directed Imagery which can easily be inferred from the client statements.

The numbers in brackets refer to session number and line numbers. The number to the left of the colon represents the session number and the number(s) to the right represent the line number. When only one number is given, it represents the session. When the range in line numbers is great (e.g., 25–37) it indicates that the material was taken from that section.

### *Formation of a Congenial Therapeutic Relationship*

Gloria initially began therapy because she knew that there was something terribly wrong but could not figure out what it was. She was in a tremendous amount of psychological pain and did not think that it was repairable so her hope was to try to relieve some of the pain so she could get through the day. Therapy took a turn for her when she became aware that the therapist was engaged in the process and cared for her (14: 72; 59: 170–173). In feeling cared for, she became vulnerable and did not know what to do about the caring (14: 14). Overtime, she became dependent on the therapist and sought his reassurance that she would not become violent but at the same time she felt guilty in asking for this validation because she did not think that it was fair given what the therapist was offering her (11: 15–17). Gloria struggled with the therapeutic relationship since it was a new experience for her not to have to fight for what she wanted, to feel cared for and that she mattered (i.e., unmet need for significance). She felt vulnerable, afraid, confused, and disarmed, but engaged in the therapy process (23: 15–17).

### *Feeling Angry toward the Therapist for Nudging Her*

Gloria soon became aware that the therapy was more than she talking and the therapist listening. The therapist became engaged and nudged her in exploring the underlying dynamics of her psychological pain and of her anger, that is, the therapist traced back her problems to their origin.

The tracing back of the problem to its origin, which was related to childhood experiences, activated anxiety and anger. Gloria became angry at the therapist for pushing her to talk about her feelings of potentially becoming aggressive and violent. She said:

> I think that you pushed me. I didn't want to talk about that, and I don't consider that fair play and you did not consider my boundaries. I had really understood that we would talk about what I wanted to talk about and go my way. I was safe when I didn't want to talk about it. I was in the process of reshaping my world. This has blown it apart completely. I don't know what the hell to do about this right now. (11: 11–35)

Gloria perceived the therapist's exploratory work as pushing her away which meant that the therapist cannot be part of her growing and that she would be on her own. She echoed this thought in saying "I'm not just sensing that I'm alone. I am alone. That's my reality" (4: 180–181).

### *Fears That Her Gains Will Be Taken from Her*

In speaking about her mother having administered phenobarbital to her when she was a child, Gloria became very angry, sad, and felt deeply hurt and betrayed (15: 7–10). A five-minute silence ensued during which she felt frightened and anxious. She also felt a growing closeness between herself and the therapist and that the therapist crossed into her world by empathically understanding her pain (15: 26) which, she said, was for her alone to bear (15: 38–40). The silence activated fear and fear generated anger. She feared that, in this closeness, the therapist would take from her what she had gained. She had for a long time craved for a relationship where both persons let the other be free. In her words, "I'm really afraid you're going to take it all away from me" (15: 83) and for "everything in the past that we've been through, all the dreams that are coming alive, the things that I want and need, I can't actually believe that you'll let me have it because no one else ever has" (15: 118–120). My experience is that "I can't have it" (15: 122). Because of her childhood experiences during which she was not validated for her feelings and needs (these were indirectly taken from her), she was predisposed to fear that what was important to her would be taken from her. This is consistent with Mahler et al. (1975) notion that a child who emerged from the "symbiotic nest" to explore the "not-mother" world, might fear that in returning to the symbiotic nest that his sense of autonomy and freedom would be taken from him.

To help Gloria experience holding on to what she had gained in the relationship and what was important to her, the therapist designed a task-directed imagery exercise (Meier & Boivin, 2011). The therapist asked her to imagine being somewhere where she could have what she wanted without the therapist taking it from her (15: 200–205). She imagined being in a flower garden and picking flowers. She then imagined that the therapist arrived and she gave him some flowers. When they were about to leave the garden, the therapist wanted to go one way but she wanted to go in a different direction and resisted until the therapist agreed to go her way. At the same time, she was afraid that the therapist, who was stronger than she, could force her to follow him. However, the therapist complied (i.e., was drawn into her projective identification of power) and they left together with Gloria leading the way. They arrived at a stranger's house, knocked on the door, and were invited in. Gloria gave them some flowers, she was invited to stay, but the therapist was not and then left. Gloria felt good being alone to do what she wanted knowing that the therapist would return because he left the flowers (15: 215–275).

The imagery exercise profoundly affected Gloria and set the agenda for the remaining therapeutic work. She spoke about her difficulties and the transformations in detail in four subsequent sessions (16, 17, 18, and 19).

First, she felt vulnerable and struggled with the therapist's positive responsiveness, gentleness, and kindness in taking her home and leaving the flowers with her. His behavior is opposite to her experiences of the past and she would have felt more comfortable had the therapist tried to take the flowers from her (16: 12–60). She was astonished that she did not have to fight to get the flowers back (i.e., what was hers) and that she could do with them what she wanted (i.e., asserted her need for autonomy). Yet she feared that he would take the flowers from her; she also feared that if he returned them to her, it would mean that he is abandoning her (16: 158, 168). But she also wondered whether "it was okay for her to keep the flowers and if it is not [is she] going to have to pay a price for keeping them. I don't know what to do when you come back. She would like him to come back because he wants to come back" (16: 207–221). The struggle is whether to believe that she is worthy of receiving good things and if she is, is there is a price to be paid for them?

Second, by holding on to the flowers and doing nothing with them, there emerged within her a part which was telling her that she should "not take the flowers. It's breaking one of my basic rules which is never to take anything from anyone and if you are going to have the flowers, you should plant them and give some of the flowers away" (17: 86–88). There was another part which was saying "but I really want the flowers; I want to keep them; they are mine; you gave them to me" (17: 45, 110). Gloria mentioned that she was always expected to give things away and if she did not give them away, she would feel very guilty. Gloria was not able to resolve this inner conflict. She stated: "I don't have an answer; I can't act on it" (17: 91–92). However, she indicated that she wants to "get that straightened out on a different level" (17: 121) and have the freedom to decide what she will do with the flowers and not "feel obligated" (17: 133). She added that the flowers are giving her a chance "to really sort out what's mine and what isn't" (17: 267–269). The struggle regarding what to do with the flowers surfaced Gloria's intrapsychic conflict between the internalized critical and demanding parent (i.e., the superego) and the needy and resisting internalized child. However, she lacked the inner resources (i.e., ego) to bring about a harmonious resolution to the conflict.

Third, Gloria chose to keep the flowers because she felt it was so important to her to keep them without understanding its importance. For her, there was a sense that the resolution of the internal conflict that she spoke about earlier (17: 91–92) is "in the flowers" without knowing how she will work it out (18: 35). As well, in keeping the flowers, she did not experience her terrible emptiness and for the first time did not experience anger at the core of her being (18: 37–47). Gloria was perplexed as to why she was still holding the flowers; she felt that she came "to a standstill" (18: 88). Yet there "was nothing beyond the flowers" (18: 334). She wondered whether holding the flowers meant that she "arrived," that this was it and something will "spontaneously happen when it's ready to happen" (18: 105–109). Her strong belief was that the coming together of the flowers was "the bringing together of everything that I had learned in order to fly, in order for the takeoff" (18: 277–279) referring to she establishing her self-identity and individuality. This also raised a question about her future career saying that she "can't be settled and unsettled at the same time – these are mutually exclusive" (20: 326–327).

### *Pulling in Opposite Directions*

The earlier therapy sessions went along relatively smoothly with both the therapist and Gloria collaboratively working toward the same goal. However, a shift gradually occurred when Gloria, feeling more confident, tried to draw the therapist into her way of thinking and relating (i.e., projective identification of power) which he resisted. According to Gloria, she and the therapist were pulling in opposite directions which resulted in a stalemate. In her view, at the urging of the therapist, she uncovered feelings about herself which left her feel upset and unsettled. She perceived that the therapist was not there for her and left her alone to deal with her feelings. According to Gloria, the therapist had his agenda and "pulled" her in his direction to which she at first complied. Gloria then decided that she will not go along with his agenda at her expense. She was not able to go along with the pull of the therapist because it would leave her unsettled. In her own words:

> There was a time when I would be anxious and I would come and talk and I would feel better. Now it's reversed. I come and talk and I feel more anxious. It's taking me longer to work things out. It's much more painful to work things out to the point of scaring me. And it just seems that if I do feel good when I come, I don't feel good when I leave. (22: 75–80)
>
> When we started out, I didn't have any idea of directions or anything like that. You would have the idea of what was going to happen and where we were going and that was okay to go along with it because I didn't have any ideas. You have these ideas and you're pushing me and the consequence of your ideas are that I'm the one who's terribly upset that it's taking me longer and longer to come back and recover. And I feel worse coming than better. (22: 135–140)
>
> My main idea at the moment is what it's doing to me. You're pulling and I'm pulling just as hard in the opposite direction in order to stay

> still, not to go in the opposite direction. I'm just staying still. I don't have anything to do but to pull back. (22: 181–186)
>
> On the one hand, you're saying to me, not verbally, like pulling me, that this has to be done. So, in one way you're pulling me and asking me to go along with that and that's okay, and you say I need it. At the same time, you're telling me that I can do all these things by myself and that I know what I need and how to use all that stuff to deal with my concerns. So, you're asking me to be two contradictory things at the same time. (22: 257–267)

In the sessions referred to above, Gloria began to rework the power struggle between her and the therapist which is a remnant of her childhood experiences with her mother who was always right and knew what was best. The therapist acknowledged her needs to participate in the therapy process. In doing so, he helped her to express an unmet need that her ideas, and she herself, were important, mattered, and significant.

### *Fights for Her Autonomy and Individuality*

After many sessions, Gloria became determined to pursue her individuality and not let the therapist prevent it from happening. She spoke about her inner turmoil, conflict, and struggle in being her own person. The steps involved in becoming her own person were (a) she felt smothered in the therapeutic relationship and needed to take her own space which she found by becoming more distant; (b) the distancing created anxiety because she did not know how the therapist would respond to her taking space; (c) she decided to assert her selfhood even if it meant that the therapist would not like her or validate her for it; (d) she wanted to know whether the therapist wanted to enter her world and liked what she was doing; and (e) she was ready to take the risk of being rejected and thereby experienced being abandoned. In her own words:

> I need some space. I don't particularly enjoy having to fight you. I see that I need more of a say in what is going on. (23: 20–39)
>
> I've been feeling very smothered lately. I want to have a look at things myself and I don't have any qualms about not knowing what to do. I just kind of want to have a look around myself and try … I feel okay with that. And I feel being smothered. And not having this space to do that. So, I know that's what I need. (23: 141–146)
>
> I've always fluctuated between being totally smothered and totally abandoned. Or being caught in the middle between the two with the other person involved being really angry. Like a lot of guilt, so it's

> been either way because of the anger. I know that the needing phase is overriding the two. I'm going nowhere if I don't have the space. (23: 153–161)
>
> I'm afraid because I don't know where you're going with all of this. I'm not back tracking. What you do is your choice, but I can't be smothered anymore. And I really know that the need is so paramount, so important. If the relationship goes, it goes. (23: 220–222)
>
> I know that distancing myself is absolutely essential for being my own person. (23: 230–231)
>
> I've distanced myself in order to look at my world and get a sense of how it works then how I wanted it to work. What I'm saying is: this is the way I want it to be for a bit while I look around and find out what all this is about. And then I'd like you to come back in. So, question one is the abandonment. It is here that either we look at the world and do the whole thing your way or you're out. That's the first part. Which leads to the second part, if it's okay the way we are right now that I look at things myself? Then the second part is when you come in whether you'll like it. That's not abandonment; it's more will you like it? But if abandonment happens you won't get a chance to like it or not like it. (23: 310–320)

### *New Territory in Living Autonomously*

Gloria mentioned that she had always had a "bodily sense" of the way she wanted to live her life and the confidence that she would achieve it. She stated:

> Where I've ended up is not new, new. I've always known deep inside that what I was looking for is a different way of being. That's probably why I've survived but I also figured that was the problem. Where I've ended up is what I always knew. I'm articulating it and living it, not as a problem but as the only way to go. (20: 186–196)

Having actually embraced a life characterized by autonomy and individuation was a new experience for Gloria and with it came joy and happiness and also the feeling of being disoriented as she had no reference points as how to live out her new found life. She gradually shifted from being other-reliant to being self-reliant. There is also a sense of emptiness and a fear of being abandoned for asserting her autonomy and individuality.

Gloria stated that she did not know what to do when she does not have to fight for what she wants as in the past she took on the survivor role. She did not know how to stop fighting. She feels vulnerable wondering when this good moment will be over and the therapist will attack her and hurt her emotionally. Gloria commented:

> A lot of energy went in undoing the old ways and learning new ways. I have a great number of life skills in those two areas [adapting and surviving]. I don't know what to do other than that. (22: 84–87)
>
> I'm on very unfamiliar ground. This is all part of moving out [of the old world and] moving into my world. (22: 55–56)
>
> I really don't know what to do in a world where I'm not fighting for survival or it's so incredibly mixed up that I'm fighting to stay equal and if I don't have to fight you on the idea of it being right and wrong and I can have it. (22: 87–90)
>
> I don't know where I fit into the world at this point in time. I grew up in a world where I had to fight to survive. It wasn't guaranteed that you'd make it through. I don't even know how to relate to the world and to what I want to do if I'm not fighting for it or fighting it. (22: 123–128)
>
> But what am I fighting for? I don't know how not to. Knowing that doesn't seem to be enough. I don't know how to stop. (22: 214–216)

She did not know where the therapist was at with her wanting to live out her life according to her preferences and wishes. She expected that he would not be supportive. She was ready to fight the therapist should he keep her from being her own person. And yet, should the therapist not block her, she would be at a loss knowing how to behave because she only learned to respond and relate to others as a fighter and as a survivor. She will not let herself be drawn into it again (i.e., ready to resist the projective identification). Regarding this, Gloria said:

> I know what I would like to expect. On an emotional level I've never known anyone who could go as far as I'm saying we have to go. And I guess the big question is why can you, when no one else I've ever known has been able to and I know how important it is for me at this point of time. I can't back off on this one that if you can't come along with this or don't want to come along with this then we're off. I mean regardless of what that means. Experientially this is a horrendously big leap. (38: 318–334)

She was concerned about the relationship, about her sense of newness and her need for emotional space with the therapeutic relationship. In the past, she experienced that others did not affirm her for her needs and feelings and she could not perceive that the therapist would be any different.

This was explored relative to trusting others and evaluating her perception. She wanted the therapist to be present and yet not present and she did not know how this would translate itself because of her need for affirmation and of her need for space (i.e., need for autonomy and being loved for asserting her autonomy). In the past she either felt smothered or abandoned by people.

> I just need an emotional space. And I need some time to get to know myself. I need some space to kind of look around. Everything is so new. And I really feel that I should have the chance to look at it first by myself. Try it out, that that kind of should be mine. On an emotional level, I have two poles, being smothered which is what I've been feeling and being totally abandoned. I don't have an experiential sense of a middle ground. (38: 117–126)

Gloria feared that in becoming autonomous she would be abandoned by the therapist and left to herself (i.e., need for connection). She was troubled by the therapist's comment that she had it within her to know how to resolve her inner conflicts and live out her life. This statement was a déjà vu experience linking it to what her father often told her. She felt that the therapist brought her to the point of being vulnerable and then copped out and betrayed her. She stated "I feel this incredible sense of betrayal. After all of this time and everything that has gone on between us, you say I know the answer" (21: 187–191). She felt that the therapist does not care for her other than for his research interests.

Gloria, however, was able to have a different understanding of what was happening in therapy and that the therapist's comment that she has the resources to live her life was not pushing her out. She recalled how she reworked her relationship with her mother. As an adult, she continued to see her mother through the eyes of a two-year old. She stated:

> It dawned on me that I suddenly knew at a very deep level that what has happened and was told was filtered through the mind of a two-year old. I link that up with being an adult and filtering through an adult's mind what had been told to the child and to the child's awareness of what was going on and ran it through an adult understanding of what happened and was, and that really brought about closure. (16: 10–20)

Although Gloria had an intellectual grasp of what was occurring in therapy, yet emotionally she was left with the fear of being pushed out and not knowing how to relate in a new way. She felt troubled in not knowing what to do with the new relationship wherein each person lets the other be.

### *Integrating the New with the Old*

At the beginning of therapy, Gloria felt divided into two worlds. The one world represented what she wanted to do and what she liked (e.g., theatre, playing piano) (i.e., inner child) and the second world represented that which she ought to do (i.e., superego) (pp. 34, 35). That is, she was conflicted between living in a conventional and the more disciplined way or to be almost completely free. She found herself moving from the one world to the other. When she was in the "want to" side, she felt guilty and when she responded from the "had to" side she felt angry. Yet she knew that to be true to herself, she had to orient her life according to her inner world (i.e., "want to" side; inner child and ego).

Gloria also became aware that, in her adulthood, she had been processing things and feelings through the eyes and heart of a two-year old, but then she suddenly was able to process the same life events through the heart and eyes of an adult. She experienced a change in her perception of past events which brought about the feelings of calm, inner peace, being more settled and being more herself (p. 26).

Gloria described the process of integration in terms of steps: (a) she learned to distinguish what was hers and what was imposed on her; (b) she learned to distinguish between being a child and being an adult; and (c) she was able to discard that which she did not want (e.g., feeling that she was damaged goods). The process brought about the feeling of inner stability (e.g., safe anchorage), shifted the focus of evaluating from that of others to self (e.g., true self), elicited self-confidence and self-acceptance, and the expectation that this will continue (e.g., confident expectation) (p. 27). She also experienced herself as being more real, energetic and creative (p. 33).

## Appreciation and Description of Psychotherapy Process

At the last therapy session, Gloria offered her summary of the therapy process in terms of phases (pp. 39, 59, and 60). These are (a) problem stating phase: this entails she knowing that there is something wrong from which she wanted relief; she thought of the therapeutic relationship as two people talking about her problem and the therapist as listening, caring, and being non-judgmental; (b) confusion phase: this was created by the therapist not acting in the way she perceived to be an expected pattern; the therapist was unexpectedly caring, accepting, and non-directive; (c) dependent phase: was brought about by she feeling secure and accepted; was in contrast to her expectations that clients are not to become dependent on therapist; (d) disentanglement phase: this represented Gloria's efforts to be her own person but feared that the therapist would not approve of her going her own way; and (e) separation and individuation phase: Gloria has a sense of being her own person without being abandoned and disowned; wants a relationship of equality.

Gloria provided an appreciation of the therapy sessions. She appreciated being able to lead the course of therapy and the therapist's skill in helping her to take the direction. She felt that she was cared for and respected; that new things were born within her and she craved to continue to experience herself at her deepest level. Lastly, she sensed that she has grown up in therapy, from being a little girl to that of a grown-up girl (p. 60).

## Termination of Therapy

Termination of a long-term relationship, including the therapeutic relationship, is always a painful experience which often brings with it a sense of insecurity, loss, and sadness. Gloria introduced the topic of termination in saying that during the past months she has been led to separate from the therapist and to pursue her own life of growth and development. She stated that she has come to the point in her life that therapy is no longer her home and that she is about to make home wherever she goes (p. 52). She added that she has separated and individuated and is her own person (p. 57). This realization brought with it feelings of sadness in leaving "home" and the feeling of apprehension about the future even though she was excited about it. The talking of it, made it real for her.

Gloria expressed her desire that the therapist play an active role in her disengaging from the therapeutic relationship which for her meant that he likes that she is disengaging and that he likes what and the way she is doing it. In taking on an active role, the therapist conveys the message that she matters and that she feels that she can come and go even though the therapist is not where she is at, yet he will be present (i.e., object constancy). In the past when she disengaged and the person, from whom she disengaged, was passive, Gloria felt that she did not matter and felt abandoned (p. 39).

Lastly, Gloria raised her concern as how to remain in contact even though she was about to go on with her life (p. 57). She wondered whether the therapist would still be there for her now that she has separated. She expressed her wish to continue the relationship but based not on dependency but on interdependency as she has grown relationally from being dependent to being interdependent (p. 60). The therapist reassured Gloria that he would be available and that she is to feel free to call him as needed.

## Conclusion

Gloria resolved her relational problems by identifying her unmet needs for autonomy, emotional bonding, and significance and by asserting them in her relationships, particularly with the therapist. Working through the transferential therapeutic relationship was an essential part of her recovery as it served as the context within which she struggled to be her true self, exercised her autonomy and dealt with the fear of being abandoned, reworked her psychic organization, and developed more efficient coping strategies and more satisfying relationship. Crucial to Gloria's reworking of her low-level borderline personality organization was she becoming aware of and asserting her needs and transforming the psychic organization which acts an essential agent in her actions and interactions.

## References

American Psychiatric Association. (1994). *Diagnostic and statistical manual of mental disorders (DSM-IV)*. Washington, DC: Author.

Bowen, M. (1978). *Family therapy in clinical practice*. New York: Jason Aronson.

Cashdan, S. (1988). *Object relations therapy: Using the relationship*. New York: Norton & Company.

Christenson, R. M., & Wilson, W. P. (1994). Separation-individuation process inventory. In J. Fischer & K. Corcoran (Ed.), *Measures for clinical practice: A source book* (2nd ed., pp. 550–552). Toronto: Free Press.

Edward, J., Ruskin, N., & Turrini (1981). *Separation-individuation: Theory and application*. New York: Gardner Press.

Fairbairn, W. R. D. (1944/1994). Endopsychic structure considered in terms of object relationships. In W. R. D. Fairbairn (Ed.), *Psychoanalytic studies of personality* (pp. 82–136). New York: Routledge.

Freud, S. (1923). The ego and the id. *Standard Edition*, *19*, 12–63.

Freud, S. (1938). An outline of psychoanalysis. *Standard Edition*, *23* (1953), 144–207.

Ivey, A. E. (1983). *Intentional interviewing and counseling*. Monterey: CA: Brooks/Cole.

Jourard, S. M. (1971). *The transparent self*. New York: D. Van Nostrand Company.

Klein, M. (1935). A contribution to the psychogenesis of manic-depressive states. In M. Klein (Ed.), *Love, guilt and reparation and other works, 1921–1945* (pp. 262–289). New York: Delacorte.

Klein, M. (1948). On the theory of anxiety and guilt. In *Envy and gratitude and other works 1946–1963* (Vol. 4, pp. 25–42). New York: Delacorte.

Klein, M. (1959). Our adult world and its roots in infancy. In M. Klein (Ed.), *Envy and gratitude and other works 1946–1963* (Vol. 4, pp. 247–263). New York: Delacorte.

Kohut, H. (1977). *The restoration of the self*. New York: International Universities Press.

Mahler, M. S., Pine, F., & Bergman, A. (1975). *Psychological birth of the human infant*. New York: Basic Books.

Masterson, J. F. (1976). *Psychotherapy of the borderline adult: A developmental approach*. New York: Brunner/Mazel.

Masterson, J. F. (1991). Comparing psychoanalytic psychotherapies. In J. F. Masterson, M. Tolpin, & P. E. Sifneos (Eds.), *Comparing psychoanalytic psychotherapies* (pp. 285–294). New York: Brunner/Mazel.

Masterson, J. F. (1993). *The emerging self: A developmental, self and object relations approach to the treatment of the closet narcissistic disorder of the self.* New York: Brunner/Mazel.
Meier, A., & Boivin, M. (1987). Self-discovery approach to counselling. *Pastoral Sciences, 6*, 145–168.
Meier, A., & Boivin, M. (1992). *A Seven phase model of the change process and its clinical applications.* Paper presented at the 8th Annual Conference of the Society for the Exploration of Psychotherapy Integration, San Diego, California, April 3.
Meier, A., & Boivin, M. (1998). *The seven phase model of the change process: Theoretical foundation, definitions, coding guidelines, training procedures, and research data.* Fifth edition. Unpublished manuscript, Ottawa, Ontario: St. Paul University.
Meier, A., & Boivin, M. (2000). The achievement of greater selfhood: The application of theme-analysis to a case study. *Psychotherapy Research, 10*(1), 57–77.
Meier, A., & Boivin, M. (2011). *Counselling and therapy techniques: Theory and practice.* London, England: SAGE Publications.
Meier, A., Boivin, M., & Meier, M. (2008). Theme-analysis: Procedures and applications. *Qualitative Research in Psychology, 5*(4), 289–310.
Meier, A., Boivin, M., & Meier, M. (2010). Working through the transference of an unresolved separation/individuation pattern: A case study using theme-analysis. In A. Meier & M. Rovers (Eds.), *The helping relationship: Healing and change in community context* (pp. 101–129). Toronto: Novalis.
Sperry, L. (1995). *Handbook of diagnosis and treatment of the DSM-IV personality disorders.* New York: Brunner/Mazel.
Winnicott, D. (1960/1965). Ego distortion in terms of true and false self. In D. Winnicott (Ed.), *The maturational processes and the facilitating environment* (pp. 140–152). New York: International Universities Press.

# Future Directions

This book presented a novel approach to psychotherapy, namely, Self-in-Relationship Psychotherapy. This approach considers it to be essential to incorporate core relational, self, and physical intimacy needs together with affect and cognitive processes in the understanding of psychological and relational problems and their resolution. The major theoretical influences in the development of Self-in-Relationship Psychotherapy and its major constructs were presented. It demonstrated how to apply Self-in-Relationship Psychotherapy to the assessment, conceptualization, and treatment of psychological and relational problems. To facilitate the assessment process, special instruments were designed to operationalize and assess each of the Self-in-Relationship Psychotherapy's major constructs. Self-in-Relationship Psychotherapy's approach in working with core needs and dealing with issues that act as barriers in working with core needs was presented. The book ends with the application of the Self-in-Relationship Psychotherapy to a young woman who struggled with psychologically separating from the emotional ties to significant others and becoming her own person.

In the future it is important to apply Self-in-Relationship Psychotherapy to different therapeutic models such as couple, family, and parent-child therapies and to assess its effectiveness to deal with the psychological and relational problems. An important goal is to determine how addressing core relational, self, and physical intimacy needs helps individuals to achieve their desired goals. In addition to determining the effectiveness of Self-in-Relationship Psychotherapy for couple, family, and parent-child therapy, it is also important to investigate the effectiveness of applying this approach to special populations such as bulimia, anorexia, drug, and alcohol addictions and to emotional disorders such as depression, generalized anxiety, obsessive-compulsive disorder, and personality disorders. An important area of investigation is to determine whether this group of problems represent compensations for unmet core childhood needs.

In addition to the clinical questions, there is also a need to research the importance of including core needs in a theory of psychotherapy. These are some of the questions that research could address: First, how do unmet core needs relate to maladaptive behaviors and to emotional problems? Second, does addressing needs and re-orienting one's life around them bring about the desired therapeutic changes? Third, in the course of normal extrauterine development, are some needs more fundamental at the beginning of development and others become important at the later stages of development? The testing of these ideas is particularly critical for Self-in-Relationship Psychotherapy since the inclusion of relational, self, and physical intimacy needs are at the core of this approach. To test these ideas, it will be necessary to develop a reliable and valid psychometric instrument that measures core needs and has the capacity to differentiate the needs.

Self-in-Relationship Psychotherapy offers a promising integrated approach to therapy. Future applications of this approach will more clearly define its unique characteristic in dealing with human problems.

# Index

Page numbers in *italics* refer to figures. Page numbers in **bold** refer to tables.